NEW BOOKS AND NEW EDITIONS OF STANDARD TEXTS

JENSEN Dis[illegible] 2nd ed £8.50/[illegible] Dairy Cattle £6.75/GALLOWAY Farm Animal Health and Disease Control £9.00/ BREAZILE Textbook of Veterinary Physiology £11.50/DELLMAN Veterinary Histology—An Outline Text-Atlas £10.50/DOUGLAS AND WILLIAMSON Principles of Veterinary Radiography 2nd ed £4.50/ JENKINS Functional Mammalian Neuroanatomy with Emphasis on Dog and Cat £9.50/HOFSTAD Diseases of Poultry 6th ed £16.00

Prices and details quoted are those current at the time of going to press but are liable to subsequent alteration without notice.

THE BRITISH VETERINARY JOURNAL

Established in 1875 this is the only monthly periodical published in Great Britain that is devoted exclusively to the study and practice of veterinary medicine and to recording scientific progress in the veterinary field throughout the Commonwealth.

In 1972 the Journal, in addition to its normal contents, is publishing three series of articles specially contributed by experts on each particular topic. The subjects of the series are: Clinical Problems in Preventive Medicine (with particular reference to intensification), Animal Health and the European Economic Community, and Conservation and Wild-Life.

published monthly annual subscription £7.00 U.S.A. and Canada $20.00

BAILLIÈRE TINDALL

Baillière Tindall
7/8 Henrietta Stree[illegible]

THE

VETERINARY ANNUAL

Editor

C. S. G. GRUNSELL, Ph.D., F.R.C.V.S.

TWELFTH YEAR

1971

BRISTOL: JOHN WRIGHT & SONS LTD.

Distribution by Sole Agents:
United States of America: The Williams & Wilkins Company, Baltimore
Canada: The Macmillan Company of Canada Ltd., Toronto

ISBN 0 7236 0317 0

PRINTED IN GREAT BRITAIN BY JOHN WRIGHT AND SONS LTD.
AT THE STONEBRIDGE PRESS, BRISTOL BS4 5NU

PREFACE

It is perhaps fitting that the Current Developments section of this year's Veterinary Annual should open with an account of the implications for the United Kingdom of the recent developments in the veterinary field in the European Economic Community. The long period during which the representatives from Britain have suffered the frustrating experience of acting as observers is coming to an end and this would be an appropriate moment at which to pay grateful tribute to the efforts made by those observers, who include the contributor of our article, to keep the profession informed of the trend of discussion in the E.E.C. It is evident that no sector of the profession will escape the effects of Britain's entry into the Common Market. The need for corporate action by veterinarians in the member states has been recognized in the formation of a European Union of Practising Veterinarians and the proposal to establish the wider-based European Federation of Veterinary Professions.

The case for the swing away from basic research to the investigation of problems of immediate importance to the livestock industry has substantial support from the contribution on the economics of animal husbandry. Using the pig as a model, the author demonstrates the pressing need to understand the evident gaps between precept and practice, and between normals established under research conditions and what happens in the field. This issue, in fact, includes two articles which both seek to understand the well-recognized vulnerability of the pig in early life. The first assembles the evidence for incriminating exposure to excessive cold as a factor in growth rate and reduced disease resistance and viability. The second is concerned with the nature of porcine immunoglobulins, their site of formation, and their levels in the dam's milk and the piglet's sera.

Two forms of abortion in sheep are discussed. In the case of Toxoplasma abortion there is evidence of widespread infection throughout the country, but accurate assessment of the importance of the disease is hampered by the limited number of centres employing the techniques required for the identification of congenital infection. Salmonella abortion, on the other hand, appears much more restricted in its distribution but here one is presented with a number of as yet unexplained epidemiological aspects of infection.

The account of Avian Salmonellosis, given by the Director of the Houghton Poultry Research Station, makes fascinating reading and, although much still needs to be done, much has been accomplished in the understanding of the disease and in the elaboration of measures to reduce the public health hazards. The co-operation of the industry in implementing these measures is clearly essential. The results of the failure of the industry to help itself are well illustrated in the short account of the background to the Newcastle Disease epidemic. The profession has an important part to play in advising on the use of the new vaccines, but the implementation of general control measures by all branches of the industry is essential if the incidence of the disease is to be reduced.

The three contributions on equine matters in this edition cover widely differing fields. In view of the shortage of British texts these should help to serve the need of the increasing number of veterinarians who find the horse section of their practices growing. The article on the ear, which is the first of a series dealing with diseases of the ear, nose, and throat, considers the subject in some depth. There is already a formidable list of equine diseases of viral aetiology and the account of their differentiation explains how epidemiological, clinical, and pathological features may be used to support laboratory diagnoses. The third contribution reports observations made on the sound vibrations produced by air flow in the respiratory tract of horses at exercise and illustrates the valuable information to be obtained by the use of comparatively simple apparatus. It is to the credit of the author that the work was carried out in the face of the limitations of general practice.

In the contribution on Fish Diseases the author draws attention to the fact that this is an area of growing importance. Quite apart from the increase in fish culture as an industry in many parts of the world, in Britain fish now rank third in popularity as household pets. A bibliography for further reading is provided.

The current developments in abdominal surgery in cattle is concerned less with surgical technique and more with seeking to explain the interesting change in the pattern of abdominal conditions in the species which has occurred in the past ten years or so.

In recent years allergic hypersensitivity has been increasingly diagnosed in canine dermatology, often at the end of a process of elimination. By collecting the substantial evidence the author of the section on Allergic Skin Conditions in the Dog has provided the information needed for more rational diagnosis.

As in previous editions the Current Literature is reviewed under the usual headings. The purpose of this section of the ANNUAL continues to be to serve as a readily available account of recent advances in the various disciplines. This year a chapter on Recent Trends in Antibacterial Therapy is included and it is intended to make this a regular feature in subsequent editions.

It has been a pleasure to collaborate with the authors to whom is owed a debt of gratitude for their painstaking work, and finally thanks are due to the publishers for the very great help they have given.

December, 1971 C. S. G. G.

CONTENTS

LIST OF PLATES

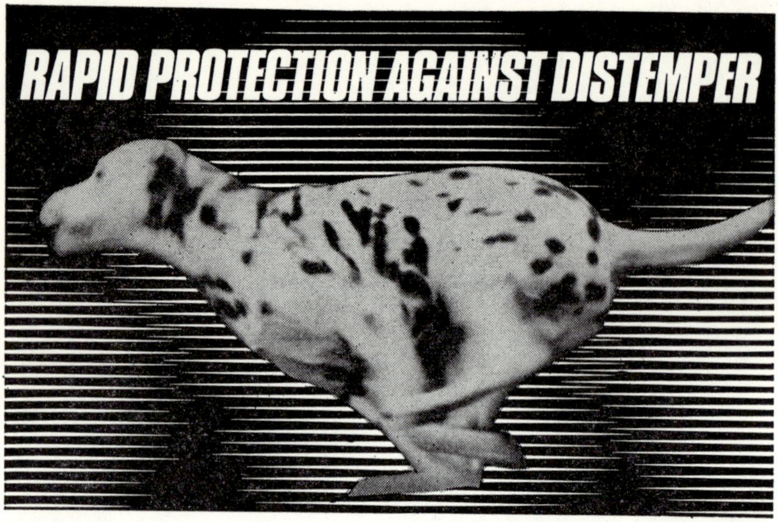
RAPID PROTECTION AGAINST DISTEMPER

Contributors and Contributions to the Veterinary Annual, 1971

DONALD P. ATTENBURROW, B.V.Sc., M.R.C.V.S., 43 St David's Hill, Exeter, Devon.

Some Observations on the Sound Vibrations produced by Air Flow in the Respiratory Tract of Horses at Exercise, 6.

W. F. BLAKEMORE, M.A., Ph.D., B.V.Sc., M.R.C.V.S., Cambridge University School of Veterinary Medicine, Wellcome Laboratory for Comparative Neurology, Madingley Road, Cambridge.

Cerebral Lipidoses and Leucodystrophies in Animals (jointly), 129.

F. J. BOURNE, B.Vet.Med., Ph.D., M.R.C.V.S., Lecturer, Department of Animal Husbandry, University of Bristol Veterinary School, Langford House, Langford, Nr. Bristol.

Porcine Immunoglobulins, 74.

E. G. C. CLARKE, M.A., Ph.D., D.Sc., F.R.I.C., Professor of Chemical Toxicology Department of Physiology and Chemistry, Royal Veterinary College, Royal College Street, London.

Poisons and Poisoning (jointly), 232.

MYRA L. CLARKE, F.R.C.V.S., Donnington, 49 Westwood Road, Tilehurst, Reading, Berks.

Poisons and Poisoning (jointly), 232.

W. R. COOK, F.R.C.V.S., Clinical Department, Animal Health Trust, Equine Research Station, Balaton Lodge, Newmarket, Suffolk.

Diseases of the Ear, Nose, and Throat in the Horse: Part I, The Ear, 12.

J. I. DAVIES, D.V.S.M., M.R.C.V.S., Divisional Veterinary Officer, Agricultural Development and Advisory Service, Ministry of Agriculture, Fisheries, and Food, Castle House, Newport Road, Stafford.

The Newcastle Disease Epidemic, 106.

F. L. M. DAWSON, M.A., B.Sc., Ph.D., M.R.C.V.S., Assistant Veterinary Investigation Officer, Veterinary Investigation Service, Ministry of Agriculture, Fisheries, and Food, The White House, Hadstock, Nr. Linton, Cambridgeshire.

Physiology and Pathology of Reproduction, 186.

J. DONNELLY, B.Sc., Senior Research Officer, Parasitology Department, Central Veterinary Laboratory, Ministry of Agriculture, Fisheries, and Food, New Haw, Weybridge, Surrey.

Arthropod Parasitology, 164. Insecticides and Control of Arthropod Parasites, 217.

ROGER EWBANK, B.V.Sc., M.R.C.V.S., Sub-department of Animal Husbandry, University of Liverpool, Veterinary Field Station, Leahurst, Neston, Wirrall, Cheshire.

The Husbandry of Laboratory Animals, 281.

T. K. EWER, B.V.Sc., Ph.D., H.D.A., M.R.C.V.S., Professor of Animal Husbandry, School of Veterinary Science, University of Bristol, Langford House, Langford, Nr. Bristol.

Animal Husbandry, 252.

T. E. GIBSON, D.V.Sc., F.R.C.V.S., F.I.Biol., Senior Research Officer, Agricultural Development and Advisory Service, Central Veterinary Laboratory, Ministry of Agriculture, Fisheries, and Food, New Haw, Weybridge, Surrey.

Helminthology, 173. Anthelmintics, 206. Drug Appendix, 228.

R. F. GORDON, D.Sc., D.V.Sc., F.R.C.V.S., Director, Houghton Poultry Research Station, Houghton, Huntingdon.

Avian Salmonellosis, 95.

E. J. JACK, M.R.C.V.S., Veterinary Investigation Officer, Ministry of Agriculture, Fisheries, and Food, Agricultural Development and Advisory Service, Veterinary Investigation Centre, Pitsford Road, Moulton, Northampton.

Salmonella Abortion in Sheep, 57.

L. P. JOYNER, B.Sc., Ph.D., F.I.Biol., Senior Research Officer, Parasitology Department, Research Service, Ministry of Agriculture, Fisheries, and Food, Central Veterinary Laboratory, New Haw, Weybridge, Surrey.

Diseases related to Protozoal Infections, 150. Chemotherapy of Protozoal Infections, 211.

S. B. KENDALL, B.Sc., Ph.D., M.R.C.V.S., A.R.C.S., F.I.Biol., Senior Research Officer, Parasitology Department, Research Service, Ministry of Agriculture, Fisheries, and Food, Weir Cottage, Bridge Road, Chertsey, Surrey.

Protozoal Infections of Poultry, 148. Fascioliasis, 181.

D. D. LAWSON, D.V.R., M.R.C.V.S., Titular Professor, Department of Veterinary Surgery, University of Glasgow Veterinary School, Veterinary Hospital, Bearsden, Glasgow.

Distichiasis in the Dog, 48.

A. C. PALMER, M.A., Ph.D., F.R.C.V.S., Assistant Director of Research, Department of Veterinary Clinical Studies, University of Cambridge School of Veterinary Medicine, Wellcome Laboratory for Comparative Neurology, Madingley Road, Cambridge.

Cerebral Lipidoses and Leucodystrophies in Animals (jointly), 129.

JOHN PASFIELD, O.B.E., M.R.C.V.S., Veterinary Adviser to Silcock and Lever Feeds Ltd., B.O.C.M. Silcock Ltd., Basing View, Basingstoke, Hants.

Implications for the U.K. of Recent Veterinary Developments in the E.E.C., 1.

H. PEARSON, B.V.Sc., M.R.C.V.S., Lecturer, Department of Veterinary Surgery, University of Bristol Veterinary School, Langford House, Langford, Nr. Bristol.

Abdominal Surgery in Cattle, 44.

W. E. PEARSON, B.Sc., B.V.Sc., M.R.C.V.S., M.I.Biol., Veterinary Adviser, W. & J. B. Eastwood Ltd., Button End, 7 Church Drive, Ravenshead, Nottingham.

Fish Diseases, 109.

A. R. W. PORTER, M.A., Barrister-at-Law, Secretary and Registrar, Royal College of Veterinary Surgeons, 32 Belgrave Square, London.

Legal Decisions and Legislation, 243.

G. R. SCOTT, B.Sc., M.S., Ph.D., M.R.C.V.S., Senior Lecturer, Centre for Tropical Veterinary Medicine, Royal (Dick) School of Veterinary Studies, University of Edinburgh Field Station, Easter Bush, Roalin, Midlothian, Scotland.

Differentiation of Viral Diseases of Horses, 138.

D. B. STEPHENS, B.V.Sc., Ph.D., F.R.C.V.S., Visitor, Agricultural Research Council, Institute of Animal Physiology, Babraham, Cambridge.

Piglet Survival, 64.

OLGA UVAROV, M.R.C.V.S., Head of Veterinary Advisory Department, Glaxo Laboratories Ltd., 39 Rodney Gardens, Eastcote, Pinner, Middlesex.

Recent Trends in Antibacterial Therapy, 225.

G. S. WALTON, B.V.Sc., M.R.C.V.S., Lecturer, Department of Veterinary Preventive Medicine, University of Liverpool Veterinary Field Station, Leahurst, Neston, Wirral, Cheshire.

Allergic Skin Conditions in the Dog, 86.

W. A. WATSON, B.V.Sc., F.R.C.V.S., Veterinary Investigation Officer, Ministry of Agriculture, Fisheries, and Food, Block 2, Chalfont Drive, Nottingham.

Toxoplasma Abortion in Sheep, 52.

S. R. WRAGG, M.A., Senior Lecturer in Agricultural Economics, University of Bristol Veterinary School, Langford House, Langford, Nr. Bristol.

Husbandry Practices and Animal Performance with special reference to Pig-keeping, 120.

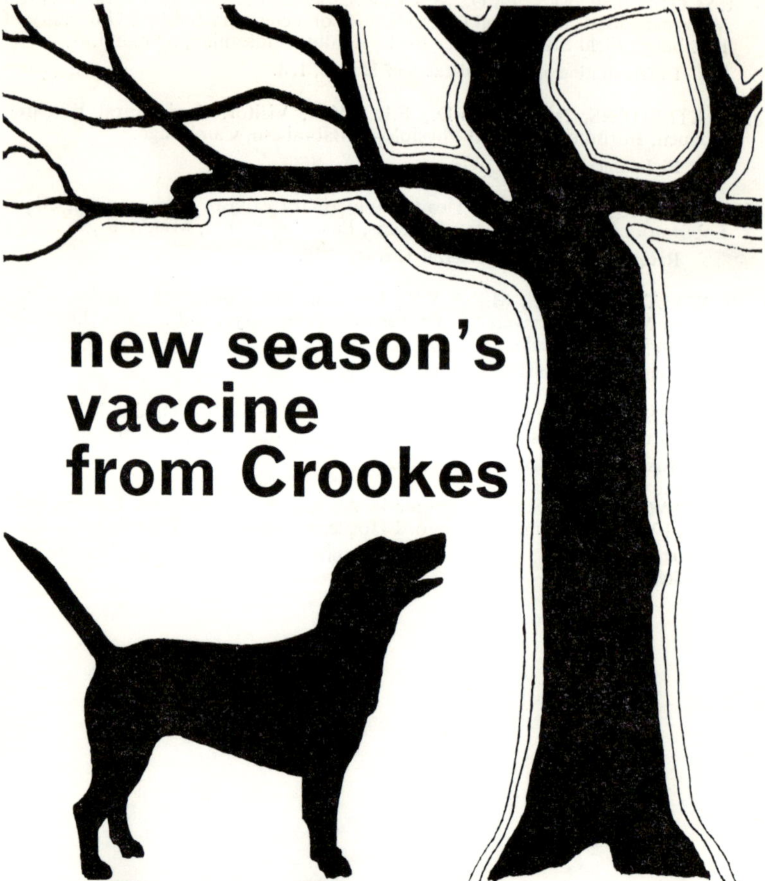

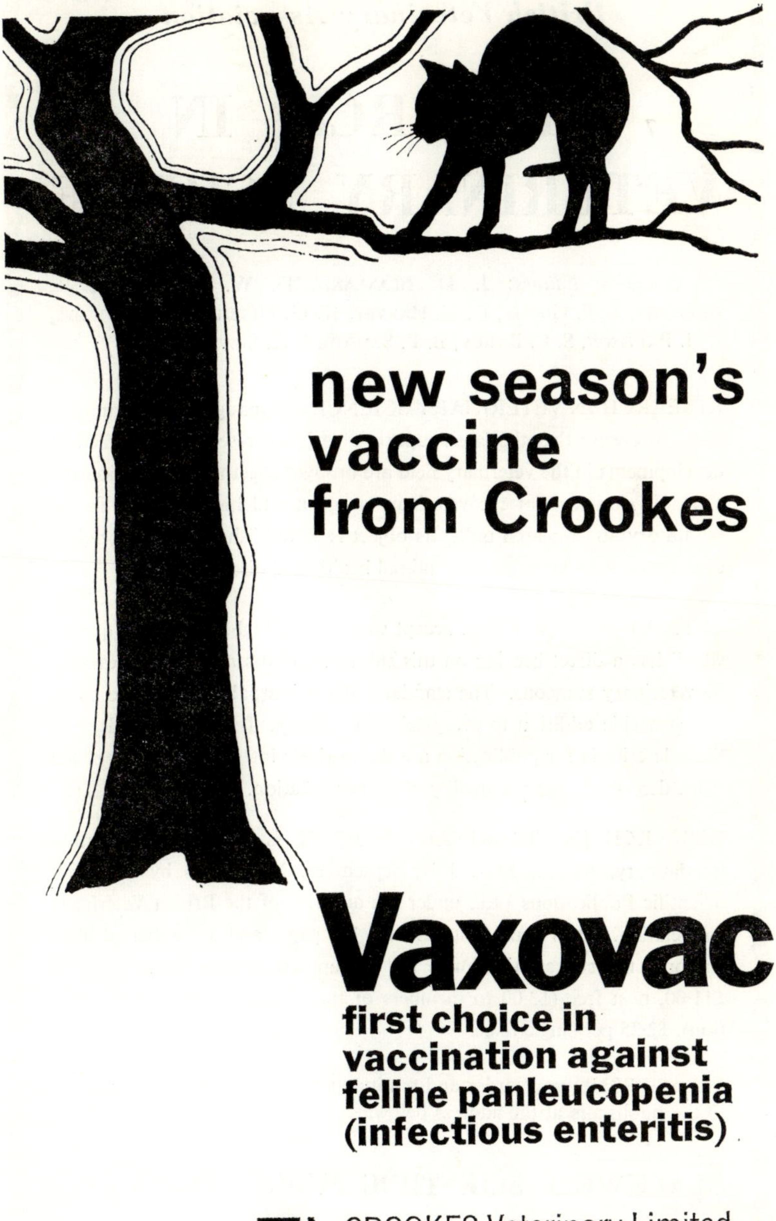
new season's
vaccine
from Crookes
Vaxovac
first choice in
vaccination against
feline panleucopenia
(infectious enteritis)
CROOKES Veterinary Limited
Basingstoke Hampshire

THE VETERINARY ANNUAL 1971

CURRENT DEVELOPMENTS

IMPLICATIONS FOR THE U.K. OF RECENT VETERINARY DEVELOPMENTS IN THE E.E.C.

John Pasfield, O.B.E., M.R.C.V.S.

An earlier paper presented to the Annual Congress of the British Veterinary Congress in 1969 (Pasfield, 1969) and reproduced in the VETERINARY ANNUAL (1969, 117) traced the progress of the Veterinary Liaison Committee since its first exploratory meeting at Aix-les-Bains in 1960, the problems it had discussed, the difficulties encountered, and the measures of agreement it had reached. This progress culminated in the four proposed Veterinary Directives of the Commission (Pasfield, 1970a, b) which have yet to be examined, and perhaps modified, by the European Parliament before becoming part of Community Law.

We in this country are still aware that, at the highest political level, the intransigent attitude of the late General de Gaulle and the veto of our earlier applications had produced an attitude somewhere between bewilderment and anger which remained unaltered until the successful Anglo-French discussions, culminating on 21 May, 1971, appeared to open the door. Whatever may have been the reasons for this marked (though welcome) change of heart, it is apparent that the concept of the General's *Europe des patries* is as implicit in the agreement to go forward on a step-by-step basis in the *esprit européen* as it is evident in the pragmatic solutions which are being adopted in order that the major concept shall go forward. The supranational European State of Monnet, Adenauer, Spaak, and Schumann must remain an ideal to be achieved through patient progress and in the fullness of time.

It now becomes important to differentiate between the private and public veterinary implications of adherence to the Community.

Whereas the terms of reference of the Liaison Committee keep it within the ambit of the Social and Economic Committee of the Commission, so that it has discussed and advised upon the harmonization of veterinary education, the equivalence of diplomas, the freedom of establishment of the veterinarian and his right to provide services in all the member states, the practice of pharmacy, and even a definition of the exercise of the Public Authority by veterinarians, it has been for the Permanent Veterinary Committee in Brussels, through its expert working parties of state veterinary officers and academicians, to formulate community law regarding the notifiable diseases of animals and their control, the standardization of diagnostic agents and their methods of application, etc., many of which are already known (though not necessarily agreed) by the veterinary authorities of this country through the Office Internationale des Epizooties, F.A.O., W.H.O., and the usual channels of information throughout the veterinary world.

The position has been complicated by the fact that, whereas British observers have attended the Liaison Committee since 1962 and have been able to report at frequent intervals, no such helpful arrangement has been possible at official level until May, 1971, so that the Ministry of Agriculture then found itself, at fairly short notice, discussing subjects such as the control of foot-and-mouth disease and rabies by vaccination and, perhaps, the adoption by the Community of the Rose Bengal plate agglutination test as a standard screening test in the control of brucellosis. No doubt in the course of time these aspects of the negotiations will be ably chronicled by Tolworth.

The Liaison Committee, meanwhile, found itself in Brussels on 23 Oct., 1969, discussing the position of the salaried veterinarian. To us this might not seem a subject for acrimonious debate. We have some 1000 assistants in practice, the great majority of whom are bound by service contracts of varying efficacy, but who practise their profession in the true and liberal sense. There are a little under 200 in research or advisory posts in commerce; these observe the ethical code and instruct the personnel of their companies in the implementation of the Veterinary Surgeons' Act. The newly formed Commercial Veterinary Services Committee of the R.C.V.S. has not uncovered reprehensible practices in this group, though 'a little cloud, no bigger than a man's hand' may be discerned in the tendency to appoint veterinarians to marketing departments in which they might develop a dual allegiance.

Such is not the case in the Community, where restricted opportunities for liberal practice have induced 800 German, 225 Belgian, 300 French, 300 Dutch, and 800 Italian veterinarians to take commercial posts varying from responsible direction to little more than qualified commercial travelling. To our self-employed colleagues of the Community this high proportion is a running sore and a subject for continuous complaint. Not only has a dual allegiance developed in many of the employees of the pharmaceutical, feeding-stuffs, and stock-raising companies: the system of contract-rearing of livestock has put them into direct competition on their clients' farms. In all this the Liaison Committee has proved rather more pious than effective. It has resolved that contracts of employment should be submitted to the national governing bodies of the veterinary profession for their approval but at present it has no means of enforcing its appeal. From this stems the practitioner resentment with the composition of the Liaison Committee and this is one of the driving forces behind the new European Union of Practising Veterinarians. The meeting in October also discussed medicated animal feeding-stuffs and noted that the delay in considering their recommendations as to control, manufacture, and distribution awaited the observations of the European Animal Feed compounders. Meantime it set up a subcommittee to continue examination of the subject.

In the context of Article 55(1) of the Treaty of Rome the Committee considered the exercise of the Public Authority by the non-salaried veterinarian. This delicate subject had been discussed at length by the

Services of the Commission, in whose opinion it was not a matter of participating in a public service or of putting one's technical knowledge at the service of the administration, but comprised two distinct and separate acts, one of technical certification and the other of the power to act independently in pursuance. It was observed that the interpretation of this clause modifying the right of establishment had proved so difficult in the case of the legal profession that, in the opinion of some authorities, that profession might have to be specifically excluded from its provisions.

On 15 Jan., 1970, the Subcommittee on Medicated Feeding-stuffs declared its anxiety at the continuous and uncontrolled use of medicinal additives and premixes and resolved that they should be subject to the same controls as were medicines themselves.

As far back as October, 1967, the *Syndicat National des Vétérinaires Praticiens Français*, at its annual Congress at Saint-Malo, announced its intention to combine the practising members in Europe into a Union of Practitioners. In pursuance of this objective it invited a number of veterinarians to attend a meeting of its Steering Committee in Paris on 19 Dec., 1968, at which the French concept of a Constitution was discussed. Representatives also attended from Denmark, Spain, and the United Kingdom, while messages of support for the project were received from Eire, Sweden, and Switzerland. When the Committee met again at B.V.A. headquarters on 29 March, 1969, the proposed constitution was further discussed, a French President, German, Italian, and British Vice-Presidents provisionally elected, and the aims of the Union more clearly expressed. These were, in short, to strengthen the hand of the practitioner in dealing with Government, other professions, agriculture, and the general public, and to make his work more widely known and respected. Further meetings of the Steering Committee took place in Brussels, Paris, Carrara, and Nancy, culminating in a first Congress of the Union at Garmisch-Partenkirchen, Bavaria, on 2 Oct., 1970. This was attended by two British delegates and the application for entry of the Society of Practising Veterinary Surgeons and the British Small Animal Veterinary Association, with a joint membership of 1855, was formally tendered and accepted. The proceedings of this Congress, sponsored by the *Bundesverband praktischer Tierärtze* and honoured by the Bavarian Government, were widely reported in Western Europe. The Union had by now begun to assume the appearance of a veterinary political weapon.

To return to the mainstream, the Liaison Committee met again in Brussels on 20 Feb., 1970, to consider the report and recommendations of the Subcommittee on Medicated Feeding-stuffs. It pursued the subject of veterinary specialization and reaffirmed its resolution that, in view of the late start made by Italian veterinary education, a period of 5 years must elapse before Italian nationals could enjoy full freedom of movement and professional establishment.

The next major event was the publication on 28 March, 1970, of the four proposed Veterinary Directives by the Commission of the E.E.C. and a recommendation to the Council of the European Veterinary Professional Association. These, in broad terms, followed the proposed Directives already promulgated for the medical and dental professions and concerned the problems debated by the Liaison Committee for a number of years. The three important directives, reproduced in the *Veterinary Record* of 31 Oct. and 7 Nov., 1970, were entitled as follows:—

1. Proposal for Directive of the Council concerning the achievement of the freedom of establishment and the right to provide services in the field of self-employed veterinary activities.

2. Proposal for Directive of the Council relating to the mutual recognition of diplomas, certificates, and other veterinary qualifications.

3. Proposal for Directive of the Council concerning the co-ordination of provisions imposed by law, regulation, or administrative action in the field of self-employed veterinary activities.

Consideration of these Directives was naturally a preoccupation of the Liaison Committee at its next meeting in Utrecht on 21 Oct. In view of its firm recommendations that the right to provide unsalaried veterinary services should be preceded by a period of adaptation for 6 months, during which time the migrant veterinarian should be employed in the country of his adoption in the sort of work he proposed to pursue and at the end of which he should satisfy an authoritative panel that he understood the language, the ethical code, and in general his responsibilities under the law, and of their resolution that the right of the veterinarian to prescribe and dispense medicaments for the treatment of animals under his care was integral to the practice of veterinary medicine, the Committee recorded its astonishment that neither of these conditions was to be found within the Directives, and asked the Economic and Social Committee to reconsider these matters. Further, it expressed its fear that a Member State, in order to give the greatest possible protection to its nationals, might transform certain independent activities into activities under the jurisdiction of the Public Authority.

It was later reported, on 3 Dec., 1970, that in the field of pharmacy the European Parliament thought a minimum period of 6 months' adaptation was a prerequisite to establishment and invited the Commission to present proposals to that effect.

A meeting of the Liaison Committee, held for the first time on the territory of an observer country, took place in London on 23 April, 1971. On this occasion some new ground was broken. A request from the European Union of Practising Veterinarians that its President should, as of right, be entitled to a seat on the Liaison Committee was rejected. A survey of the social security of the practising veterinarian in the Community and of the provisions available from his own profession for disablement, sickness, retirement, or death indicated that Great Britain was poorly organized in this respect. On the other hand, the visiting delegates were clearly impressed by the solidity and stability, and yet the flexibility of the British system, and it may be that one of the best things we have to offer to an enlarged Community is our ability to co-operate, accommodate, and still keep our powder dry.

In the meantime the concept of a European federation of veterinary professions was afoot. If this was the brainchild of the Federal German Republic's *Tierärzteschaft* the drafting of its provisional constitution was left to the United Kingdom. After these statutes have been considered and commented upon by the other national veterinary bodies of Western Europe it is hoped to launch the new Federation on the occasion of the 10th Federal German Veterinary Congress at Wiesbaden, 11–15 Sept., 1972.

The most recent meeting of the Veterinary Liaison Committee in Brussels on 21 Oct. was to have been devoted to a consideration by the 4 applicant countries of the proposed Veterinary Directives in the light of certain observations made by a Head of Division of the Social and Economic Committee, E.E.C. At this meeting the observers from Eire and Denmark made their several contributions. A fortunate meeting of the Joint Officers Committee R.C.V.S.–B.V.A. some days earlier enabled the British delegation to circulate an authoritative paper on our own points of view and this document was taken as a basis for discussion. It became clear, however, at a very early stage, that some of the sacred cows of the V.L.C. were due for slaughter. In particular, the suggested period of 6 months' adaptation as a prerequisite for the migrant veterinarian in the receptor country (which did not figure in the relevant proposed Directive) was rejected by the Social and Economic Committee as inimical to the spirit of the Treaty of Rome. The mutual equivalence of diplomas as a point of harmonization leading to the freedom of movement of veterinarians was thrown back to the Liaison Committee for further consideration. Probably the only constructive information to come down from the Commission was that it seemed likely that some way would be found to allow the legal profession to move freely in terms of Articles 52 and 55, and that if such an intractable problem could be solved the medical and para-medical professions need not be dismayed.

On balance, therefore, the V.L.C. is less sure of itself than it was five years ago. Its two main weaknesses have been pinpointed: it has no power or influence in the upper echelons of the Services of the Commission (a weakness which will be still further apparent as our own Animal Health Division enters fully into the Permanent Veterinary Committee), and its unanimous opinion, as in the matter of the Period of Adaptation, appears to carry no weight, which was certainly not what the V.L.C. was given to understand at the time of the Italian educational difficulty. The new European Union of Practitioners has observed these things and is vocally dissatisfied. It is interesting to speculate that, if the E.U.P.V.S. decides to co-operate wholeheartedly with the proposed European Federation of Veterinary Professions, these two bodies could bring a great accession of strength to the V.L.C. to the benefit of all those exercising the veterinary profession independently.

On the credit side we have been assured that, after 1 Jan., 1973, when the Six have become the Ten, things will alter for the better. There is even a hint of re-negotiating the Treaty, and a very broad hint indeed that one full member is worth any number of observers. We, with ground to lose and not much to gain, must take the European view and decide what it is we have to offer.

REFERENCES

Pasfield, J. (1969), *Vet. Rec.*, **85**, 568.
— — (1970a), *Ibid.*, **87**, 539.
— — (1970b), *Ibid.*, **87**, 579.

SOME OBSERVATIONS ON THE SOUND VIBRATIONS PRODUCED BY AIR FLOW IN THE RESPIRATORY TRACT OF HORSES AT EXERCISE

Donald P. Attenburrow, B.V.Sc., M.R.C.V.S.

The act of ventilation of the lung results in a reciprocal flow of air in the respiratory tract. This flow of air produces sound within the respiratory tract. A recently developed technique allows selective detection and permanent recording of those sound vibrations that result from the respiratory airflow in the trachea of the equine during all forms of exercise in the open field.

This contribution presents part of the data gathered by the application of a telemetric stethoscope to 60 clinically normal horses exercised at the canter and gallop. The data are evaluated by well-established physical techniques and are briefly discussed under the following headings: (1) reproduction of the sounds as sound, (2) graphical representation of the sounds, (3) the amplitude envelope, (4) the relationship of the respiratory sound to limb movement, (5) the inspiratory time constant.

Materials and Method

The technique illustrated in *Fig.* 1 includes the use of an audio-vibration transducer, radio transmitter and receiver, pre-amplifier, and tape recorder.

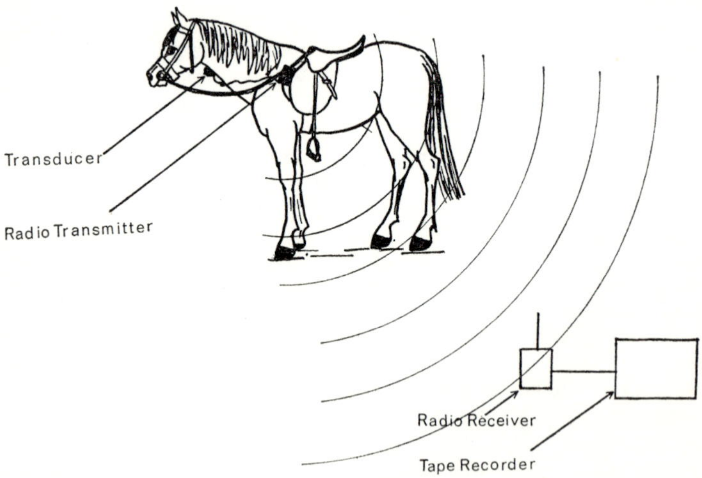

Fig. 1.—Showing the use of an audio-vibration transducer, radio transmitter and receiver, and tape recorder.

The selective detection of the sound at source is achieved by the specialized construction of the transducer, the applicator casing, and the method of application. The device does not respond to nor record any of those ambient sounds associated with a moving horse in an open field. The audio-vibration transducer is applied externally to the skin overlying the region of the third and fourth tracheal ring. The technique does not involve surgical interference or removal of hair. The data may be reproduced as sound or in graphical form, by the use of an ink jet writer.

Table I gives a breakdown of the subjects from which recordings have been taken. The height varies from 16·3 h.h. to 12·2 h.h. The subjects were exercised in a wide circle and in a straight line. They were ridden in the normal manner with normal tack. An assessment of the past health and condition of each subject was obtained from the owner or manager. The condition of each subject at the time of recording was assessed by clinical examination in the traditional manner.

Table I.—NUMBERS AND TYPES OF HORSES EXAMINED

	TYPE				TOTAL
	Thoroughbred	Light Hunter	Heavy Hunter	Pony	
No. of horses	14	27	4	15	60

REPRODUCTION OF THE SOUNDS AS SOUND

Tape recordings of respiratory sounds were made as follows: at the walk, trot, canter, canter (high blowing), and gallop. It was found that the sounds produced at the canter and gallop had a marked rhythm and regularity. In contrast, the respiratory sounds at the walk and trot have a less easily recognizable rhythm. It was noted that the sounds of expiration appeared louder than those of inspiration.

A recording of the horse 'high blowing' at the canter demonstrates the effect of this particular nostril movement upon the expiratory sounds.

GRAPHICAL REPRESENTATION OF THE SOUNDS

The sound signals stored on magnetic tape may be fed into an ink jet writer (Mingograf). This instrument responds to the electrical output of the tape recorder and traces out on paper a graphical representation of the sounds. The Mingograf paper is marked both vertically and horizontally in millimetres. The chart speed is such that 200 mm. is equivalent to 1 second. Measurements along the horizontal axis are measurements in time. The amplitude or loudness is measured on the vertical axis. It is therefore possible to measure (1) the variations in amplitude of the sounds that occur during the period of inspiration and during the period of expiration, (2) the difference between the amplitude of the sounds of inspiration and expiration, (3) the duration of inspiration and expiration, (4) the respiratory rate, and (5) any abnormalities that occur. (*Plates I–V.*)

Fig. A is a Mingograf of the sounds produced during one respiratory cycle of a horse exercised at the canter. It clearly demonstrates the amplitude and duration of the sounds produced during the period of inspiration and the period of expiration. Between one inspiration and the following expiration, and between expiration and the next inspiration, there is a period of zero or near-zero sound.

Fig. B is a Mingograf of the recording of a horse 'high blowing' when exercised at the canter.

The Amplitude Envelope

Fig. C is a Mingograf of the sounds which are produced during one respiratory cycle of a horse exercised at the canter. To demonstrate what is meant by the term 'amplitude envelope', the maximum amplitudes (plus and minus) that occur within the respiratory cycle are joined by a black line. It will be seen that the envelope of the sounds produced during inspiration reaches a maximum at the mid-point of this period. The amplitude envelope of the inspiratory sound tends often to be fusiform, but can be diphasic. The maximum amplitude of the sound produced during expiration is reached at or very shortly after the beginning of this period. The amplitude envelope of the expiratory sound is overall typically cone-shaped and is also diphasic. The diphasic nature of the amplitude envelope of the expiratory sound is a constant feature of all respiratory excursions examined at the canter and gallop. The recorded maximum amplitude of the expiratory sound at the canter is typically twice that of the inspiratory sound. It will be demonstrated that the diphasic nature of the expiratory envelope is related to weight-bearing by the limbs.

Fig. D is a typical Mingograf of the sound which is produced during one respiratory cycle of a horse exercised at a slow gallop. It is seen that the amplitude envelope differs slightly from that of the respiratory sound produced at the canter (*Fig. A*), the differences being: (1) the maximum amplitude of the inspiratory sound tends to occur at the beginning of inspiration, (2) the amplitude envelope of the expiratory sound is diphasic but the cone shape, typically seen at the canter, is not so obvious at the gallop.

Fig. E is a typical Mingograf of the sounds which are produced during one respiratory cycle of a horse exercised at a fast gallop. It will be seen that the amplitude of the sounds produced during inspiration and expiration are approximately equal.

The Relationship of the Respiratory Sound to Limb Movement

The breathing frequency of 22 horses was measured by telemetry in the various kinds of motion by Dietmar Specht in 1965. His observations led him to suggest that because of the nature of some of his recordings there was a relationship between the respiratory cycle and the limb movement. The present investigations show that Specht's suggestion is correct. By counting the number of strides in a given interval of time (stride rate), and by counting the number of recorded respirations in that given interval of time, it was possible to establish that the striding rate was equal to the respiratory rate. By watching the limb action and listening to the sound from the receiver it was also possible to establish that each stride was associated with one respiratory cycle.

To determine accurately the very close relationship between the respiratory cycle and the cycle of limb movement it is necessary to record the precise moments when a particular limb strikes and leaves the ground. This has been

PLATE I

RESPIRATORY SOUND MEASUREMENT IN HORSES

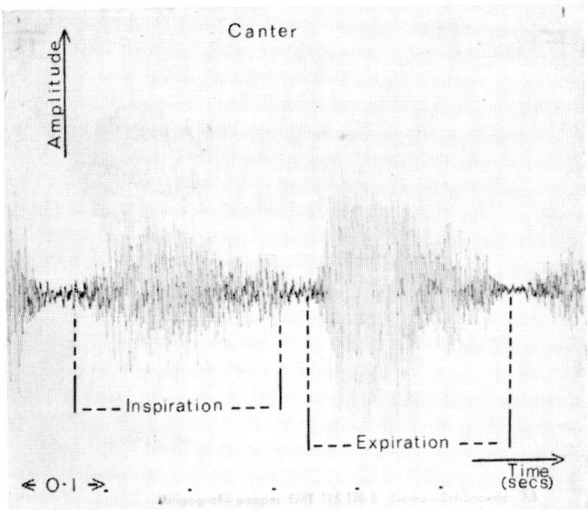

Fig. A.—A graphical representation (Mingograf) of the sounds produced during one respiratory cycle within the trachea of the equine exercised at the canter.

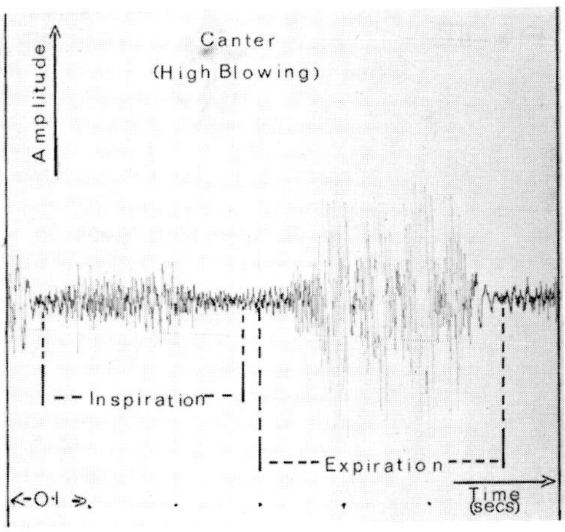

Fig. B.—A graphical representation (Mingograf) of the sounds produced during one respiratory cycle within the trachea of the equine exercised at the canter. This horse is 'high blowing'.

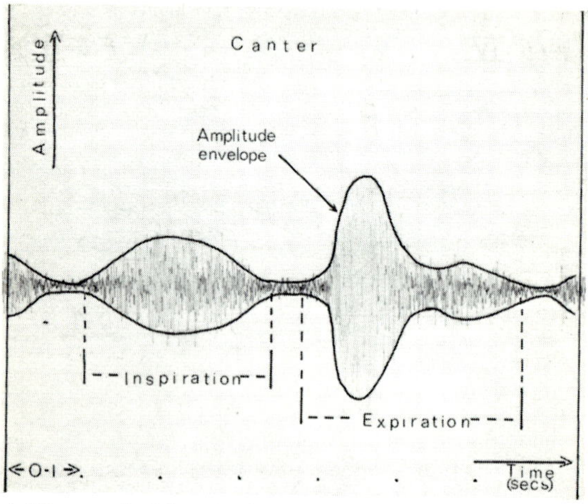

Fig. C.—A Mingograf of the sounds which are produced during one respiratory cycle of a horse exercised at the canter.

RESPIRATORY SOUND MEASUREMENT IN HORSES—*continued*

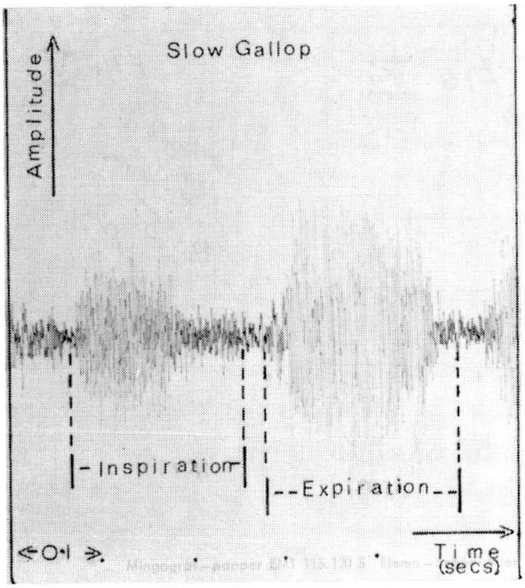

Fig. D.

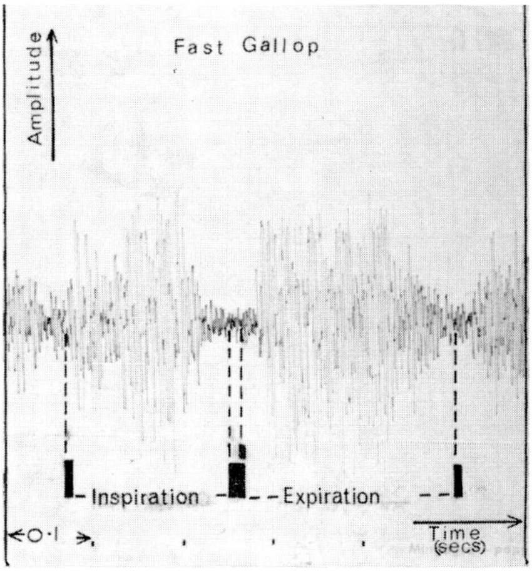

Fig. E.

Fig. D.—A graphical representation (Mingograf) of the sounds produced during one respiratory cycle within the trachea of the equine exercised at the slow gallop.

Fig. E.—A graphical representation (Mingograf) of the sounds produced during one respiratory cycle within the trachea of the equine exercised at the fast gallop.

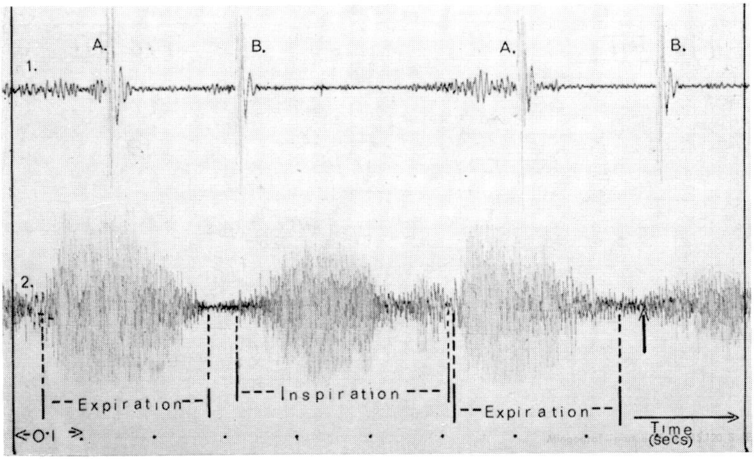

Fig. F.—A graphical representation (Mingograf) showing data simultaneously transmitted from the horse exercised at the canter. On this Mingograf, signal A on the upper trace indicates the precise moment that the leading leg strikes the ground and signal B indicates the precise moment that it leaves the ground. The lower trace is a graphical representation of the sounds produced during respiration which were recorded simultaneously on a second channel on the same tape.

PLATE IV

RESPIRATORY SOUND MEASUREMENT IN HORSES—*continued*

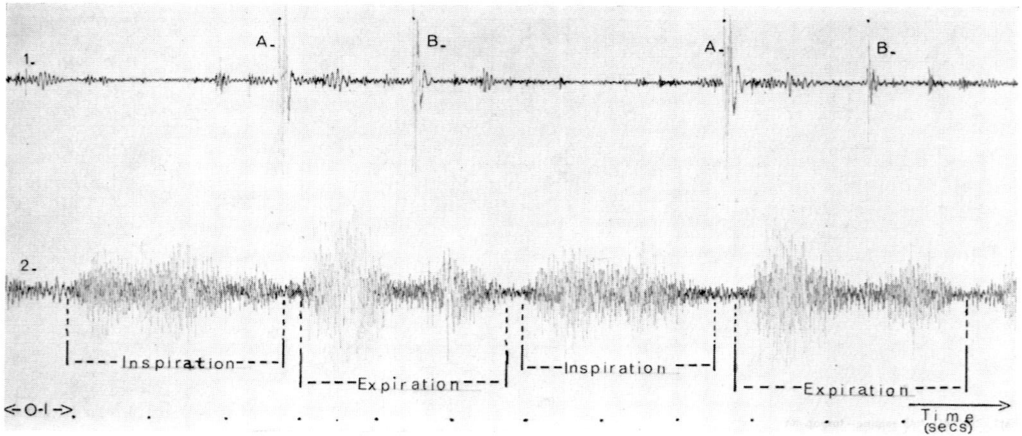

Fig. G.—A graphical representation (Mingograf) showing data simultaneously transmitted from the horse exercised at the canter. The lower trace is a graphical representation of the sounds produced during respiration which were recorded simultaneously on a second channel on the same tape.

RESPIRATORY SOUND MEASUREMENT IN HORSES—*continued*

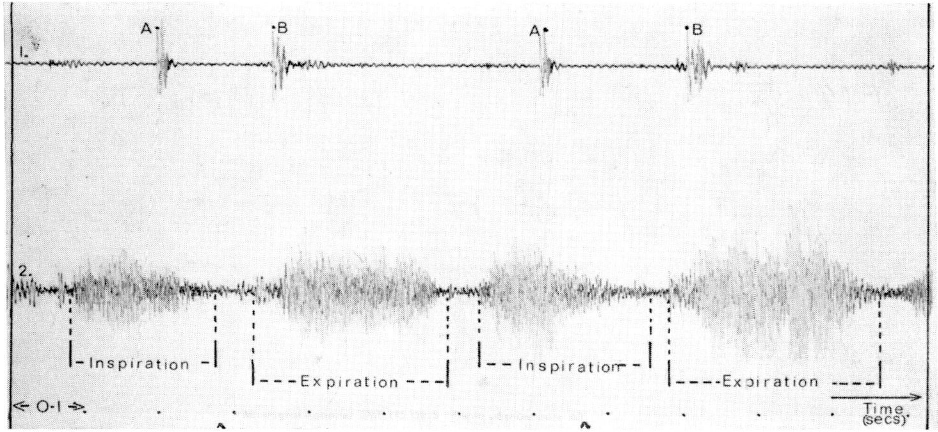

Fig. H.—A graphical representation (Mingograf) showing data simultaneously transmitted from the horse exercised at the canter. The lower trace is a graphical representation of the sounds produced during respiration which were recorded simultaneously on a second channel on the same tape.

done by attaching to the foot a make-and-break switch that makes when the foot strikes the ground and breaks when the foot leaves the ground. The signals produced by the contacts at these instants are transmitted by a telemetry channel separate from that channel which is transmitting the respiratory sounds. The results are recorded simultaneously on separate channels of the same tape.

Figs. F–H show data simultaneously transmitted from a horse exercised at the canter. On the Mingograf shown as *Fig. F*, signal A on the upper trace indicates the precise moment that the leading leg strikes the ground and signal B indicates the precise moment that it leaves the ground. The time measured between signal A and signal B is the exact time that the leading leg is bearing weight during one complete stride. The lower trace is a graphical representation of the sounds produced during respiration which were recorded simultaneously. By comparing the signals on the upper trace with those on the lower trace it is seen that the leading foreleg strikes the ground in the middle of expiration and leaves the ground at the beginning of inspiration.

On the tracing shown as *Fig. G*, signal A on the upper trace indicates the precise moment that diagonally opposite limbs strike the ground and signal B indicates the precise moment that they leave the ground. The time measured between signal A and signal B is the exact time that diagonals were bearing weight during one complete stride. It will be seen that diagonals struck the ground just before the beginning of expiration and left the ground in the middle of expiration.

On the Mingograf shown as *Fig. H*, signal A on the upper trace indicates the precise moment that the hind-leg diagonally opposite the leading foreleg strikes the ground and signal B indicates the precise moment that it leaves the ground. The time measured between signal A and signal B is the exact time that the hind-leg (diagonally opposite the leading foreleg) is bearing weight during one complete stride. It will be seen that the hind-leg diagonally opposite the leading leg strikes the ground in the middle of inspiration.

In the precise relationship that exists at the canter, between the respiratory cycle and the cycle of limb movement the constant features are:—

1. Inspiration begins at the moment when the leading foreleg leaves the ground, that is when the period of suspension begins.

2. Only half the inspiration period is completed whilst the horse is in suspension as the hind-limb diagonally opposite to the leading fore-limb strikes the ground at the middle of inspiration.

3. The diagonally opposite limbs strike the ground just before the first phase of expiration begins.

4. The leading fore-limb strikes the ground just before the second phase of expiration begins.

Physiological functions such as coughing and swallowing and some clinical conditions may and do cause interruptions in this relationship.

Inspiratory Time Constant (*Fig.* 2)

The sounds produced by respiratory airflow in the trachea of the 60 horses exercised at the canter and gallop were recorded, and from these recordings Mingografs were produced of each horse exercised at the canter and of 40 of these horses exercised at the gallop.

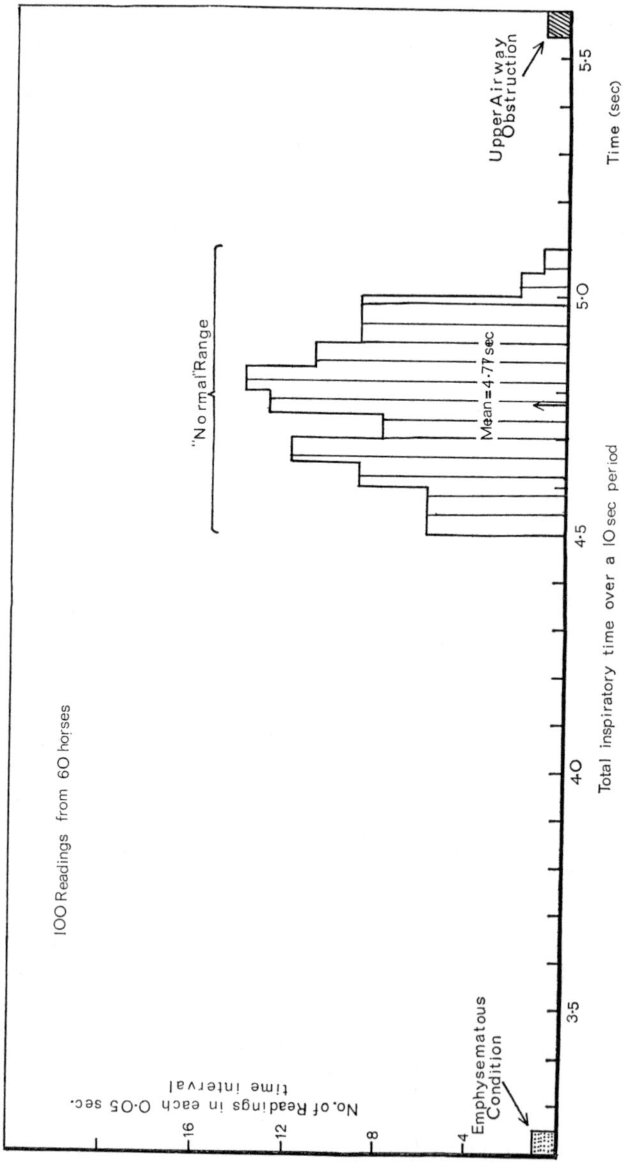

Fig. 2.—A histogram from 100 measurements at the canter and gallop, each measurement being the total time spent inspiring in any 10-second period.

A 10-second period was marked off on each Mingograf and the duration in time of the inspiratory sound of each inspiratory period contained in the 10-second period was measured and totalled. It was found that although these Mingografs included recording of respiratory rates that varied from 96 to 145 per minute, and the height of the horses recorded varied from 12·2 to 16·2 h.h., the total time spent inspiring during the 10-second period is a constant at 4·77 seconds with a standard deviation of + or − 3 per cent. Variations from this constant normally only occur when the subject coughs, swallows, or clears the nostrils.

This constant would appear to be an interesting physiological phenomenon. Its possible significance when related to clinical conditions of the respiratory tract is suggested by the following recordings of 2 horses:—

1. A horse suffering from emphysema of the lung was recorded at the canter. The inspiratory time of this horse in a 10-second period was 3·71 seconds.

2. A pony with a clinical obstruction of the left nostril was recorded at the canter. The inspiratory time of this pony in a 10-second period was 5·70 seconds.

Acknowledgements.—I should like to thank Dr. Flack, of the Physics Department, Exeter University, for his untiring interest and help, Mr. Roberts, M.R.C.V.S., of the Equine Research Station, Newmarket, for his considerable encouragement, and the members of the Exeter Riding Club and all those horse-owners in my practice without whose help and patience this work would not have been possible. Telemetric Link by Lustraphone Ltd.

REFERENCE

Specht, Dietmar (1965), *Telemetrische Untersuchungen der Atemfrequenzen von Reitpferden in allen Gangarten und beim Springen*, Inaugural Dissertation, University of Berlin.

DISEASES OF THE EAR, NOSE, AND THROAT IN THE HORSE

PART I: THE EAR

W. R. Cook, F.R.C.V.S.

INTRODUCTION

In one article, or even in three, it is not possible to give an account of every aspect of ear, nose, and throat disease in the horse. Emphasis will be placed, therefore, on the practical matters of diagnosis and treatment and a bibliography provided for more detailed study. The subject will be introduced in three parts. Part I, which follows, will describe diseases of the ear, but Parts II and III, in later editions of the VETERINARY ANNUAL, will refer to diseases of the nose (nasal chamber and accessory sinuses) and throat (pharynx, larynx, trachea, and oesophagus). The aim is to compile a short text on a subject which has not previously been covered as an entity.

The diseases are classified on an aetiological basis and will be commented upon in each section in the same order, i.e., congenital defects, diseases caused by trauma and foreign bodies, those caused by infection (bacterial, viral, and fungal), parasitic and neoplastic diseases; diseases caused by nervous dysfunction (paralysis, paresis, neuralgia, or hypersensitivity), allergy, and diseases caused by management (nutrition or hygiene). General observations on domestication as a fundamental cause of diseases of the ear, nose, and throat in the horse have been made by Cook (1971).

ANATOMY

The ear consists of three natural divisions: external, middle, and internal. The surgical anatomy of the ear is illustrated by *Figs.* 3–11.

The anatomical nomenclature adopted is that used by Sisson and Grossman (1945). Some clinical aspects of the anatomy and physiology of the equine ear have been commented upon by Cook (1966a, b), and anatomical illustrations of clinical interest are also available (Cook, Campbell, and Dawson, 1968; Cook and Tompsett, 1968). Chors (1928) describes the anatomy and histology of the inner ear and Eggston and Wolff (1947) comment on the comparative anatomy of the ear.

CLINICAL EXAMINATION

General anaesthesia is necessary for otoscopy of the external ear and for most radiographic examinations. Endoscopy of the Eustachian tube diverticulum (guttural pouch), an essential part of all middle-ear examinations, may be carried out in the majority of cases without anaesthesia but general anaesthesia is necessary for some diagnostic problems of this region and for most therapeutic techniques.

Literature is available on the choice of instrument for endoscopy of the middle ear (Cook, 1970a) and on the technique of endoscopy (Cook, 1970b).

The radiography of the petrous temporal bone and its anatomical relations is illustrated in atlas form by Schebitz and Wilkens (1968). The radiology of the horse's ear is described by Cook (1970c, 1972).

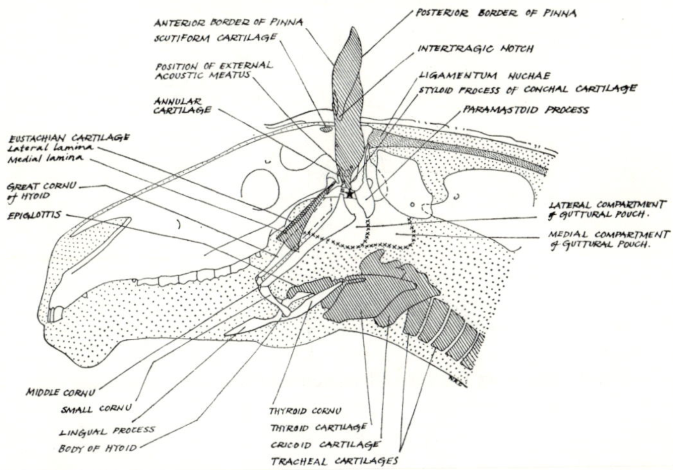

Fig. 3.—To show the basic anatomy of the external ear and Eustachian tube diverticulum (guttural pouch) in relation to the remainder of the osseous and cartilaginous skeleton. The star, under the styloid process, marks the area in which a pain reflex can often be elicited, in the presence of mycosis of the guttural pouch.

External Ear

Congenital Defects

Temporal Teratoma (*dentigerous cyst*).—Ectopic molar teeth sometimes develop in the temporal region, in association with either the squamous temporal or the petrous temporal bone (*Figs*. 4, 11).

The clinical signs of a subcutaneous swelling anterior to the base of the external ear in a young horse, accompanied by a discharging sinus about half-way up the anterior border of the conchal cartilage, are sufficiently characteristic to permit a tentative diagnosis (*Fig*. 4). Clinical signs may be present in a foal of a few weeks old, though the case may not be presented for examination until the horse is 2 or 3 years of age or even older. Confusion might arise in rare cases where there is no sinus or no swelling or where the sinus discharges, not on the outside of the pinna, but at a point within the external auditory meatus. Under these conditions, the disease could be mistaken for an abscess of the external ear (*see below*, Otitis Externa) though the prolonged discharge of mucopus should, in itself, help differentiation. However, a positive diagnosis can be made by radiography, taking radiographs in two planes in order to establish the position of the teratomatous tooth (Cook, 1970c). Sometimes more than one tooth is present. *Fig*. 5 illustrates a specimen demonstrated by Jennings (1960). The dense radio-opacity of dental tissue allows the tooth and its location to be identified in relation to the squamous or petrous temporal bone. The injection of a

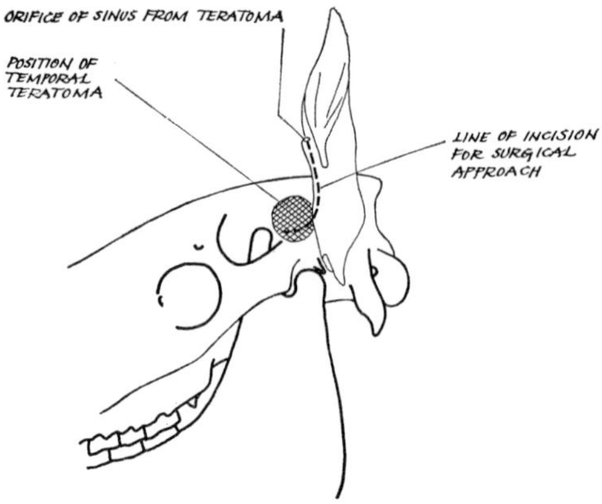

Fig. 4.—Showing the surgical anatomy of temporal teratomata.

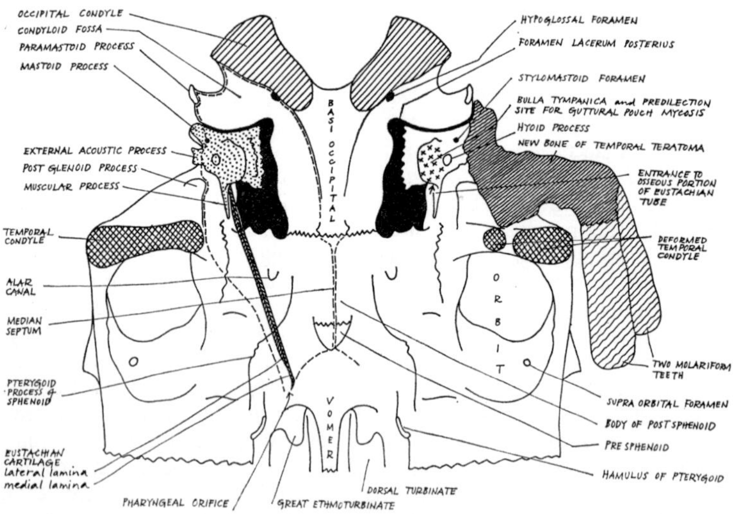

Fig. 5.—Diagrammatic view of the base of the skull to show, on its right side, the normal anatomical relations of the petrous temporal bone and, on its left side, one particular instance of a temporal teratoma. The specimen came from a 15-year-old Clydesdale gelding (Jennings, 1960) and illustrates the great size that these defects can achieve if surgical removal is not effected when the animal is young. In this particular case there was no cranial invasion, but the new bone formation had blocked the left external auditory meatus and there was deformity of the left temporomandibular articulation.

contrast medium into the sinus tract may provide some additional information, though this is probably unnecessary in most cases. An assessment of the number and distribution of the abnormal teeth is of value when it comes to planning their surgical removal. In older horses the teratoma may perforate the temporal bone and invade the cranial cavity (Dewar, 1903) and it is necessary to be aware of this prior to surgery. It seems that not every teratoma in the temporal region results in the formation of an aural sinus. Walley (1889) gives the case record of a 16-year-old carthorse in which a temporal teratoma invaded the cranium and was drawn attention to by a disturbance of the C.N.S., there being no external swelling discernible and no sinus formation.

Treatment should be directed towards the surgical resection of the epithelial lining of the cyst and the tooth or teeth which it contains. After irrigating the cyst cavity with 0·5 per cent cetrimide* solution, a probe should be placed in the sinus tract to identify its course. A vertical skin incision is made from the tract orifice down to a point level with the zygomatic process and then curved anteriorly and horizontally in order that a skin-flap can be reflected from the region anterior to the base of the ear (*Fig*. 4). Bone gouges, chisels, and a hammer may be required to sculpt free the more firmly embedded teeth from their temporary alveoli or to remove bone.

Following removal of the tooth or teeth, the 'socket' should be curetted and any loose bone fragments removed. The cyst wall, with its inner epithelial lining and outer fibrous thickening, is now removed *in toto*. The cyst may have various branches. Bone haemorrhage can be controlled by the use of gelatin sponge.† Dead space is occluded in the usual way and the skin-flap sutured, leaving a drainage tube in position below the most ventral point of the incision. The tube can be removed after 6 or 7 days. If all abnormal tissue has been resected, complete healing should take place without persistent sinus formation.

During surgery, the presence of the auriculopalpebral branch of the facial nerve and the most dorsal section of the parotid salivary gland should be remembered (*Fig*. 7) and damage to these structures avoided. The scutiform cartilage of the ear (*Fig*. 3) must be closely related to the site of the teratoma though its fate and involvement with the condition have not been studied. Surgery on the young animal probably carries a better prognosis than if it is delayed, as the larger the tooth grows the greater the risk of cranial involvement (*Fig*. 5).

Dermoid Cyst.—This is less common than a dentigerous cyst but may occur in the same site. Clinical signs are similar, though there will be less swelling. Radiography allows the two conditions to be differentiated and the use of contrast medium will facilitate assessment of the sinus ramifications. Treatment is by surgical removal of the epithelial lining and fibrous capsule, as for a dentigerous cyst.

Congenital 'Paresis' of the Pinna.—The familiar lop-eared condition is looked upon as a feature of interest though of no particular importance and is often thought to indicate a horse of kind and placid temperament. However, the ears of a lop-eared horse lack muscular control and adopt the same

---

* Cetavlon, I.C.I. Pharmaceuticals.

† Sterispon, Allen & Hanburys Ltd.

position as a previously normal ear that has become paralysed, i.e., the pinna falls into the horizontal position, its long axis transverse to the spine (*Fig.* 6 A). It is possible that this may be associated with a bilateral defect of the motor nerves, i.e., the anterior and posterior auricular branches of the facial nerve (*Fig.* 7), or of the extrinsic auricular muscles themselves. Some lop-eared horses are unable to rotate their ears forwards into the 'pricked-up' position and, at fast exercise, the ears flop about in an uncontrolled manner due to head movement. It is a matter for further observation as to whether all lop-eared horses are incapable of 'laying-back' their ears. It is possible that this function is still retained in some lop-eared horses, but the general inability of a lop-eared horse to lay back its ears may have contributed to the belief that these horses have a placid temperament.

Diagnosis of the condition presents no problem and it is debatable whether one is justified in listing this as a disease, in that the condition causes the horse no apparent harm. There is no other sign of facial palsy and, though it is not possible to judge the ability to hear by observing movement of the pinna, it has never been suggested that these horses are deaf. The auricular nerves and muscles in these cases might, however, repay study, as also might an examination of the auditory nerves.

Traumatic Diseases

Open Wounds.—Wounds of the external ear are not common but can be of some cosmetic importance. Careful suturing is required and general anaesthesia will be necessary. Cleaning and débridement should be carried out as indicated but tissue should be preserved as far as possible. If the wouud has resulted in both epithelial surfaces of the pinna being torn, each side will require individual suturing, using a fine needle and interrupted sutures of stainless steel or monofilament nylon. To preserve the shape of the pinna and to avoid cicatricial deformity, the torn pinna may be 'splinted' by means of a sheet of X-ray film applied to each side of the ear and sutured in position after shaping (Heinzer, 1968).

The cosmetic 'cropping' of horses' ears is, fortunately, no longer fashionable.

Frost-bite.—In some climates the apices of the pinna, where there is little subcutaneous tissue, are exposed to damage by frost-bite. The ragged appearance of the ear can be improved by surgery, both ears being 're-pointed'. In order that the ears should be symmetrical, a plastic template may be used (Hecht, 1964). The cut edges are sutured and tetanus anti-toxin should be given, as with all operations of this type.

Chronic Granuloma.—Neglected wounds in mobile regions of the horse's body where there is a paucity of skin frequently produce exuberant granulation. At the base of the concha these may be treated by the application of copper-sulphate powder at 4-day intervals, by surgery, or, in persistent cases, by radiotherapy (Silver, 1963). Neglected or poorly healing skin wounds may initiate recurrent fibroma (sarcoid) formation (Cotchin, 1960).

Necrosis of the Conchal Cartilage.—This may occur as the result of open wounds and infection. A sinus forms in association with the lesion and surgical excision of the necrotic tissue is necessary. Necrosis may be a sequel to severe bruising of the cartilage and twitches should not be applied to the base of the ear.

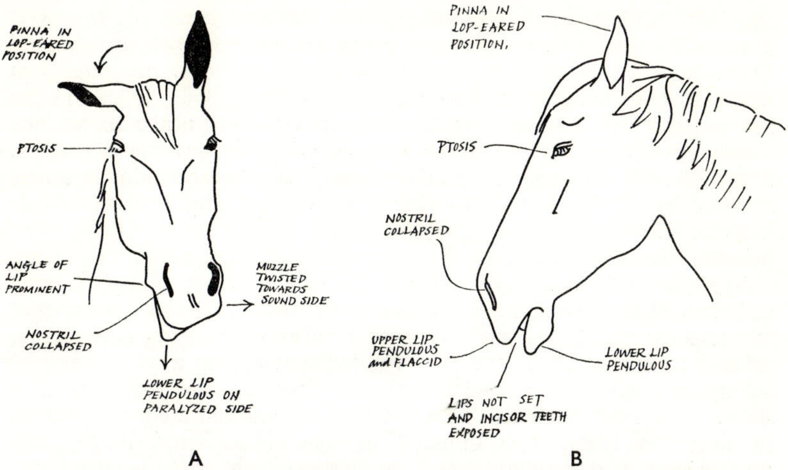

Fig. 6.—To show the clinical signs associated with paralysis of the facial nerve (cranial VII). A, Unilateral paralysis of the facial nerve, as caused by intracranial, intratemporal or, possibly, by extratemporal damage close to the stylomastoid foramen. B, Diagram taken from a photograph of a 6-year-old gelding showing bilateral facial palsy. When the paralysis is bilateral the lower lip droops to such an extent that the incisor teeth are exposed to view. Also the muzzle is slack and both nostrils are collapsed but the upper lip is not twisted.

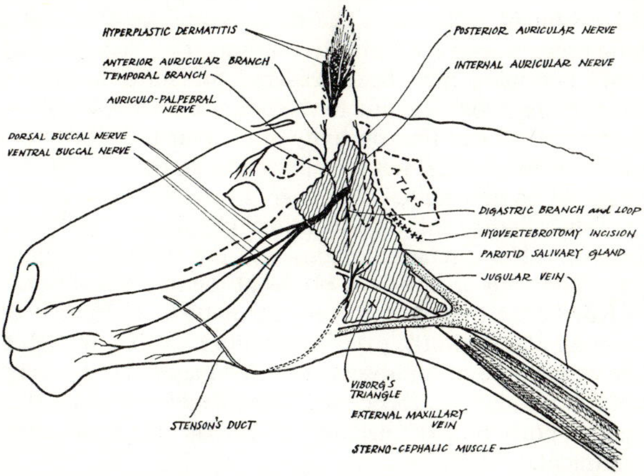

Fig. 7.—Showing the peripheral distribution and anatomical relationships of the facial nerve (cranial VII). The parotid salivary gland is variable in size and is shown here at its largest, filling Viborg's triangle ventrally. In some cases its ventral edge coincides with the line of the sternocephalic tendon, as in *Fig.* 10. Diverticulotomy may be effected by a ventral (Whitehouse) approach, by a ventrolateral approach dorsal to the external maxillary vein in Viborg's triangle, or by a dorsolateral (hyovertebrotomy) approach as shown in the diagram.

Foreign Bodies in the External Auditory Meatus.—There are no known reports in the literature of foreign bodies in the horse's external ear. However, it seems that these do occur and may require careful otoscopy before they are discovered. Messervy (1971) has encountered a Dartmoor pony that was shown to have a tight spiral of cellophane, 8·00 cm. long, lodged in the peritympanic region of the meatus. Head shaking in a vertical plane was the presenting sign and the pony showed neither otorrhoea nor torticollis. A foreign body was suspected as the cause of lateral headshaking in a case reported by de Ban and Jones (1971), though not confirmed (*see* Otitis Externa, *below*).

Infective Diseases

Hyperplastic Dermatitis of the Pinna.—A vegetative lesion occurs frequently and often bilaterally on the concave surface of the pinna. These circumscribed, unpigmented, focal, and slightly raised plaques which often coalesce are referred to by owners as 'warts'. The lesion resembles a white bacterial colony on a dark culture medium (*Fig.* 7). Histologically, they have been shown to be areas of chronic hyperplastic dermatitis and are not neoplastic (Binninger and Piper, 1968), although one worker (Thomsett, 1970) describes the condition as a 'papillomatosis'. In most cases, the lesion appears to be asymptomatic. Occasionally, horses seem to resent the affected ear being handled, but this head-shyness may have resulted from previous handling or attempts at treatment. Owners tend to notice this lesion in a horse which is an established 'head-shaker', but it is difficult to be certain whether there is any relationship.

The aetiology is not fully understood. A virus infection or chronic irritation from biting flies has been suspected but the lesions persist for long periods. Eight affected horses which were observed over a period of 2 years still had the lesions at the end of this time (Binninger and Piper, 1968).

No useful treatment is known. The topical application of corticosteroid and antibiotic preparations are ineffective and their application may increase head-shyness. Tattooing may be considered for show horses, where the lesion becomes more noticeable due to the practice of clipping short the long hairs that normally grow in the concavity of the pinna. This 'treatment' has not been tried but the result, if not the ethics, should be satisfactory. General anaesthesia would be necessary. A simpler 'treatment' is to cover the areas with boot polish or indian ink or discontinue clipping.

Otitis Externa.—The discharge of pus into the external auditory meatus has been described with an overflow of pus at the intertragic notch (*Fig.* 3), causing the hair below the notch to become matted. The pus is thought to originate from an abscess in the external auditory meatus, though this is not proved. The occurrence of an abscess may, or may not, be associated with symptoms of head-shaking or torticollis. Treatment involves local cleaning of the cartilaginous portion of the meatus and perhaps the application of some antibiotic ointment.

Chronic otitis is not a problem in the horse as it is in the dog. The possibility of a teratomatous condition should be considered if persistent otorrhoea is encountered (*see* Temporal Teratoma). Alternatively, a rare cause of purulent otitis externa is an ascending infection from an otitis media associated with guttural pouch mycosis (Bjorklund and Pälsson, 1970) or empyema of the guttural pouch (Durante, 1949).

Ulcerative otitis externa is uncommon but 1 case has been described recently by de Ban and Jones (1971). Clinical signs comprised the sudden onset of head-shyness, with head-shaking in the stable and one ear held most of the time in the lop-eared position. The head-shaking took the form of a side-to-side movement, i.e., lateral rotation as seen with otitis externa in the dog. Torticollis was not observed but an aural discharge was present, as indicated by matting of hair at the intertragic notch (Jones, 1971). Excess wax was present in the left ear and, after cleansing, a discrete ulcer was found. The symptoms resolved following cleansing of the ear and a single application of an antibiotic and corticosteroid ointment.*

Fungal Otitis Externa.—Fungal spores can be isolated from the external auditory meati of apparently healthy horses when the meati themselves are dusty and contain excess wax but are not otherwise diseased. Under conditions of domestication, where the horse is stabled and in close contact with decaying vegetation (hay and straw), it is not surprising that spores are present, though no proper studies have been made and it is not known whether a mycelium forms,† or whether the spores cause any trouble in the external ear itself. The contamination is mentioned because, *if* the ear drum becomes damaged, spores could enter the tympanic cavity of the middle ear and, in this way, be responsible for starting a true mycosis which would be seen endoscopically when the infection spreads from the tympanic cavity to the guttural pouch. This hypothesis as to the cause of guttural pouch mycosis requires further investigation. It could be one reason why the predilection site for guttural pouch mycosis is close to the osseous Eustachian tube and bulla tympanica (*Fig*. 5). Another hypothesis is to assume the presence of a primary mycosis of the tympanic cavity, arising from an ascending infection (*see* Otitis Media).

From the diagnostic point of view, the first hypothesis is of interest as it emphasizes the necessity for developing a technique to examine the osseous portion of the meatus and the membrana tympani. Unfortunately, the equine ear drum is smaller and more inaccessible than that of either man or dog and an entirely satisfactory technique has not yet been developed. The presence of ceruminous discharge in the depth of the meatus and the difficulties of removing this without causing haemorrhage complicates the issue. Wax may be softened by the use of a saturated solution of sodium bicarbonate or a few drops of hydrogen peroxide. Cleaning of the meatus prior to otoscopy can also be carried out using an aural douching syringe,‡ with its nozzle placed close to the osseous meatus, though without completely blocking the canal.

Following cleansing of the meatus by fluid irrigation and the use of cotton-wool swabs on applicators, a forward (direct) viewing fibrelight endoscope§ of external diameter not exceeding 4 mm. is used for otoscopy, in conjunction with an infant human bronchoscope (*Fig*. 8). Under general anaesthesia the bronchoscope is first introduced into the meatus so that its tip engages in the

---

* Tetra-delta Suspension, Upjohn Ltd.

† In man otomycosis results in the formation in the meatus of masses of material like wet blotting-paper, varying in colour from white through brown to black (Hall and Colman, 1969).

‡ Down Bros., Mayer, & Phelps Ltd.

§ Resectoscope, Down Bros., Mayer, & Phelps Ltd.

mouth of the external acoustic process. Warm water is pumped into the osseous portion of the meatus, using the ventilation tube on the bronchoscope. If the light-carrying rod is omitted, this provides for a two-way flow of fluid. A convenient apparatus for supplying a continuous flow of warm and, if necessary, medicated water is a compressed-air pump of the type designed for horticultural use.* The endoscope is introduced down the bronchoscope and

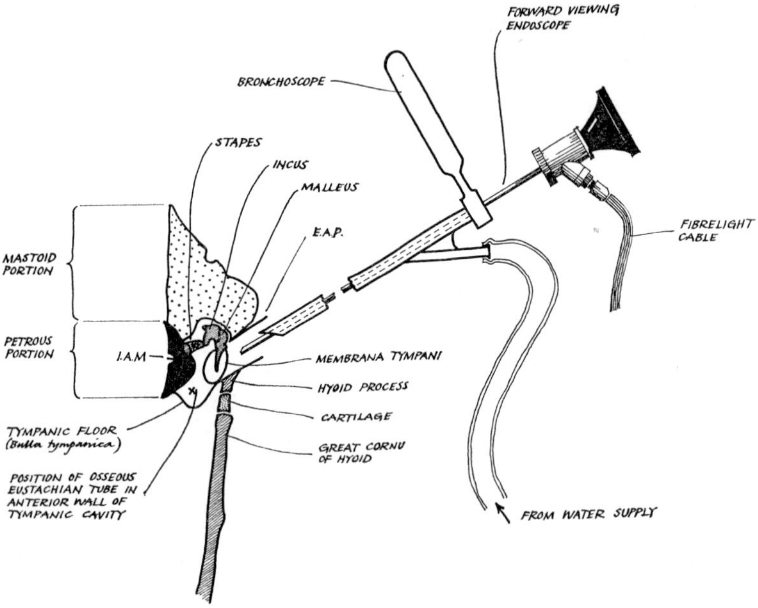

Fig. 8.—Diagrammatic transverse section through petrous temporal bone showing the anatomy of the tympanic cavity and the technique of otoscopy using a forward-viewing fibrelight endoscope. The muscular process, tympanic floor, hyoid process, and external acoustic process develop from membrane and the petrous temporal bone (the petromastoid portion) develops in cartilage.

the region of the membrana tympani examined using an ‘underwater’ technique. Any haemorrhage that has previously been precipitated by the application of cotton-wool swabs for removal of wax is, in this way, washed away continuously and the ‘misting-up’ problem of the endoscope is also solved.

Experience with this technique needs to be gained before it can be properly assessed. As yet, comment cannot always be made with certainty on the health or otherwise of the membrane. That rupture of the ear drum in the horse does occur, however, has been shown, at post-mortem examination, by Bjorklund and Pälsson (1970).

Parasitic Diseases

Parasitic Otitis Externa.—

1. *Psoroptic ear mange* (*Psoroptes cuniculi*): Psoroptic mange mites have been found in profusion in the external auditory meatus of 1 horse recently

* Associated Sprayers Ltd.

(Cook and Barnett, 1971). The otoscopy was being carried out as part of a routine examination though the horse was showing no symptoms of otitis and neither were there any accompanying skin lesions elsewhere in the body. Head-shaking was not present. Following this Peace (1971) carried out routine otoscopy of about 12 horses which were being anaesthetized for other purposes and found ear mites, bilaterally, in 2 horses. The mites were not identified. None of these horses was showing signs of aural discomfort and, again, the condition was apparently asymptomatic.

Reports of psoroptic mites in the ears of the horse, ass, mule, sheep, goat, and rabbit are not uncommon. The ear mite *Psoroptes cuniculi* (synonym: *Psoroptes hippotis*) shows no tendency to invade other parts of the body yet often appears simultaneously in both ears, generally confined to the lower part of the meatus, where they can be seen as small, white, moving objects. The presence of these mites is not always asymptomatic and aural discharge, head-shaking, rubbing, and epileptiform symptoms have been reported in the species affected (O'Connor, 1957). If itching is present, it is said to occur only when the animal becomes heated. A horse may shake its head and rub the ears against fixed objects. The disease can sometimes be recognized by these signs and the falling of hair in the upper parotid region (Hutyra, Marek, and Manninger, 1946). The literature does not record whether the head-shaking caused by ear mites is a rotation of the head on its long axis (as shown by dogs) or whether it is the more familiar head-nodding, precipitated by slow exercise, with movement of the head and neck in a vertical plane.

Diagnosis can be made by the direct examination of swabs collected from the depth of the meatus but is more certain using a forward-viewing fibrelight endoscope and the technique already described. A canine otoscope with a long speculum may be tried but it is doubtful whether a sufficiently good view would be obtained of the depth of the meatus. General anaesthesia will be essential for either method. Treatment is by the application of benzyl benzoate or benzene hexachloride, repeated two or three times at weekly intervals.

Under practice conditions, a retrospective diagnosis of ear mites is likely to be made if symptoms of head-shaking disappear following the application of a parasiticide. Such results are, unfortunately, rare.

2. *Ear ticks*: In arid areas of the U.S.A., the Spinose ear tick (*Otobius megnini*) is a cause of head-shaking in the horse (Tarshis and Ommert, 1961). Affected horses show torticollis and head-shaking. They may become unmanageable, rolling about the ground in an effort to allay the irritation caused by these ticks. Diagnosis is by naked-eye examination of the concave surface of the pinna. Treatment is by the application of an organic phosphate insecticide, combined with a silica aerogel.

Neoplasia

Papilloma of the Pinna.—Viral papillomata are common, especially in foals and yearlings. A tentative diagnosis can generally be based upon the tumour's clinical appearance, many of them being pedunculated. However, caution is advisable before giving a firm prognosis on what an owner may lightly dismiss as an 'angleberry', especially with the sessile type. A biopsy examination should be carried out, in cases of doubt, in order to differentiate this condition from fibroma and the more serious recurrent fibroma (sarcoid).

Treatment of the viral papilloma is not often indicated, as spontaneous regression generally occurs with the passage of time and the danger of disfiguring deformities of the ear following premature surgical removal can be avoided.

The application of elastic bands or other ligatures to the base of pedunculated warts is sometimes warranted as an economic therapy in preference to surgery. The technique needs to be used with caution, however, and progress kept under observation. Antitetanus therapy should not be omitted as the slow necrosis of tissue is generally associated with sepsis. Horses have contracted tetanus and died whilst undergoing this line of treatment.

Recurrent Fibroma (Sarcoid) of the Pinna.—The external ear is part of the common integument and is therefore subject to the same diseases that affect skin in general. It would not be appropriate here to include a dissertation on all skin diseases in the horse but important diseases should be mentioned. The recurrent fibroma (sarcoid) is such a disease and, when it affects the skin of the ear, it is necessary to recognize its true nature and not to mistake it for something more benign. Diagnosis is based on examination of biopsy material. Treatment of a sarcoid on or near the ear must be with caution. Surgical removal is associated with the risk of recurrence and, with the general 'shortage' of skin in this area, closure of the surgical wound may be difficult and accompanied by heavy cicatrix formation with deformity of the ear. Autologous grafting of sarcoid tissue (Voss, 1969) might be considered or radiotherapy using radon seeds (Silver, 1963).

Melanoma of the Parotid Region.—The parotid salivary gland is one of the predilection sites for equine melanomata and this should be remembered when subcutaneous enlargements of this area occur, especially in a grey horse. The disease is mostly seen in aged horses and tends to run a clinically benign course over a long period (Cotchin, 1960), though facial paralysis and epistaxis are possible complications from a parotid lesion and a concurrent retropharyngeal lesion has been seen, causing dysphagia and dyspnoea. Treatment should consist of masterly inactivity. Attempts at surgical removal of the melanoma are likely to be not only unsuccessful but actively unhelpful due to the diffuse nature of the lesion.

Nervous Dysfunction

Congenital 'Paresis' of the Pinna—see 'Congenital Defects'.

Facial Paralysis.—The anatomy of the facial nerve is well illustrated by Barone (1964). The extrinsic muscles of the ear are one of many groups of facial muscles that might be affected, unilaterally or bilaterally, following damage to cranial nerve VII. Involvement of the aural branches is generally, though not always, accompanied by damage also to the palpebral and buccal branches and implies a point of damage, close to the stylomastoid foramen of the petrous temporal bone (extratemporal), within the bone itself (intratemporal) or centrally (intracranial). The auriculopalpebral branch of the facial nerve is given off from the parent trunk immediately after it emerges from the stylomastoid foramen (*Fig.* 7). The clinical signs of facial paralysis are easily recognized in the horse (*Fig.* 6), though identification of the cause may require careful radiography, endoscopy of the guttural pouch, and other techniques. In human medicine, various electrical tests of conductivity and excitability are employed to decide whether the paralysis is a non-degenerative or a degenerative one (Hall and Colman, 1969). Adoption of these techniques and a closer assessment of tear secretion in veterinary medicine would enable a more accurate prognosis to be formed and more effective treatment to be given.

Unilateral facial paralysis affecting the ear, eyelids, and muzzle can be a sequel to guttural pouch mycosis in which the lateral compartment of the pouch becomes 'walled-off' with fibrous tissue and an abscess develops in the compartment (*see* Subparotid Abscess). Under these conditions, the nerve is damaged as it courses close to the styloid process of the conchal cartilage to which the mucosa of the lateral compartment is attached (*Fig.* 3). Unilateral facial paralysis is not a constant feature of subparotid abscess and can accompany cases of guttural pouch mycosis that do not show this feature. One pony showed evidence of intermittent facial palsy affecting the right ear, eye, and muzzle, in conjunction with scar formation in the roof of the right guttural pouch (Cook, 1966c), and another showed unilateral facial paralysis of 4 weeks' duration affecting the ear, eye, and muzzle in conjunction with severe incoordination as the presenting sign of guttural pouch mycosis. Nine months later an intermittent facial paresis was still present. At post-mortem examination the hyoid was fused to the petrous temporal bone. It would be interesting to know whether the damage to the facial nerve in these cases is extratemporal or intratemporal. Finally, guttural pouch mycosis may cause facial palsy indirectly due to the exostoses which this disease frequently causes in the region of the external acoustic process (*Fig.* 9).

Other causes of facial palsy in the horse affecting the ears include parotid melanoma and fracture of the petrous temporal bone (*see below*).

Bilateral facial palsy indicates intracranial damage and is generally accompanied by other more serious signs of C.N.S. disturbance. A 6-year-old gelding has been seen, however, in which bilateral facial palsy was the only sign present (*Fig.* 6 B). It is possible that, in this case, the paralysis was induced by exposure to an extreme of temperature. The horse had been stabled, during a heat wave, in a poorly ventilated loose box with a corrugated-iron roof. The paralysis was present for 12 months. In some cases low temperatures appear to cause facial paralysis, e.g., a cold wind blowing on a horse's heated skin or standing for long periods in a cold stable (Hutyra and others, 1946). Unilateral central paralysis from an intracranial lymphosarcoma has been reported (von Pick and Puschner, 1970).

Treatment of facial paralysis depends on removal of the cause, e.g., relief of surrounding pressure from oedema, abscess formation, exostoses, etc. In veterinary practice, this generally implies simple anti-inflammatory methods coupled with the passage of time. Surgical decompression techniques, as used in human medicine, are not employed. Prognosis depends on cause but there is a lack of published information on the duration of even the simpler forms of facial paralysis. In man, regeneration of the nerve, if it occurs at all, is at the rate of 0·25–4 mm. per day. Depending on the point of injury, recovery may take 4–9 months (Ballenger, 1969). In more than one horse, recovery has been observed as long as 12 months after onset.

Tetanus.—An erect ear carriage, i.e., the pinna in a vertical position (*Fig.* 3), is one of the more advanced signs of tetanus, generally accompanied by retraction of the eyelids and flaring of the nostrils.

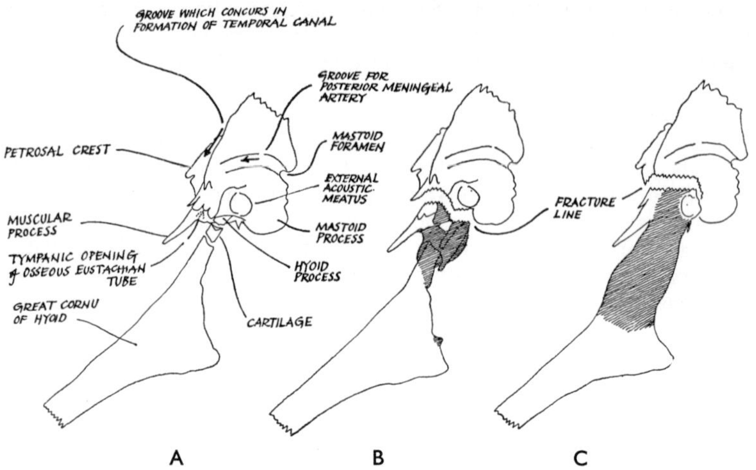

Fig. 9.—Lateral views of petrous temporal bone and great cornu of hyoid. A, A healthy articulation, showing the detailed anatomy of the petrous temporal bone. B, Fusion of the great cornu and petrous temporal bone with a heavy bone callus medially and some exostoses laterally. The fusion was accompanied by a fracture of the petrous temporal bone along the line indicated, though without separation. These bone changes were found at autopsy of a 9-year-old hunter gelding that had a healed guttural pouch mycosis lesion of the related pouch. Clinical signs had been of epistaxis initially, followed by persistent dysphagia. C, Fusion of great cornu with fractured petrous temporal bone. Lesion found at routine autopsy of a 30-year-old Thoroughbred stallion (Miller, 1960). As with B there was no separation at the fracture line and the bones are shown 'exploded' for the purpose of demonstration only.

Middle Ear

The middle ear comprises the tympanic cavity, the Eustachian tube, and its ventral diverticulum, the guttural pouch. For convenience the diseases of all three parts will be described together. The function of the guttural pouch has been the subject of much conjecture (Gratzl, 1934a) but remains an enigma.

Congenital Defects

Tympany (*Emphysema*) *of the Guttural Pouch.*—It may be a coincidence but there seems to be some predilection for this condition to occur in fillies rather than in colts. Three cases observed by the writer have all been fillies and so also was a case seen by Vaughan (1959) and others, in the literature, reported by Holmes (1962), Wheat (1962), and O'Connor (1971). The condition has been described by many other authors, though without individual case records being cited. An exception to the incidence of published reports being in female Equidae is the case quoted by Sisson and Grossman (1945).

The condition is thought to be caused by some congenital defect of the pharyngeal orifice which allows excess air to enter but not to escape from the affected guttural pouch. Membranous flaps attached to the medial lamina of the Eustachian cartilage have been incriminated as the cause, as also has muscle paralysis and inflammation of the pharyngeal orifice (Hutyra and others, 1946).

The problem first arises in foals. The exact nature of the defect has not yet been satisfactorily described. The writer has been unable to identify any organic defect of the pharyngeal orifice or vestibule and is inclined to think that this is a functional defect. Air accumulates and produces a characteristic non-inflammatory and non-painful swelling in the parotid region of the same side. Due to the strapping effect of the sternocephalic tendon and the thickness of the parotid salivary gland, the tissues below the tendon become more distended than those above (*Fig.* 8). Percussion indicates that the swelling is gaseous in nature, as the whole area resonates like a drum. Due to the laxity of the median septum, the accumulation of air also causes some swelling to occur on the unaffected side (*Fig.* 10). Clinicians should be cautious, however, in assuming that the condition is bilateral. The writer has not encountered anything but unilateral tympany, the side affected being that on which the greatest swelling was present. Raker (1971) reports having seen 2 foals with bilateral tympany.

Diagnosis presents no particular difficulties. The swelling fluctuates from day to day as some air generally escapes at intervals through the pharyngeal orifice. Diagnosis can be confirmed by passing a Neilsen catheter into the affected side via the nasal chamber and noting the immediate collapse of the swelling. If a bilateral condition is present it would, presumably, require both pouches to be catheterized before the tympany disappeared completely. Lateral radiography shows the presence of a grossly dilated cavity, the emphysematous pouch having stretched both caudally and ventrally (Cook, 1972). Sisson and Grossman (1945) cite a yearling colt in which the pouch stretched 30 cm. posterior to the ventral tubercule of the atlas and had a capacity of nearly 7 litres, though one as large as this must be rare. Secondary infection of the diseased pouch is commonly present, to a varying degree, but gross empyema of the cavity does not occur. Dysphagia (difficulty in swallowing) and inspiratory snoring due to obstruction of the epipharynx may occur when the degree of tympany is severe.

Treatment by surgical entry into the affected pouch (diverticulotomy) through a ventral approach (Whitehouse, 1957) and either blunt dissection aimed at enlarging the pharyngeal orifice or resection of mucous membrane meets with variable success (Wirstad, 1951; Holmes, 1962; Wheat, 1962, 1966). A more satisfactory treatment is to disregard the pharyngeal orifice and create a fistula in the median septum, allowing the diseased guttural pouch to communicate freely with the healthy side, from where normal escape of air can take place (Cook, 1966b). The median septum can be identified without difficulty following a ventral diverticulotomy and a piece 2 or 3 cm. square removed. The surgical approach in this condition is relatively simple as the pouch extends ventrally, lateral to the larynx, and lies closer to the skin than normal (*Fig.* 10).

Recently, the writer has created a fistula in the median septum by diathermy, without resort to diverticulotomy. A 90-cm. length of stiff wire, insulated except at each end by a sheath of rubber tubing, was passed into the healthy guttural pouch via the nasal chamber. The distal tip was bent slightly to facilitate introduction and, once inside, the wire was rotated so that the deflection pointed the tip medially. With the endoscope in the diseased pouch the tip of the wire could be manipulated in such a way that it touched the median septum. The proximal tip was then connected to the diathermy electrode and cautery applied until a small window had been created. The above technique was used successfully on a 2-month-old Thoroughbred filly foal. Some tympany returned temporarily for 4 or 5 days postoperatively

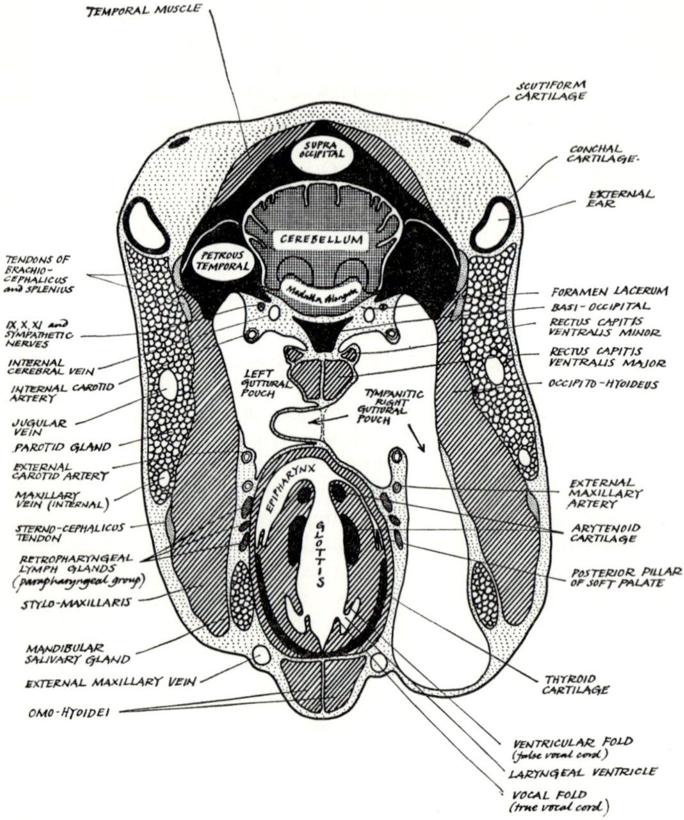

Fig. 10.—Diagrammatic transverse section through a horse's head just posterior to the vertical rami of the mandible. The left side of the head shows the more or less normal anatomy of the region, with the exception that the median septum of the guttural pouch is deflected from its correct position (indicated by the dotted lines). The right side shows a reconstruction of the early changes that occur during tympany of the guttural pouch. When the tympany becomes greater the larynx would be deflected towards the left of midline, causing a hard swelling in the ventral half of the head; the right guttural pouch spreads across to cause a tympanitic swelling above this, following compression of the left guttural pouch. The epipharynx becomes even more obstructed and snoring or inspiratory dyspnoea may occur. It should be noted that, when the guttural pouch is of normal size, its ventral portion does not occupy Viborg's triangle.

due to the postoperative swelling in the septum obstructing the window. When the swelling regressed tympany did not recur. This technique is now regarded as the one of choice for this condition, as it is simple to execute and requires no diverticulotomy.

An alternative approach to the problem, which also avoids the need for diverticulotomy, is to operate through the nostril and make a fistula between guttural pouch and epipharynx at the median pharyngeal recess. The fistula is created at the same point as it sometimes occurs spontaneously during the course of a guttural pouch mycosis. A small bronchoscope, lubricated externally, is introduced up the nasal chamber on the opposite side to that of the affected pouch and its distal tip placed in the pharyngeal recess. A trocar, such as a long intramedullary pin, is now introduced up the shaft of the bronchoscope and advanced into the diseased pouch. This manœuvre should, ideally, be carried out under endoscopic observation, with the endoscope in the diseased pouch. The slightly diagonal position of the bronchoscope in the nasal chamber and pharynx will ensure that the fistula connects with the diseased side. Having created an opening the trocar is withdrawn. The fistula opening can be enlarged by diathermy using a wire as already described. Prevention of tympany by creation of a fistula at the pharyngeal recess appears to be satisfactory from a practical point of view though there is one objection to the technique on theoretical grounds. The presence of a fistula between the epipharynx and the guttural pouch might be akin to a permanently patent Eustachian tube. In man this causes the patient to hear his own voice (autophony) with painful distinctness and other sounds, too, roar in the head. The one Thoroughbred filly operated on as a foal with this technique went into training as a 2-year-old, and appeared normal. A check examination carried out when the filly was a yearling suggested that the fistula had closed but, nevertheless, tympany had not returned. In the middle of its 2-year-old season the filly incurred a fractured pelvis and euthanasia was carried out. Post-mortem examination of the guttural pouch confirmed that the pharyngeal fistula had healed. In view of this it is difficult to understand why tympany had not returned. There was no relevant macroscopic defect observed in either the pharyngeal orifice or the related pharyngeal musculature.

Intermittent tympany of the guttural pouch in an aged pony has been encountered and was associated with a fractured hyoid bone (*see below*).

Traumatic Diseases

Fracture of the Petrous Temporal Bone.—In spite of its name (Gk. *petra*, a rock), the bone is frequently fractured following accidents during which a horse, generally an unbroken yearling, rears up on its hind-legs and falls over backwards. In fact it is only the petrosal portion of the bone that contains the labyrinth or internal ear which is dense (*Fig*. 8). This forms the medial wall of the tympanic cavity but, apart from the roof of the tympanic cavity, the remainder of the middle ear is formed of membrane bone and is not particularly strong.

Fracture of the petrous temporal bone may be associated with one or more of the following signs: haemorrhage from the external ear, circling, torticollis, ataxia, facial paralysis, recumbency, or coma. If damage was limited to the petrous temporal bone, the prognosis would not necessarily be fatal but, in the majority of cases, this fracture is accompanied by multiple fractures involving the base of the skull (basi-occipital bone) and other regions. Diagnosis of a fractured petrous temporal bone is, therefore, mostly arrived at during a post-mortem examination. In life, diagnosis would depend on a careful radiographic examination under general anaesthesia. Clicking sounds from the ear may be made when the horse is feeding, caused presumably by bone movement associated with the proximity of the temporomandibular joint (*Fig.* 5).

Pathological and undisplaced fractures of the petrous temporal bone can remain undetected during life, only to be discovered at post-mortem examination. This type of fracture is accompanied by fusion of the great cornu of the hyoid to the petrous temporal bone (*Fig.* 9 B, C). The fusion of the hyoid and petrous temporal bone is thought to be the primary lesion and the one that ultimately causes the secondary fracture. The fracture is presumed to occur due to the abnormal stresses placed upon the petrous temporal bone when there is no longer a proper articulation with the hyoid apparatus at the hyoid process (*Fig.* 9 A). The fusion is caused, in the first instance, following the severe inflammatory reaction in this region that accompanies an attack of guttural pouch mycosis. Alternatively, it could, conceivably, be a geriatric change, as bilateral fusion has been seen on one occasion (Cook, 1966c).

The fracture line divides the petrous temporal bone obliquely in a lateromedial direction, with the muscular process, the bulla tympanica, and, sometimes, the external auditory meatus fused to the great cornu with a heavy bone callus (*Fig.* 9 C), i.e., the tympanic portion of the petrous temporal bone that develops embryologically in membrane separates from the petromastoid portion that is developed in the cartilaginous ear capsule. There is no sign of a reparative process at the fracture line. The lesion illustrated in *Fig.* 9 C was found at the routine post-mortem examination of a 30-year-old Thoroughbred stallion (Miller, 1960). The subject was a valuable horse whose veterinary history had been under close observation throughout its life. One clinical sign that could, conceivably, have been associated with this lesion was this horse's extreme shyness about the mouth. Introduction of the bit was difficult and examination of the mouth impossible, the horse seeming to resent opening its mouth or having its tongue handled. It is possible that this manipulation would have caused movement of the hyoid apparatus, on which the tongue is suspended (*Fig.* 3), and pain at the fracture site. (This same shyness has been a feature of other horses that have had a known history of guttural pouch mycosis, some of which have had similar bone lesions, e.g., *Fig.* 9 B.) The second sign shown by this particular horse, when in training, was a sudden refusal to move when being exercised. The horse would stand motionless, for minutes at a time, with head raised as though it was looking at something in the sky. It is pure speculation, however, as to whether this trait was caused by the ear lesion as there is no means of knowing whether the fracture and bone callus was present during its early years in training.

A variety of other pathological fractures and exostoses of the petrous temporal bone occurs in conjunction with guttural pouch mycosis (Cook, 1966a; Cook and others, 1968). The hyoid bone may or may not also be affected. Fusion of the great cornu and petrous temporal bones can occur without there being, at post-mortem examination, any signs of fracture of either bone. The lesion is generally a sequel to guttural pouch mycosis and may be accompanied by clinical signs of ataxia, dysphagia, or facial paralysis.

Fractures of the Great Cornu of the Hyoid Bone.—The literature on hyoid fractures has been reviewed recently (Cook, 1968). Fractures may be traumatic in origin, following the same type of accident that causes fracture at the base of the skull, or they may be pathological fractures, secondary to guttural pouch mycosis or retropharyngeal lymph-node abscesses. Clinical signs include epistaxis, dysphagia, and pharyngeal swelling. Diagnosis is confirmed by endoscopy of the pharynx and guttural pouches, manual palpation of the pharyngeal region via the mouth, and radiography in two planes.

Spontaneous repair may follow traumatic fractures but recovery would, presumably, be more rapid if surgical fixation of the fracture site was possible. There are no reports in the literature of this having been undertaken.

A 20-year-old pony mare that had a long-standing repaired fracture above the muscular angle of the great cornu, with a heavy bone callus around the fracture site fusing the hyoid to the petrous temporal bone, developed such a fibrous reaction in the pouch that the pharyngeal orifice became almost completely stenosed. As a result of this, mucus accumulated in the pouch and, at post-mortem examination, twelve chondroids were present, together with 250 ml. of mucopurulent exudate. The clinical signs shown by this pony were parotid swelling with occasional tympany of the guttural pouch and some respiratory stertor, but nasal discharge was scanty and intermittent. Extension of the head for manipulation of the larynx caused extreme discomfort; the pony reversed rapidly, became ataxic, and fell over. This reaction may, again, have been caused by sudden pain following attempted movement of an ankylosed hyoid-petrous temporal joint.

Fracture of the Occipital-sphenoid Junction.—Fractures of the base of the skull (i.e., the roof of the guttural pouch) occur most frequently in young animals that have fallen over backwards. It is a matter for speculation as to whether this injury is the result of indirect trauma from the region of the poll, or whether it occurs following sudden contraction of the powerful ventral straight muscles of the neck that insert on the basilar tubercles (Cook, 1970c). Both factors may be involved. The fracture generally occurs at the suture line between the basi-occipital and the body of the post-sphenoid (*Figs.* 5, 11), where the skull is also weakened by the large foramen lacerum anterius.

Clinical signs are of recumbency and nasal haemorrhage, the blood escaping into the guttural pouch and then into the respiratory tract. Diagnosis is normally confirmed at post-mortem examination but ante-mortem diagnosis would be possible by lateral and ventrodorsal radiography.

Foreign Bodies in the Guttural Pouch.—

1. *Bullets, shrapnel*: These used to be occasional causes of guttural pouch empyema in army horses during the 1914–18 War, but the presence of air-gun pellets and other ballistics cannot be entirely ruled out even today. Sudden pharyngeal swelling accompanied by dysphagia and the development of a mucopurulent nasal discharge occur. Diagnosis is by radiography, preferably in two planes to indicate the position of the foreign body. Treatment is by surgical removal, via the pharyngeal orifice or through a diverticulotomy incision.

2. *Drainage catheters*: Rubber catheters that have been inserted into the guttural pouch for drainage of empyema problems sometimes break and portions of them are left in the cavity. Clinical signs are of a persistence of the nasal discharge and of a discharging sinus tract at the site of the diverticulotomy. Diagnosis is by endoscopy and/or radiography (Cook, 1972).

The catheter can be removed via the nasal chamber. Under general anaesthesia a well-lubricated adult-size oesophagoscope (external diameter 20 × 16 mm. and length 43·0 cm.) is introduced up the ventral meatus and, by direct vision, guided into the guttural pouch on the same side. The cartilaginous medial lamina of the pharyngeal orifice can be identified and the tip of the oesophagoscope guided lateral to this into the pouch. The

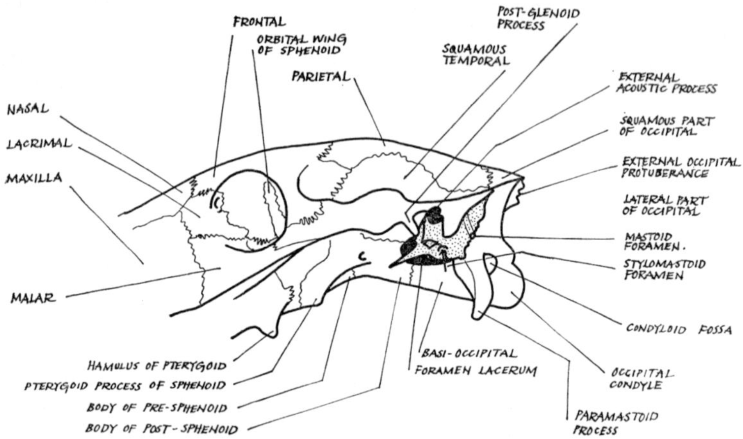

Fig. 11.—Lateral view of skull showing the osseous relationship of the petrous temporal bone.

foreign body is withdrawn using long-handled crocodile forceps (working length 50 cm.).

3. *Food material*: Chronic dysphagia and the return of food material at the nostril can be caused by the presence of a pharyngeal/guttural pouch fistula. Such a fistula is thought most likely to occur following simultaneous rupture of a retropharyngeal lymph-node abscess into both the guttural pouch and the epipharynx (Cook, 1968). The fistula forms just anterior to the oesophageal entrance and, during swallowing, food material becomes impacted into the guttural pouch. Diagnosis can be made by lateral radiography, as the food material results in a characteristic cloudy density of the guttural pouch region (Cook, 1972). Endoscopy of the affected guttural pouch may be difficult as the food blocks the objective prism and prevents vision. Alternatively, an oesophagoscope can, under general anaesthesia, be inserted into the affected guttural pouch, giving a direct view of the cavity and its contents.

The guttural pouch should be washed free of food material using a two-way system. A Neilsen catheter is introduced up the oesophagoscope to provide a continuous flow of water from a compressed-air pump or mains supply. This irrigation is carried out under general anaesthesia with the cuff of the endotracheal tube well inflated and the poll raised. Subsequently an attempt should be made to close the pharyngeal fistula, via a laryngotomy approach. To maintain anaesthesia at this stage additional thiopentone might be given, or the endotracheal tube might be inserted via a temporary tracheotomy incision. Alternatively, the endotracheal tube might simply be withdrawn completely for periods of about 7 minutes at a time. The edge of the fistula should be freshened prior to suturing with chromic catgut. Solid food should be withheld for at least a week postoperatively.

Infections

Otitis Media.—Strictly speaking, this term includes infections and inflammation of any part of the middle ear and therefore includes the guttural pouches. However, for the present the remarks below refer to the tympanic cavity only.

Bacterial and maybe fungal infections of the tympanic cavity probably occur in the horse, though this is not yet fully substantiated. It is similarly hypothetical as to whether these are ascending infections from the pharynx via the Eustachian tube, or whether they are descending via the external ear. The former seems the most likely source of infection in an animal like the horse that is so liable to respiratory infections.

Nothing is known about diseases of the osseous portion of the Eustachian tube (*Fig.* 9) that connects the tympanic cavity anteriorly (*Fig.* 8) with the cartilaginous portion of the tube and its diverticulum, the guttural pouch. It seems probable, however, that this capillary-sized tube, 6–7 cm. long, does become inflamed (salpingitis) and therefore blocked during the course of respiratory infections. This could lead to a number of diseases developing in the tympanic cavity, about which we have yet to learn.

Septic Otitis Media.—Sepsis of the tympanic cavity has followed the premeditated rupture of the ear drum and irrigation of the guttural pouch through the middle ear with an iodine solution.* This technique was used for the treatment of guttural pouch mycosis in a 2-year-old Thoroughbred filly. In effect, the mycosis of the guttural pouch cleared up rapidly following this one irrigation, though the filly developed a temporary sepsis of the middle ear, signs of which were first noticed 7 days after treatment. Attention was drawn to the problem by ataxia of the hind-quarters, followed by ataxia of the forelegs 3 days later and complete loss of balance with falling on two occasions. Following each fall the filly stood immediately and without difficulty. In addition, head-shaking was present, taking the form of lateral rotation similar to that shown by a dog with otitis. The head was also held with the affected ear lower than the healthy one (torticollis). After 1 week, the severe ataxia resolved and over the next month disappeared completely. Pressure on the fenestra vestibuli, or even penetration, with disturbance of the semicircular canals of the inner ear was presumably responsible for the ataxia and loss of balance. The filly made a satisfactory recovery from the primary condition and also from the septic otitis media. At no time was nystagmus present and the filly showed no tendency to circle in one direction. A check examination carried out 16 months later revealed no abnormality other than a small cicatrix across the cartilaginous Eustachian gutter near its upper end. Limb movement was normal and there was no ataxia, though slight and transient torticollis was detected once.

The unusually rapid disappearance of the mycelium following one irrigation of the tympanic cavity in the foregoing case tends to support the hypothesis that guttural pouch mycosis may be secondary to a primary mycosis of the

---

* Dermevan, Evans Medical Ltd.

tympanic cavity. As the ear drum appeared to be intact prior to treatment, the route of infection was presumably an ascending one, via the osseous Eustachian tube.

The above hypothesis is lent some support by the case history of a 15-year-old stallion with guttural pouch mycosis, surveyed by Bjorklund and Pälsson (1970). The left-sided guttural pouch lesion gave rise to pyrexia, inappetence, abnormal head posture, head-shyness, and, eventually, a left-sided purulent otitis externa. Post-mortem examination revealed a perforation of the membrana tympani and, presumably, a septic otitis media. The otitis externa appeared to be secondary to an otitis media, but whether the inflammation in the tympanic cavity occurred before or after the changes in the guttural pouch is an open question. Otitis media has also been encountered in conjunction with empyema of the guttural pouch (*see below*).

Catarrh or Sepsis of the Guttural Pouch (*Diverticulitis*).—A catarrhal diverticulitis probably accompanies most infections of the respiratory tract, though a specific diagnosis of this entity will not be made unless endoscopy is carried out (Gratzl, 1934b, 1936, 1966). Parapharyngeal lymph-node abscesses associated with *Streptococcus equi* infection burst into the cavity but satisfactory drainage of pus will occur in most cases.

The clinical signs of a parapharyngeal lymph-node abscess will be those of a severe pharyngitis. In the early stages pyrexia might be present, followed by dysphagia and coughing with the return of food material down the nostrils. There may be episodes of choking. The head will be held low and in extension and there may be some soft-tissue swelling dorsal to the larynx. Palpation of the area will be resented and coughing will be precipitated by the manipulation. Salivation may be excessive and the animal might nibble a small wisp of hay over a long period without being able to swallow. Initially there will be no evidence of a purulent nasal discharge.

Endoscopy reveals a soft-tissue swelling in the roof of the nasopharynx (epipharynx) and the dorsal half of the larynx may not be visible. The guttural pouches show a similar 'hummocky' appearance on the floor of the guttural pouch with obliteration of such landmarks as the external carotid artery and the glossopharyngeal and hypoglossal nerves. At this stage there may be no free pus in the cavity of the pouch. Lateral radiography shows a gross thickening of the soft tissue in the region of the parapharyngeal lymph-nodes.

When the abscess matures and ruptures into the adjacent guttural pouch, symptoms begin to regress. The owner may associate the lessening of the cough and other symptoms with the first appearance of a purulent nasal discharge, as pus drains from the guttural pouch.

Treatment should be directed towards encouraging the lymph-node abscess to burst. Warm fomentations of the throat and friars' balsam inhalation might help. Systemic antibiotic therapy should be avoided if possible and reliance placed on general nursing. The affected animal may be able to eat grass better than hard food and periods of grazing will also help to overcome dehydration brought on by any reluctance or inability to swallow fluids.

Empyema of the Guttural Pouch.—If pus fails to drain from the guttural pouch following maturation of a lymph-node abscess as described above, empyema occurs and, in the passage of time, the retained pus becomes inspissated, i.e., converted into a dry cheesy material. Over a period of years this inspissated material may become pressed into ovoid concretions, so-called 'chondroids'.

With the decline in the incidence of strangles over the past 20 years, empyema of the guttural pouch has become a comparatively rare disease. In the past 10 years the writer has encountered 4 cases only: 2 have been horses (a 12-year-old Thoroughbred and a 15-year-old half-Thoroughbred) with bilateral inspissation of pus, and 2 others were 20-year-old ponies with unilateral chondroid formation. The description below relates to the bilateral inspissation problem and chondroid formation is dealt with later.

Clinical signs include a bilateral purulent nasal discharge and abnormal prominence of the parotid salivary glands. Inspiratory stertor at rest is caused by obstruction of the epipharynx and, because of this swelling in the roof of the pharynx, the larynx may not be viewable endoscopically. The head is held low and in a position of extension. The horse may have an apprehensive facial expression and show the 'whites' of its eyes excessively. Poll flexure may be resented, but there is no sensitivity to digital palpation in the parotid region immediately below the conchal cartilage (*see* Guttural Pouch Mycosis). Salivation may occur with transient episodes of choking due to epipharyngeal obstruction. The nasal discharge is sometimes malodorous. The 12-year-old Thoroughbred showed a bilateral purulent otitis externa which presumably was associated with secondary rupture of the ear drum and an otitis media. This mare also showed signs of head-shaking whilst at rest, with lateral rotation of the head.

Endoscopy shows severe nasopharyngeal obstruction with the escape of liquid pus from both pharyngeal orifices. Standing endoscopy of the guttural pouch is not possible as the gross pharyngeal swelling prevents an endoscope being introduced into the guttural pouch. Under anaesthesia this may be possible but viewing will be interfered with by the presence of pus. The lack of a normal air space and the inability to detect the normal landmarks is, in itself, of diagnostic value. Lateral radiography confirms the absence of air in the guttural pouch. The dense radio-opacity caused by inspissated pus shows a slightly flocculent pattern, though this is less marked than the mottled pattern caused by the presence of food material (Cook, 1972). If the retained pus is still fluid, a fluid level with an air space above may be demonstrable by lateral radiography with the horse in the standing position.

In the absence of facilities for radiography or endoscopy, a diagnosis of empyema might be confirmed by placing a urethral catheter, as used for mares, in the suspected pouch and observing what fluids, if any, drain away. Irrigation of the pouch would be necessary, however, if the pus was at all inspissated. A simple guttural pouch cannula with an internal bore of 12 mm. can be constructed from copper tubing, complete with the distal deflection necessary for inserting the cannula into the guttural pouch of the conscious horse (Cook, 1970a). A Neilsen catheter can be passed into the guttural pouch through this tube which then allows a free two-way flow of fluids. Due to the danger of irrigating fluids being inhaled in the conscious standing horse, this technique should not be used except under general anaesthesia with an endotracheal tube in position.

Treatment involves drainage of the abscess cavity and reduction of the associated inflammatory reaction in order that the normal evacuation of mucus through the pharyngeal orifice can be re-established. If the pus is still fluid it should be possible to carry out this drainage satisfactorily through the pharyngeal orifice and render a diverticulotomy unnecessary. In the first instance, the fluid content of the pouch should be evacuated entirely, using a two-way catheter as already described, with the horse under endotracheal anaesthesia and the poll raised above the level of the nostril. Catheters specifically designed for irrigation of the guttural pouch (modified Gunther's catheters) are available, in two sizes, as standard items in Germany (Cook, 1970b). If an operating table is available, the head can be allowed to hang over the edge of the table during irrigation.

Simple evacuation of pus may be sufficient to reduce the inflammatory swelling and to restore the physiology of the pouch to normal. In a long-standing case a self-retaining 40-cm. balloon catheter* may be inserted, under general anaesthesia, through the pharyngeal orifice and left in situ for a few days to assist further drainage, the anterior end of the catheter lying in the common meatus of the nasal chamber. The catheter is introduced, under endoscopic observation from the opposite side of the pharynx, using a piece of wire as a stylet to enable the catheter to be guided into the pouch. When the catheter is in position the cuff, now in the guttural pouch, is inflated with a requisite amount of sterile water (e.g., 30 ml.) and the wire with-drawn.

If the pus is inspissated the above irrigation technique will be unsatisfactory as the inspissated material is too solid to be flushed out easily. External drainage of the pouch through a diverticulotomy incision is required. Various approaches are possible, i.e., the ventral approach (Garm, 1946; Whitehouse, 1957), ventrolaterally through Viborg's triangle (O'Connor, 1957), or dorso-laterally via a sub-atlantal (hyovertebrotomy) approach (O'Connor, 1957). As the empyema is often bilateral, the ventral approach is preferred as this permits both sides to be drained through the one skin incision, ventral to the larynx. A long-handled spoon is useful for digging out the dried pus.

Because of the pre-existing obstruction to the airway in this condition it is important that, before a general anaesthetic is administered for either diagnosis or treatment, a tracheostomy is carried out under local anaes-thesia in the standing position. If a tracheostomy for a permanent tracheotomy tube is created, this allows for direct tracheal intubation and, by keeping the endotracheal tube away from the pharynx, facilitates pharyngeal endoscopy and irrigation techniques. The severity of pre-anaesthetic airway obstruction can be judged by lateral radiography.

Bilateral empyema of the guttural pouches, with the retention of liquid pus, has been encountered in an 11-year-old Thoroughbred brood mare that was shown to have a round-cell sarcoma originating from the base of the skull and invading the air space of the epipharynx and both guttural pouches. The tumour mass completely obstructed the left pharyngeal orifice and partially obstructed the right. Clinical signs were similar to those described above with the addition of several episodes of epistaxis following a history of a blow on the poll during air transit.

Empyema of the lateral compartment only is encountered as a sequel to guttural pouch mycosis (*see* Subparotid Abscess, *below*).

---

* Warne Balloon Catheter, William Warne & Co. Ltd.

Subparotid Abscess (empyema of the lateral compartment).—Strangles abscesses occasionally occur in the subparotid lymph-nodes which are embedded in the parotid salivary gland. These abscesses mature and discharge, in most cases, on to the skin surface. A diagnosis can be based on bacteriological examination of the pus. However, a more chronic form of subparotid abscess occurs as a sequel, sometimes considerably delayed (e.g., 12–20 months), to the condition of guttural pouch mycosis (Cook, 1966c) and, in these cases, the abscess discharges internally. A hemispherical swelling appears in the parotid region ventral to the base of the conchal cartilage, caused by the accumulation of inspissated pus in the 'walled-off' lateral compartment of the guttural pouch. The abscess discharges internally from a sinus which connects with the remainder of the pouch. Drainage is poor, however; the walled-off pus becomes inspissated and a chondroid might form. The eventual discharge of pus into the pharynx results in a chronic pharyngitis and persistent coughing may be present. Facial paralysis affecting the ear, eye, and muzzle may also occur.

A tentative diagnosis can be made by endoscopy and radiography of the guttural pouch. Diagnosis is confirmed by exploratory surgery of the swollen area and release of the inspissated material. The abscess cavity can be approached by a skin incision parallel to the posterior border of the most dorsal section of the parotid salivary gland (*Fig.* 7). The gland should be reflected forwards to expose the pus in the lateral compartment of the pouch, anterior to the paramastoid process. The initial skin incision is the same as the hyovertebrotomy approach to the guttural pouch (O'Connor, 1957), though here it is the medial compartment of the pouch that is entered. Alternatively, an incision has been made directly through the salivary gland to reach a subparotid abscess and, although the principle seems faulty, satisfactory repair followed drainage of the abscess and a salivary fistula did not form. It is possible that the gland was already inactive due to the sepsis medially.

Chondroid in the Guttural Pouch.—This condition is still encountered, though rarely. Two cases seen have both been small and aged ponies. The clinical signs are as for empyema, the formation of chondroids merely being a long-term sequel to an empyema or some other pathological change in the pouch that has resulted in partial or perhaps complete occlusion of the pharyngeal orifice.

Lateral radiography, under anaesthesia, with the patient in lateral recumbency, is probably the best way to demonstrate these concretions of inspissated pus. If radiographs are taken in the standing position, the chondroids are not observed as they lie below the accompanying fluid level of pus. Alternatively, the chondroids can be identified endoscopically after irrigation of the pouch and drainage of fluid pus. Fractures of the great cornu may accompany this problem (*see above*).

A collection of small chondroids may be treated using trypsin and an irrigation technique as already described. Alternatively, the chondroids might be broken up mechanically, using crocodile forceps and/or a high-pressure jet of water introduced from a mains supply via a two-way catheter. However, these techniques may prove difficult to carry out and external drainage through a diverticulotomy incision is probably more satisfactory.

A midline skin incision is made as for a laryngotomy. Blunt dissection lateral to the larynx permits exposure of the thickened guttural pouch mucosa which is now punctured lateral to the external carotid artery, the pharyngeal (X) and glossopharyngeal (IX) nerves. The opening need only be made large enough to admit the passage of a pair of whelping forceps, though the wound can be enlarged to admit the operator's hand, if necessary. The chondroids can be removed by forceps or by spoon. The latter will be quicker if there are large numbers of small chondroids. The mucosa can subsequently be coapted except at a point of entry for a drainage catheter. The skin wound is partially closed.

Guttural Pouch Mycosis.—This potentially fatal condition first described by Rivolta (1868) is by far the most common disease of the guttural pouch, though it has been recorded only sporadically in the literature until recently (Cook, 1966a, 1968; Cook and others, 1968). Most of the previous references are from Scandinavian workers (e.g., Ekelund, 1910; Buer, 1942). In the past 10 years the writer has encountered over 50 cases.

The most common clinical signs are fairly characteristic, i.e., intermittent epistaxis occurring generally in a resting animal and/or dysphagia with coughing during eating and the discharge of food material down both nostrils. Other signs associated with interference with the cervical sympathetic nerve supply, the inner ear, and eye also occur, though less commonly, e.g., Horner's syndrome (ptosis and nasal congestion); vertigo; conjunctivitis, and corneal opacity or ulceration. In order of decreasing frequency of occurrence the clinical signs are epistaxis, dysphagia, parotid pain, torticollis, nasal catarrh, head-shyness, abnormal respiratory noise at exercise, sweating and shivering, transient ataxia (? vertigo), ptosis, nasal congestion, recurrent conjunctivitis and photophobia, corneal opacity, epiphora, colic, and facial paralysis. Attention may be drawn to the disease by the presence of one or more of the above signs, though asymptomatic guttural pouch mycosis is also thought to be possible.

The similarity of many of these signs to those shown by horses with grass sickness and periodic ophthalmia should be noted. Whilst the writer was at the Glasgow Veterinary School a number of horses were admitted as suspect grass-sickness cases but these proved, on investigation, to have guttural pouch mycosis. Similarly, 1 horse with symptoms suggestive of periodic ophthalmia was admitted and also proved to have a long-standing cicatrix in the guttural pouch on the same side as the affected eye (Cook, 1966c).

The pathogenesis of guttural pouch mycosis is not understood but a recent case suggests that it may be the end-result of a pathological process that has been present for as long as 6 or 7 years. A 9-year-old Thoroughbred brood mare, presented with dysphagia and epistaxis, was shown to have a mycelium in the right guttural pouch. Further inquiry into the history of this mare revealed that, since she came out of training as a 3-year-old, she had been liable to intermittent attacks of corneal opacity of the right eye. Five or six episodes had been observed over an almost equal number of years. Each attack had lasted about 48 hours and one such episode was observed whilst the mare was under treatment at the Equine Research Station, Newmarket.

A tentative diagnosis can often be arrived at from the history, supported perhaps by the presence of abnormal sensitivity to digital palpation below the conchal cartilage on the affected side (*Fig*. 3). Diagnosis is a relatively simple matter following endoscopy of the guttural pouch. The typical lichenous lesion and/or scar formation can be generally observed, without difficulty, in the predilection site in the roof of the guttural pouch, close to the point of articulation of the great cornu of the hyoid bone with the petrous temporal bone (*Fig.* 5). Pharyngeal endoscopy is also helpful in some cases (Cook, 1966a). Difficulty may be experienced in confirming a diagnosis if endoscopy is carried out in the very early stages of the disease, i.e., when haemorrhage from the guttural pouch is occurring in the absence of a detectable mycelium (*see case report cited under* Vestibular Dysfunction, *below*). Lateral and ventro-dorsal radiography of the guttural pouch and base of the skull may assist in assessing the extent of bone changes that are present in cases of long standing.

In the absence of exact knowledge concerning the aetiology, treatment has been empirical. Recovery can occur spontaneously, without treatment. This factor, combined with the difficulties of carrying out controlled experiments, makes it impossible to assess any particular line of therapy. Aetiological hypotheses include a guttural pouch mycosis that is secondary to one of the following: otitis media, an aneurysm of the internal carotid, middle meningeal, or internal maxillary artery, fracture of the petrous temporal or hyoid bone, arthritis of the atlanto-occipital or hyoid-petrous temporal joint, lymphadenitis of the suprapharyngeal glands, and phlebitis of the venous relations of the foramen lacerum, i.e., the ventral cerebral vein, middle meningeal vein, and cavernous or petrosal sinuses. The petrous temporal bone has been graphically described as lying in a venous bed and, in man, stagnation of blood in these sinuses is thought to be a factor causing a comparable disease known as the 'jugular foramen syndrome' (Eggston and Wolff, 1947).

The impression given is that local irrigation of the guttural pouch with a fungostat* and trypsin† in 100 ml. of sterile saline is worth while. The horse must be anaesthetized and placed in dorsal recumbency for treatment, in order that the fluid remains in contact with the mycelium on the roof of the pouch for at least 30 minutes. Following irrigation, the pouch is drained and 100 ml. of a non-irritant iodine solution‡ are left in the pouch for 5 minutes. Treatment is repeated at intervals of 4–7 days and four or five medications could be necessary. On one occasion a mycelium has been bathed, under endoscopic observation, with a 4 per cent solution of formol saline (40 ml.) for 30 minutes. The outcome was satisfactory.

Oral potassium iodide therapy is often given daily as a supportive treatment for about 3 weeks in the hope that, when excreted through the respiratory-type mucosa of the guttural pouch, it will have a beneficial effect. Alternatively, 30 g. sodium iodide have been given intravenously at weekly intervals. As yet no horse has developed a scurfy skin, as occurs sometimes with iodism in cattle.

If fibrous thickening has been gross, corticosteroid and antibiotic therapy has been used in the hope of reducing the danger of permanent nerve damage. A systemic fungostat such as griseofulvin§ would appear, on theoretical grounds, not to be indicated in this condition as it is said, by the manufacturers, to be excreted solely through keratin. As there is no keratin in the columnar

* Nystan (3 mega, non-sterile), E. R. Squibb & Sons, Ltd.
† Tryptar (100,000 I.U. trypsin), Armour Pharmaceutical Co. Ltd.
‡ Dermevan, Evans Medical Ltd.
§ Fulcin, I.C.I. Pharmaceuticals.

ciliated mucosa of the guttural pouch this line of therapy seems unlikely to be useful though, in practice, there is perhaps no harm in trying it in the hope that excretion is not quite as specific as it is said to be.

The fungostatic antibiotic amphotericin B* has been used systemically for mycoses in man but its administration is complicated and accompanied by risk of toxicity. It has not been used systemically by the writer, but daily nebulization of the guttural pouch with this material has been given recently through an indwelling balloon catheter. (*For the method of insertion of these catheters see section on* Empyema of the Guttural Pouch.)

Various attempts have been made to carry out local irrigation therapy on the conscious horse. A great deal depends on the degree of co-operation one gets from the horse. By definition, these horses tend to be rather head-shy and catheterization of the guttural pouch during consciousness may be less easy than it is on other horses. Indwelling balloon catheters (inserted under general anaesthesia) have been used, however, and also various catheters designed to spray fluids on to the roof of the pouch, e.g., the compressed-air pump with its normal spray attachment suitably lengthened and its distal tip smoothed down. A long-stemmed anaesthetic spray† might also be used for this purpose inserted down a cannula placed in the guttural pouch. Unfortunately, this spray has the slight disadvantage that it will not function properly if the stem is pointing upwards. It could be used in conjunction with a simple chin prop of the type recommended for endoscopy (Cook, 1970b). The method of choice for local therapy is nebulization. A Wright's nebulizer is attached to an oxygen cylinder at one end and the proximal end of the balloon catheter at the other. With the horse standing in stocks, two 90-minute periods of inhalation can be given daily for 7 or 10 days. The material used for nebulization has been a 2-oz. sterile saline solution containing 3 ml. of a 2½ per cent suspension of natamycin.‡ Nebulization with amphotericin B§ has also been tried, using twice-daily administration of 50 mg. in 2 oz. of sterile water. It is thought that the simple passage of air into the guttural pouch may, in itself, be beneficial as the humidity and temperature of the diverticulum is lowered and conditions made less favourable for fungal growth. The catheter is left patent therefore between treatments, thus providing both drainage and ventilation. The proximal end of the catheter should lie just within the anterior nares in order to cause minimal discomfort.

Surgical ligation of the internal carotid artery on the affected side is feasible but of no avail in preventing fatal haemorrhages, as the circle of Willis provides such effective collateral circulation. Surgical removal of the diphtheritic membrane can also be effected via a ventral diverticulotomy, but this procedure carries with it the considerable risk of precipitating a fatal haemorrhage.

Puncture of the ear drum and irrigation of the tympanic cavity and pouch with fungostatic solutions is a line of treatment that justifies further investigation. The 1 case treated in this manner responded encouragingly and this therapy may prove to be both more effective and more economic than others.

---

* Fungizone Intravenous, E. R. Squibb & Sons Ltd.
† Down Bros., Mayer, & Phelps Ltd.
‡ Pimafucin, Brocades Ltd.
§ Fungizone Intravenous, E. R. Squibb & Sons Ltd.

The external acoustic meatus should be first washed well with 0·5 per cent cetrimide* solution and dried by tampons and aspiration in order that the drum be punctured under more or less clean conditions. The drum is ruptured using a sterile hypodermic needle and fluids are subsequently pumped through the middle ear and out into the guttural pouch using a Higginson enema pump with the vulcanite nozzle pressed firmly into the meatus. Alternatively, an aural douching syringe can be correctly sited, by touch, in the mouth of the osseous external auditory meatus. Following irrigation, the meatus should be plugged with a cotton-wool swab impregnated with antibiotic. Bulla osteotomy, as recommended occasionally for otitis media in the dog (Spreull, 1964), may be worth consideration in the horse if the disease really does start in the tympanic cavity.

There is no useful treatment for the haemorrhage caused by this disease, other than the replacement of blood loss, as it occurs, by transfusion. The need for this should be anticipated if previous haemorrhages have been severe or if the horse is already seriously anaemic. In an emergency, cross-matching of blood is unnecessary if previous transfusions have not been given.

Apart from the above measures, horses should be nursed carefully, with vitamin and iron supplement as required. All food should be well damped and fed at ground level, or the horse should be turned out to graze as it may be able to eat grass better than hard food. Straw bedding should be replaced by peat or wood chips to reduce stable dust to a minimum.

Neoplasia

Primary neoplasia of the petrous temporal bone has not been reported, though there are descriptions of guttural pouch neoplasia (Bitzan, 1933; Kuscher, Pommer, and Kment, 1944; von Heipe and Thieme, 1956). The writer has encountered a round-cell sarcoma of the guttural pouch that also affected the epipharynx (nasopharynx). Such tumours that do occur in this region seem likely to be malignant. Those reported have been sarcoma (2) and carcinoma (2). Cotchin (1960) comments on the metaplasia of epithelium that must occur to produce a squamous-cell carcimoma in a region that, in health, is lined with stratified, columnar, ciliated epithelium.

Clinical signs are of nasal catarrh and, if ulceration occurs, the discharges are blood-stained. A tentative diagnosis is based on endoscopy and radiography and confirmed by biopsy examination. The tumour may be sited in a region of the pouch that is not the predilection site for guttural pouch mycosis and this assists in differentiation.

Treatment is difficult, though radiography using radon seeds might be considered (Silver, 1963), if histological reports indicate that the tumour is likely to be radiosensitive.

INNER EAR

Vestibular Dysfunction.—Knowledge of inner-ear disease in the horse is scanty. Clinical signs of vertigo are not frequently recognized but do occur and may be more common than is at present realized. The filly cited above (*see* Septic Otitis Media) that developed vestibular dysfunction following a known disease of the middle ear showed ataxia similar to that associated with the 'wobbler' syndrome though the history and the presence of head-shaking,

* Cetavlon, I.C.I. Pharmaceuticals.

aural discharge, and torticollis made differentiation easy in this particular case. However, ataxia unassociated with irrigation of the middle ear has been encountered as an early sign in many cases of guttural pouch mycosis and is often, though not always, accompanied by torticollis.

In 1 particular case, the ataxia was such that, during a comparatively mild haemorrhage, the horse fell down. The horse remained down for 45 minutes, then stood again without difficulty, and walked home, though it continued to drip blood from both nostrils all night. Endoscopy of the affected guttural pouch 7 days later revealed a small area of mucosa dorsally in the most caudal region of the medial compartment that was covered by a blood-stained frothy fluid. It was presumed that a mycelium was hidden by this fluid though the lesion in this case was posterior to the bulla tympanica. Local irrigation of the pouch with fungostatic and enzyme solution was carried out under general anaesthesia. No further episodes of haemorrhage occurred and the horse was presumed to have recovered, though there was no opportunity to carry out a check endoscopy. The horse completed a season's hunting and performed creditably in four point-to-point races. Epistaxis recurred 8 months later and was again accompanied by serious ataxia and rapid recumbency, though total blood-loss was slight. A further epistaxis a few days later was fatal.

Post-mortem examination showed the presence, in the same guttural pouch, of an extensive mycelium and an eroded aneurysm of the internal carotid artery. The tympanic cavity contained altered blood though it was not obviously abnormal in other respects. The internal ear was not examined. This was an atypical case of guttural pouch mycosis but it raises a number of interesting questions. Was the ataxia caused by nerve pain in the roof of the guttural pouch or could it have been associated with intracranial haemorrhage around the acoustic nerve or intratemporal haemorrhage into the tympanic cavity, causing pressure effects on the fenestra vestibuli and disturbance of the semicircular canal?

A 9-year-old in-foal mare with guttural pouch mycosis and anaemia showed serious ataxia, for the first time, 10 minutes after the slow administration of 40 mg. acepromazine maleate* intravenously in preparation for endoscopy.

Severe ataxia may also accompany bone changes affecting the hyoid and petrous temporal bones. From the above it can be seen that vertigo, bulbar neuralgia, or anaemia is a possible cause of ataxia associated with guttural pouch mycosis and that this disease, fracture of the petrous temporal bone, and other diseases of the base of the skull should be regarded as a differential diagnosis for the ataxia caused by spinal cord defects, diseases of the vertebral column, and disorders of the cerebellum. The clinical signs of cerebellar and vestibular disease can be similar and difficult to differentiate. Anatomically the two sites are closely related and the same disease may well produce dysfunction of both parts, hence the use of the clinically descriptive term, 'cerebello-vestibular syndrome' (Palmer, 1970). However, an example of an equine ataxia produced by a cerebellar rather than a vestibular dysfunction is the disease of Arab horses known as 'cerebellar hypoplasia' (Dungworth and Fowler, 1966) or 'progressive cerebellar degeneration' (Cook and Palmer, 1971). The clinical signs occur in foals or yearlings and comprise

---

* Acetylpromazine Injection, Boots Pure Drug Co. Ltd.

head tremor, ataxia, and partial blindness. It seems probable that this is an hereditary disease of the Arab breed.

In man vestibular function can be tested by observing nystagmus stimulated by cooling the labyrinth (caloric test). This test has been applied to the sheep (Palmer, 1958) and a recent report refers to its use in the horse (Lahunta and others, 1970) but further experience is probably necessary before the results can be correctly interpreted.

Deafness.—Little is known about deafness in the horse. Bilateral deafness is likely to be noticed, though no references to well-documented cases have been discovered. Unilateral deafness will probably pass unnoticed as also will partial bilateral deafness. Subjective assessment is ruled out in all species except man. A possible diagnostic test for deafness would involve sophisticated telemetry of electro-encephalographic responses to sound.

Chors (1928) describes degenerative changes of the cochlear nerve in about half of all horses examined, with atrophy first of ganglion cells followed by degeneration of the cochlear nerve fibres peripherally and centrally. The aetiology is obscure but senile, toxic, and hereditary factors are mentioned. Clinically, the cochlear degeneration is not considered to be significant, though a partial deafness is thought to occur. The vestibular nerve is reported to be unaffected by these degenerative changes.

The importance to ethology of the sense of hearing awaits study. The suggestion has been put forward that certain instances of disobedience may be overcome by plugging the external ears (Hobson, 1971).

REFERENCES

BALLENGER, J. J. (1969), *Diseases of the Nose, Throat and Ear*. Philadelphia: Lea & Febiger.

DE BAN, N. E., and JONES, A. K. (1971), 'Ulcerative Otitis Externa in a Horse', *Vet. Rec.*, **88**, 342.

BARONE, R. (1964), *Anatomie des Equides Domestiques*, vol. III. Lyons: Laboratoire d'Anatomie, École Nationale Vétérinaire.

BINNINGER, C. E., and PIPER, R. C. (1968), 'Hyperplastic Dermatitis of the Equine Ear', *J. Am. vet. med. Ass.*, **153**, 69.

BITZAN (1933), quoted by COTCHIN, E. (1956).

BJORKLUND, N. E., and PÄLSSON, G. (1970), 'Guttural Pouch Mycosis in the Horse. A Survey of 7 Cases and a Case Report', *Nord. VetMed.*, **22**, 65.

BUER, A. W. (1942), 'Mycosis of the Guttural Pouch in the Horse', *Skand. VetTidskr.*, **32**, 593.

CHORS, P. (1928), 'The Anatomy, Histology and Pathology of the Inner Ear of the Horse', *Arch. Ohr.-, Nas.- u. KehlkHeilk.*, **118**, 1.

COOK, W. R. (1966a), 'Observations on the Aetiology of Epistaxis and Cranial Nerve Paralysis in the Horse', *Vet. Rec.*, **78**, 396.

— — (1966b), 'Clinical Observations on the Anatomy and Physiology of the Equine Upper Respiratory Tract', *Ibid.*, **79**, 440.

— — (1966c), Fellowship Thesis, 'Observations on a Mycotic Disease of the Guttural Pouch in the Horse', R.C.V.S. Library.

— — (1968), 'The Clinical Features of Guttural Pouch Mycosis in the Horse', *Vet. Rec.*, **83**, 336.

— — (1970a), 'Instrument Specifications for Equine Rhinolaryngoscopy', *Ibid.*, **87**, 429.

— — (1970b), 'Procedure and Technique for Endoscopy of the Equine Respiratory Tract and Eustachian Tube Diverticulum', *Equine vet. J.*, **2**, 137.

— — (1970c), 'Skeletal Radiology of the Equine Head', *J. Am. vet. Radiol. Soc.*, **11**, 35.

— — (1971), 'The Cause of Ear, Nose and Throat Disease in the Horse', *Br. Racehorse*, **33**, 327.

COOK, W. R. (1972), 'Radiology of the Equine Ear', *J. Am. vet. Radiol. Soc.*, in the press.
— — and BARNETT, S. F. (1971), unpublished material.
— — CAMPBELL, R. S. F., and DAWSON, C. (1968), 'The Pathology and Aetiology of Guttural Pouch Mycosis in the Horse', *Vet. Rec.*, **83**, 422.
— — and PALMER, A. C. (1971), 'Arab Cerebellar Disease' *Ibid.*, **88**, 200.
— — and TOMPSETT, D. H. (1968), 'Anatomical Models prepared by Corrosion Casting', *Med. biol. Illust.*, **18**, 183.
COTCHIN, E. (1956), 'Spontaneous Neoplasms of the Upper Respiratory Tract in Animals', *U.I.C.C. Monograph Series*, **1**, 30.
— — (1960), 'Tumors of Farm Animals', *Vet. Rec.*, **72**, 816.
DEWAR, J. R. U. (1903), 'Dermoid Cysts', *J. comp. Path. Ther.*, **16**, 127.
DUNGWORTH, D. L., and FOWLER, M. E. (1966), 'Cerebellar Hypoplasia and Degeneration in a Foal', *Cornell Vet.*, **56**, 17.
DURANTE (1949), quoted by HUTYRA, F., and others (1946).
EGGSTON, A. A., and WOLFF, B. (1947), *Pathology of Ear, Nose and Throat Conditions in Man.* Baltimore: Williams & Wilkins.
EKELUND (1910), quoted by BUER, A. W. (1942).
GARM, O. (1946), 'Empyema of the Guttural Pouch of Horses and its Treatment', *Skand. VetTidskr.*, **36**, 401.
GRATZL, E. (1934a), 'Investigations into the Function and Morphology of the Guttural Pouch in the Live Horse', *Wien. tierärztl. Mschr.*, **21**, Nos. 3 and 4, p. 65.
— — (1934b), 'Pharyngitis (Angina) in Domestic Animals, with Special Reference to the Horse', *Tierärztl. Rdsch.*, 15 January, p. 97.
— — (1936), 'An Investigation of Diseases of the Guttural Pouch', *Tierheilkunde und Tierzucht*, **54**, 373.
— — (1966), 'Diseases of the Guttural Pouch', in *International Veterinary Encyclopaedia* (ed. DALLING, T.), p. 1189. Edinburgh: Green.
HALL, I. S., and COLMAN, B. H. (1969), *Diseases of the Nose, Throat and Ear.* London: Livingstone.
HECHT, P. (1964), 'Equine Ear Trim', *MSU Veterinarian* **24**, (1), 35.
HEINZER, C. D. (1968), 'Equine Surgery, Variation in Technique', *Mod. vet. Pract.*, **49**, 36.
VON HEIPE, T. H., and THIEME, E. (1956), 'A Primary Squamous Cell Carcinoma of the Guttural Pouch', *Berl. Munch. tierärztl. Wschr.*, **169**, 72.
HOBSON, G. (1971), 'Plugged Ears for Obedience?', *Vet. Rec.*, **89**, 223.
HOLMES, R. A. (1962), 'Anatomy and Pathology of the Guttural Pouches of the Horse', *Mod. vet. Pract.*, **43**, 45.
HUTYRA, F., MAREK, J., and MANNINGER, R. (1946), *Special Pathology and Therapeutics of the Diseases of Domestic Animals.* Vol. 3, *Diseases of the Skin*, p. 626. London: Baillière, Tindall, & Cox.
JENNINGS, S. (1960), unpublished communication. (British Veterinary Association Congress.)
JONES, A. K. (1971), personal communication.
KUSCHER, A., POMMER, A., and KMEMT, A. (1944), 'Neoplasia of the Guttural Pouch', *Tierärztl. Wschr.*, 18 February, p. 53.
LAHUNTA, A., DE JEFFERSON, D. A., GEARY, J. C., and LOWE, J. E. (1970), 'Granuloma Compressing the Brain of a Pony', *Cornell Vet.*, **60**, 622.
MESSERVY, A. (1971), personal communication.
MILLER, WM. C. (1960), personal communication.
O'CONNOR, J. J. ed. (1957), 'Operations on the Head and Neck', in *Dollar's Veterinary Surgery.* London: Baillière, Tindall, & Cox.
O'CONNOR, J. P. (1971), 'A Case of Tympany of the Guttural Pouch', *Ir. vet. J.*, **25**, 11.
PALMER, A. C. (1958), 'A Test for Vestibular Function in Sheep', *Br. vet. J.*, **114**, 307.
— — (1970), 'Pathogenesis and Pathology of the Cerebellovestibular Syndrome', *J. small Anim. Pract.*, **11**, 167.
PEACE, C. K. (1971), personal communication.
VON PICK, M., and PUSCHNER, H. (1970), 'Central Facial Paralysis in a Case of Lymphosarcoma in the Horse', *Tierarztl. Wschr.*, **83**, 249.
RAKER, C. W. (1971), 'The Relationship of the Guttural Pouch to Upper Respiratory Conditions', *Proc. Am. Ass. Eq. Pract.*, p. 250.
RIVOLTA, S. (1868), quoted by BUER, A. W. (1942).

SCHEBITZ, H., and WILKENS, H. (1968), *Atlas of Radiographic Anatomy of Dog and Horse*. Berlin: Parey.

SILVER, I. A. (1963), 'The Treatment by Radiotherapy of Proliferative Lesions in the Horse', *Proc. Br. Eq. vet. Ass.*, p. 49.

SISSON, S., and GROSSMAN, J. D. (1945), *The Anatomy of the Domestic Animals*. Philadelphia: Saunders.

SPREULL, J. S. A. (1964), 'Treatment of Otitis Media in the Dog', *J. small Anim. Pract.*, **5**, 107.

TARSHIS, I. B., and OMMERT, W. D. (1961), 'The Spinose Ear Tick in the Horse and other Animals', *J. Am. vet. med Ass.*, **138**, 665.

THOMSETT, L. R. (1970), 'Differential Diagnosis of Skin Diseases of the Horse', *Equine vet. J.*, **2**, 46.

VAUGHAN, L. C. (1959), personal communication.

VOSS, J. L. (1969), 'Transmission of Equine Sarcoid', *Am. J. vet. Res.*, **30**, 183.

WALLEY, T. (1889), 'Odontoma of the Temporal Bone of a Horse, with Consequent Cerebral Softening', *J. comp. Path. Ther.*, **2**, 152.

WHEAT, J. D. (1962), 'Tympanites of the Guttural Pouch of the Horse', *J. Am. vet. med. Ass.*, **140**, 453.

— — (1966), 'Selected Clinical Cases', *Proc. Br. Eq. vet. Ass.*, p. 62.

WHITEHOUSE, A. W. (1957), in *Dollar's Veterinary Surgery* (ed. O'CONNOR, J. J.). London: Baillière, Tindall, and Cox.

WIRSTAD, H. P. (1951), 'Tympanites of the Guttural Pouch in Foals', *Nord. VetMed.*, **3**, 87.

ABDOMINAL SURGERY IN CATTLE

H. Pearson, B.V.Sc., M.R.C.V.S.

The most remarkable aspect of abdominal surgery in cattle during the past 20 years has been the shift of emphasis from the reticulum to the abomasum. The incidence of reticulitis has declined so rapidly that it is now sometimes regarded as a disease of minor importance. By contrast, abomasal disorders have become increasingly important as a cause of gastro-intestinal illness in dairy cattle, but fortunately displacements now appear to be less common than during the mid-sixties and this may be due to the use of less intensive feeding systems in dairy herds.

Right and left displacements of the organ have generally been regarded as separate entities, justifiably perhaps in view of their differing symptoms and mortality-rates, but Pearson (1964) suggested that they might be different manifestations of the same disease with more severe symptoms in right displacement because of dehydration and hypochloraemia resulting from stasis of fluid in the abomasum.

In an exhaustive investigation of abomasal function in dairy cows, Svendsen (1969) showed that ruminal fluid may affect the motility of the abomasum by direct action on the mucosa. Fluid taken from the rumen of a cow after a 15-lb. concentrate feed (crude protein minimum 13 per cent, raw fat minimum 3·5 per cent, and crude fibre maximum 9 per cent) and introduced by catheter into the recipient abomasum caused a decrease in abomasal motility. Ruminal fluid after hay feeding had no effect. The volatile fatty acid (V.F.A.) content of the ruminal fluid after concentrate feeding was markedly increased and the effect of a solution of V.F.A. was therefore tested. Above a certain concentration abomasal motility was reduced. Raised levels of V.F.A. in the abomasum, which normally contains very little, could result either from increased levels in the ruminal fluid or from an accelerated flow of ingesta into the abomasum or a combination of both.

The effect of varying diets on abomasal gas production was then determined. Hay had little effect but 3 lb. of concentrates almost doubled the production of abomasal gas and 15 lb. caused a fourfold increase in gas formation. This increased gas production was shown to be due to an increased flow of ingesta into the organ. Irrespective of the diet, the *p*H of the abomasal contents remained constant.

By reducing abomasal motility and inflating the organ with gas, Svendsen succeeded in reproducing displacements of the abomasum to the left and to the right, in non-pregnant, hay-fed cows which had not recently calved. His observations suggested that left displacement may occur when the rumen is reduced in size, and right displacement when the rumen is more distended, thus confirming the view of Neal (1964) that diminution in the size of the rumen is a prerequisite of left abomasal displacement. The experiments also proved that the dehydration and alkalosis associated with right displacement could be entirely explained by sequestration of secreted abomasal fluid in the isolated abomasum.

A subsequent paper (Svendsen, 1970) described the effects on the abomasum of feeding grain in the form of rolled barley. Within 2 hours of a 5-kg. grain feed, the abomasum became distended with fluid at a time when the V.F.A. concentration of its contents was at a peak. The author suggested that the decreased abomasal motility could be caused by an increased absorption of V.F.A. and is therefore directly comparable with ruminal atony in rumen acidosis. In both cases, the cause is an increased concentration of undissociated ions resulting, in the rumen, from a fall in *p*H, and in the abomasum, from increased V.F.A. concentration. The author concludes that the feeding of large quantities of easily digestible carbohydrate may result in abomasal atony and distension of the organ with gas and fluid which are exactly the conditions required experimentally to produce left or right abomasal displacement. Svendsen's work thus confirms the views of Pinsent, Neal, and Ritchie (1961) and of Dirksen (1962) that abomasal displacement starts with an atony of the abomasum which then dilates with fluid and gas.

The effect of grain feeding on the motility of the caecum has also been investigated (Svendsen and Kristensen, 1970), and again motility was inhibited as the V.F.A. concentration increased. The authors suggest that the atony in grain poisoning, abomasal displacement, and caecal dilatation may be related to an increase in the concentration of undissociated V.F.A. in the digesta of that particular part of the gastro-intestinal tract, with a resulting increase in the absorption of V.F.A. In the rumen, the concentration of undissociated V.F.A. is increased because of acidosis caused by lactic acid fermentation; in the abomasum, the V.F.A. are in undissociated form because of the low abomasal *p*H. The fact that increased concentration of undissociated V.F.A. increases the absorption rate and simultaneously inhibits the motility of that particular section of bowel may suggest a physiological regulatory mechanism to facilitate better utilization of food. Beyond a certain level, however, the atony becomes complete and illness develops.

The continuing importance of traumatic reticulitis is reflected in a paper by Neal and Edwards (1968), describing 53 cases of vagus indigestion in 32 of which evidence of reticulitis was demonstrated at operation or autopsy. Curiously, none of these animals had shown the characteristic symptoms of pain associated with reticulitis, and, as the lesions were always on the right wall of the reticulum, the authors suggest that the absence of such symptoms may be due to the fact that only visceral peritoneum is involved, the parietal peritoneum remaining unaffected.

In 21 cases, the abomasum was grossly distended with food material in the form of finely ground rumen contents of porridge-like consistency. In all cases, the distension was confined to the fundus, the cranial portion of which was adherent in most instances to the reticulum. This leads the authors to suggest that the impaction is due to dysfunction of the fundus rather than to functional stenosis of the pylorus. Six cases of vagus indigestion were associated with positional changes of the abomasum, 3 to the right and 3 to the left. The primary disorder in such animals is not clear. Rumen distension could result from occlusion of the reticulo-omasal orifice caused by displacement of the abomasum, which could equally damage branches of the vagus nerve and so interfere with motor function of the forestomachs. A third possibility is prior injury of the nerve resulting in both rumen distension and abomasal atony.

The decreased incidence of recurrence in right displacement of the abomasum following pyloroplasty or pyloromyotomy (Verschooten and others, 1970) suggests that spasm of the pylorus may supervene in cases of abomasal dilatation. Functional pyloric stenosis or pylorospasm could not be demonstrated at laparotomy but 22 cases out of 34 recovered uneventfully after division of the pyloric musculature. The mortality-rate following conventional repositioning and emptying of the abomasum is not stated, but the incidence of recurrence is apparently considerably reduced if the pylorus is sectioned. Corroboration of this work would provide an interesting analogy between the abomasum and the simple stomach of the dog (Funkquist and Garmer, 1967).

Hutchins, Blood, and Hyne (1957) recognized three syndromes as complications of traumatic reticulitis: (1) indigestion due to adhesions, (2) diaphragmatic hernia, (3) pyloric stenosis. All three were attributed to the mechanical effects of reticular adhesions. In the first two, symptoms of ruminal hypermotility, bradycardia, and systolic cardiac murmur were described. Neal and Edwards (1968) found the cardiac symptoms to be uncommon in their series.

The dearth of recorded cases of diaphragmatic hernia does not substantiate a close association with traumatic reticulitis, but the fact that vagus indigestion and diaphragmatic rupture have certain symptoms in common has led other workers to attribute these symptoms to vagal dysfunction. Guay, Lamothe, and Pelletier (1969) described the successful repair of a diaphragmatic rupture in a cow and postulated vagal involvement because of rumen hypermotility and bradycardia of 34 per minute. There were extensive adhesions in the cranioventral abdomen but not arising from the reticulum. De Moor, Verschooten, and Desmet (1969), describing a similar operation, found no hypermotility but chronic ruminal tympany. Troutt and others (1967) also recorded 3 cases all of which showed chronic bloat without hypermotility; 1 animal had concurrent traumatic reticulitis. These authors suggest that diaphragmatic defects occur in cattle often enough to be considered seriously in differential diagnosis whenever chronic ruminal tympany is encountered. The diagnosis is confirmed by rumenotomy: in most recorded cases of acquired hernia, the defect affects the lower third of the right side of the diaphragm with herniation of the reticulum into the thorax. Successful repair is reported either by resection of the seventh or eighth rib or through a paramedian laparotomy. Midline laparotomy gives equally good exposure.

Whether the symptoms of vagus indigestion, and indeed rupture of the diaphragm, are directly comparable with those described by Hoflund (1940) following experimental section of some branches of the vagus nerve, or whether they result from the mechanical effect of peri-reticular adhesions as suggested by Hutchins and others (1957), is still open to doubt, particularly in view of the continuing reports of abomasal impaction unassociated with reticular or abomasal adhesions. Merritt and Boucher (1967) record the successful treatment of 3 such cases and maintain that in the absence of peritoneal adhesion the prognosis is good. The term 'impaction' in this context may be confusing. Neal and Edwards (1968) described abomasal contents of porridge-like consistency and found that a positive diagnosis of impaction by percussion could not be made in any instance. Other authors have found the abomasum to be sufficiently enlarged with dry and impacted ingesta to be identified by ballottement (Pope, 1961; Jones and Pirie, 1962; Baker and Lewis, 1964; Merritt and Boucher, 1967).

Postoperative recovery in such animals suggests that vagus nerve involvement cannot always be implicated in cases of abomasal 'impaction'. The findings of Verschooten and others (1970) indicate that pylorospasm also may contribute to abomasal dilatation, but this may be a manifestation of vagal dysfunction.

REFERENCES

Baker, G. J., and Lewis, M. R. W. (1964), *Vet. Rec.*, **76**, 416.

Dirksen, G. (1962), *Dilatation, Displacement and Torsion of the Abomasum in Cattle.* Berlin: Parey.

Funkquist, B., and Garmer, L. (1967), *J. small Anim. Pract.*, **8**, 523.

Guay, P. Lamothe, P., and Pelletier, R. (1969), *Can. vet. J.*, **10**, 191.

Hoflund, S. (1940), *Svensk. Vet. Tidskr.*, **45**, Suppl. 15, 322.

Hutchins, D. R., Blood, D. C., and Hyne, R. (1957), *Aust. vet. J.*, **33**, 77.

Jones, R. S., and Pirie, H. M. (1962), *Vet. Rec.*, **74**, 582.

Merritt, A. M., and Boucher, W. B. (1967), *J. Am. vet. med. Ass.*, **150**, 1115.

de Moor, A., Verschooten, F., and Desmet, P. (1969), *Vet. Rec.*, **85**, 87.

Neal, P. A. (1964), *Nord. VetMed.*, **16**, Suppl. 1, 361.

— — and Edwards, G. B. (1968), *Vet. Rec.*, **82**, 396.

Pearson, H. (1964), *Ibid.*, **76**, 1429.

Pinsent, P. J. N., Neal, P. A., and Ritchie, H. E. (1961), *Ibid.*, **73**, 729.

Pope, D. C. (1961), *Ibid.*, **73**, 1174.

Svendsen, P. (1969), *Nord. VetMed.*, **21**, Suppl. 1.

— — (1970), *Ibid.*, **22**, 571.

— — and Kristensen, B. (1970), *Ibid.*, **22**, 578.

Troutt, H. F., Fessler, J. F., Page, E. H., and Amstutz, H. E. (1967), *J. Am. vet. med. Ass.*, **151**, 1421.

Verschooten, F., Oyaert, W., de Moor, A., and Desmet, P. (1970), *Vet. Rec.*, **86**, 371.

DISTICHIASIS IN THE DOG

D. D. Lawson, D.V.R., M.R.C.V.S.

The name 'distichiasis' means a double row of eyelashes and is therefore more appropriate when applied to man than to the dog which has eyelashes normally only on the upper eyelids. In all other respects, however, the condition in man and dog appears to be virtually identical.

The known incidence in the dog is very much higher than in man where a frequency in the order of 1 in 100,000 patients is reported (Duke-Elder, 1963). The veterinary literature on distichiasis is brief and does not contain any definite indication of incidence, but check of records shows an incidence of approximately 1 in 1000 or even as high as 1 in 200 has been found in a recent survey. Detailed examination of dogs which were anaesthetized for other purposes has revealed that cases which may have only one or two extra lashes present, and may not show sufficient irritation for the owner to report, occur much more frequently than is generally recognized.

The breed distribution of distichiasis is wide and includes Pekingese, Poodles, Boxers, Spaniels, Collies, Pugs, Alsatians, and Terriers, and presumably other breeds are also affected (Smythe, 1958; Magrane, 1965; Halliwell, 1967; Startup, 1969; Bedford, 1971).

The extra lashes emerge from the orifices of the meibomian glands, which can be seen as a regular row of 20–25 circular openings on the conjunctival edge of both upper and lower-lid margins. In the dog some of the extra hairs arise from the conjunctival surface at points a short distance inside the line of the meibomian gland orifices and these hairs may represent an abnormal extension of the normal hair cover of the eyelids and are abnormal in position and direction of growth only.

Hairs from both sites will contribute to the eye irritation because their tips impinge on the cornea and bulbar conjunctiva.

In the region of the nasal canthus the skin is normally free of hair cover, which thins out and stops clear of the skin mucous junction, but it is not uncommon to find dogs in which this zone of hairless skin does not occur and hairs are present all the way to the conjunctiva. Fortunately these hairs do not appear to cause irritation or damage to the eye, probably because of the protection afforded by the membrana nictitans.

In man where distichiasis occurs it is claimed that these extra lashes replace the meibomian glands either completely (Mann, 1957; Duke-Elder, 1963) or partially (Duke-Elder, 1963), the meibomian glands having become modified to take on hair-bearing function. Embryologically this is claimed to represent heterotypical differentiation of the meibomian glands which are modified sebaceous glands. Where partial function of the meibomian glands is retained, some secretory activity is preserved together with the growth of hairs from the site.

In the dog it is possible to demonstrate the secretory function of the meibomian glands by expressing material from the orifices and, although in the very badly affected parts of the eyelids it may not be possible to produce this secretion, it is very much more common to find that large amounts of meibomian gland secretion can be produced from orifices which also carry ectopic hairs. Where secretion cannot be obtained, the typical meibomian gland orifices may also be poorly represented. No cases of total absence of the row of meibomian glands have been reported in the dog.

The size of the extra lashes varies very considerably and although in some cases they are sufficiently large to be detected by naked-eye examination if seen in profile against the sclera, it is much more common for them to be sufficiently small that their identification is difficult, even when a powerful hand-lens is used (Smythe, 1958; Magrane, 1965; Startup, 1969). The fine lashes may hold a small droplet of mucus or tear on the lid edge and this feature is often more readily seen than the fine hairs themselves. Detailed inspection of the lid edges, using an operating microscope, at up to $\times 25$ magnification, reveals that many fine, unpigmented, distichiasis lashes pass unnoticed where lower degrees of magnification are employed. Not uncommonly only the tip of the hair projects above the surface and its presence is revealed only when the area is stroked gently by a fine metal rod and the lash is made to move.

In common with hairs at other sites on the body the distichiasis lashes are capable of withstanding a considerable degree of traction when the hairs are still undergoing active growth. At some later time the ability to withstand plucking is reduced and the hairs become sufficiently loose that they are readily removed by forceps. Close inspection of the site from which the hair has been easily removed will often reveal that the tip of a new, replacement hair is already visible. These young hairs are not readily removed by plucking and the shaft of the hair may break resulting in the contoured tip being replaced by a ragged end which is liable to be even more irritating to the eye than was the original tip.

Distichiasis lashes may be single or multiple with some three or four hairs emerging from a single orifice, but this multiplicity of hairs is not evident until the individual hairs are removed and counted. Not infrequently the most obvious hair may be easily removed by plucking, but the remaining hairs that protrude less are firmly attached and when finally removed, following electrolysis, may be found to have a total length that is some five to ten times greater than the length of hair visible above the surface.

The total number of points from which these lashes emerge on the lid edges varies greatly. In some dogs only a few extra lashes are found, perhaps only a total of two on the four eyelids, but very many more, up to perhaps 30–40 lashes, have been found on one eyelid, with a total count for the four lids in excess of 100 (Magrane, 1965).

Where large numbers of lashes are found they tend to occur in rows, but these are often not very regular in arrangement.

The degree of irritation that they produce varies markedly and is more or less proportional to the numbers of extra lashes present. Where only a few hairs impinge on to the eye the dog may show no evidence of irritation, especially if the hairs are of a soft flexible type. Where large numbers of hairs rub on the eye marked epiphora occurs and in more severe cases gross thickening of the superior bulbar conjunctiva can occur or corneal excoriation and oedema, or corneal ulceration may result (Startup, 1969). The most commonly encountered sign is epiphora and in all dogs where this occurs, or where persistent irritation is reported, careful scrutiny for distichiasis should be made. The signs of irritation most often are seen for the first time in dogs under 1 year of age, but the onset of signs may not be noted until the dog is much older—even some 6 or 7 years. This variation in age of presentation is not readily explained and, although the young cases are considered to be hereditary in origin, the concept that cilia can develop spontaneously along the lid margin as a result of chronic irritation has been put forward to explain the late cases (Halliwell, 1967; Startup, 1969).

Various forms of treatment have been described (Smythe, 1958; Magrane, 1965; Startup, 1969; Bedford, 1971) including the plucking out of lashes, destruction of the lash follicles by electrolysis, and the excision of parts of the lid edge either as a partial tarsal plate excision or as a lid-splitting and excision procedure.

1. Cutting the abnormal lashes flush with the surface gives immediate, but short-lasting relief since the hairs regrow within a short period.

2. Epilation by plucking with forceps also gives prompt relief, but if lashes break, as they are likely to, and the very short lashes grow up and project, irritation will recur.

3. Epilation by electrolysis employs a fine needle electrode (cathode) which is inserted into the lash follicle and a small direct current is passed to a large plate electrode applied to the body surface. The production of free hydrogen at the needle electrode produces a fine foam which is the visible evidence of the tissue destruction that is being caused. Sufficient damage to destroy the lash follicle and to prevent regrowth of the hair is produced.

Where only a few lashes occur it is the method commonly suggested as the method of choice. It is, however, not always easy to direct the electrode into the follicle because of difficulty in holding the lid and uncertainty in determining the direction that should be followed to pass it to the lash follicle. If the follicle is effectively destroyed the lash can be removed by epilation forceps, with the minimal use of force. If the follicle has not been destroyed this loosening of the hair will not occur and repeat electrolysis is necessary.

Electrolysis may require to be repeated because of 'regrowth' of lashes which presumably arise from untreated or undestroyed follicles.

Good results can be obtained if considerable care is exercised and sufficient magnification employed to assist with lash detection and electrode placement. Some damage to the epithelial surface occurs, but this is seldom sufficient to be detected by the owners and even where very extensive epilation has been carried out no cases of scarring distortion have occurred, contrary to reports elsewhere (Startup, 1969).

4. Partial tarsal plate excision is aimed at excising a V-shaped strip from the lid edge, sufficient to remove both the cilia and the meibomian glands, although the shallow wedge of tissue must remove only part of the meibomian glands.

This procedure is advised where an extensive or complete row of cilia occurs. No suturing is employed and haemorrhage is controlled by application of adrenaline. If an excessive amount of tissue is removed a secondary entropion may follow scar contraction (Fuchs, 1903; Smythe, 1958; Bedford, 1971).

5. Lid-splitting and partial excision is a more radical version of tarsal plate excision, with the tarsal plate split to a depth of some 6 mm. approximately 2 mm. from the inner edge of the lid and the strip removed by cutting in at

right-angles through the conjunctiva. The defect is sutured closed after suitable control of haemorrhages. This procedure is prone to cicatricial contraction, distortion of the eyelid edge, and resultant long-term failure (Fuchs, 1903, Bedford, 1971).

BIBLIOGRAPHY

Bedford, P. G. E. (1971), *J. small Anim. Pract.*, **12**, 11.

Berens, C. (1949), *The Eye and its Diseases*, p. 356. Philadelphia: Saunders.

Duke-Elder, S. (1963), *Textbook of Ophthalmology*, Vol. 3, Part 2, p. 873. St. Louis: Mosby.

Fuchs, E. (1903), *Textbook of Ophthalmology*, pp. 537, 786. New York: Appleton.

Halliwell, W. H. (1967), *J. Am. vet. med. Ass.*, **150**, 874.

Magrane, W. C. (1965), *Canine Ophthalmology*, p. 59. London: Baillière, Tindall, & Cassell.

Mann, I. (1957), *Developmental Abnormalities of the Eye*, p. 381. London: British Medical Association.

— — (1963), *Development of the Human Eye*, p. 268. London: British Medical Association.

Smythe, R. H. (1958), *Veterinary Ophthalmology*, pp. 159, 187. London: Baillière, Tindall, & Cox.

Sorsby, A. (1964), *Modern Ophthalmology*, Vol. 4, p. 768. London: Butterworths.

Startup, F. G. (1969), *Diseases of the Canine Eye*, p. 92. London: Baillière, Tindall, & Cassell.

TOXOPLASMA ABORTION IN SHEEP

W. A. Watson, B.V.Sc., F.R.C.V.S.

History and Distribution of the Disease

Toxoplasmosis is the result of infection by a protozoan parasite *Toxoplasma gondii*. This organism was first found in North African rodents and described by Nicolle and Manceau (1908). The isolation from the brain of a child (Wolfe, Cowen, and Page, 1939) and the development of an effective serum antibody test by Sabin and Feldman (1948) stimulated considerable medical interest in the disease.

The possible association between toxoplasma infection and ovine abortion was first noted in the United States (Cole and others, 1954). In the same year Hartley, Jebson, and McFarlane (1954), in New Zealand, described characteristic necrotic lesions in ovine placentae and organisms resembling *T. gondii* were observed in sections. Since that time toxoplasmosis has been recognized as the most important known cause of ovine abortion in New Zealand (Hartley and Marshall, 1957), and it has been recorded in Great Britain (Beverley and Watson, 1959), Australia (Osborne, 1959), Canada (Hulland and Tobe, 1961), Ireland (Crowley, 1964), and Russia (Galuzo, 1965).

Serological surveys of sheep in Great Britain indicate that the infection is widespread. In Yorkshire 66 per cent of normal lambing ewes were shown to have a dye-test titre of 1 : 16 or more, with infection more prevalent in the grassland and wold flocks than in the hill flocks (Beverley and Watson, 1961). In Yorkshire and North-west England more detailed examinations of aborted material have shown toxoplasmosis to be one of the most frequently diagnosed causes of ovine abortion for a number of years (Beverley and Watson, 1962; Archer and others, 1971; Archer, Beverley, and Watson, 1971). Figures produced nationally do not give a true indication of the importance of toxoplasmosis, as the use of the techniques necessary for the demonstration of congenital infection is confined to a limited number of laboratories. Diagnoses also tend to be made on samples of material from individual cases of abortion rather than on a flock basis.

Aetiology

The causative organism found in acute infection is crescent-shaped or ovoid, $4–7 \times 1{\cdot}5–3\ \mu$ in size, with one end rather pointed and the other rounded. The nucleus is spherical and situated near the rounded end. It is an obligatory intracellular parasite which multiplies by binary fission and probably also by internal budding. When the host develops a resistance, toxoplasma is eliminated or encysts in various tissues. Such cysts may remain dormant for many years.

The life cycle of the parasite has been further elucidated by the demonstration of resistant oocyst forms in the faeces of infected cats and schizogonic and gametogonic stages in the intestinal epithelium. These observations indicate that the parasite should be classified as a coccidian (Hutchinson, 1965; Work and Hutchinson, 1969a, b; Hutchinson and others, 1970). The significance of these findings in sheep remains to be assessed.

Epidemiology

Congenital transmission of toxoplasmosis occurs in sheep and the placenta of a sheep aborting from the disease contains many thousands of organisms. The placentae of sheep giving birth to live lambs may also be infective. It is likely that predators or scavengers transfer infection over a wide area from this type of material as the parasite may remain viable in the foetus or placenta for several days. There is no evidence that the parasite is present in the milk, urine, or vaginal discharge of aborting sheep. Experimentally, sheep may be infected by subcutaneous, intranasal, intravenous, intraperitoneal, or oral inoculation.

Symptoms

Although nervous symptoms, apparently associated with localization of the parasite in the brain, have been described in sheep (Olafson and Monlux, 1942; Zlotnik, 1959), experimental inoculation produces no evidence of a systemic reaction other than a transient pyrexia with abortion or the birth of congenitally infected live lambs. Toxoplasma infection in early pregnancy will produce foetal resorption with apparent infertility (Jacobs, 1961). In late gestation a live lamb is born, often accompanied by diseased membranes, whilst a non-immune ewe, infected in mid-pregnancy, usually aborts or retains the dead foetus in utero until full term, when it is passed as a mummified lamb. Ewes challenged before mating do not have infected foetuses or placentae (Hartley, 1961; Watson and Beverley, 1971a).

Whilst toxoplasma is frequently isolated from sporadic cases of abortion (Beverley and Watson, 1961; Beverley and Mackay, 1962) the disease can on occasion cause heavy losses, particularly in self-contained non-immune flocks. Details of outbreaks in three such flocks have been recorded by Watson and Beverley (1963, 1971b). In these the parasite was recovered from the products of conception in 23 of 33 instances in the absence of other abortion pathogens. Serological examinations indicated that infection was widespread in all ages of sheep. The detailed examination of foetal material showed that the organisms could be more readily isolated from tissues in a reasonable state of preservation than from those undergoing degeneration.

Pathology

Foetus

The macroscopic changes caused by congenital toxoplasmosis in the lamb are not pathognomonic. Occasionally grey foci may be seen macroscopically in the foetal cerebrum and microscopically these areas show focal or diffuse round-cell infiltrations. Toxoplasma pseudocysts may be found near these areas or in other parts of the brain free of any inflammatory reaction. Small inflammatory lesions are sometimes seen in the lungs, heart, or liver (Beverley and others, 1971).

Placenta

The characteristic lesions are multiple, fine, white or yellow foci 1–2 mm. in diameter in the cotyledons (*Plate VI, Fig. A*). These are often calcified and have a gritty consistency. They are most readily seen if the foetal membranes have been washed in saline, when the normal villi spread and float, exposing foci in the deeper parts of the cotyledon. The lesions occur at varying depths and differ in size (*Plate VI, Fig. B*). Except for a slight oedema the intercotyledonary areas are normal.

Microscopically the earliest changes are a focal, mononuclear infiltration, with hyperplasia of the trophoblastic epithelium. Later, there is coagulative necrosis and calcification. Toxoplasmas may infrequently be seen on section as terminal colonies (*Plate VII, Fig. C*). When they are found, they are usually in a villus in the early stages of reaction near to a necrotic area. As necrosis progresses, the organisms lose their morphology and become unrecognizable. Histopathological confirmation of toxoplasmosis depends upon the recognition of the placental lesions rather than on the identification of the parasite (Beverley, Watson, and Payne, 1971).

Immunity

Serological surveys of the sheep populations in a number of countries have been undertaken, using the dye test developed by Sabin and Feldman in 1948. The demonstration of heat-stable antibody remaining after the heating of serum at 56° C. for up to 2 hours is a better indication of infection than some arbitrary level of dye-test antibody in untreated serum. Heat-stable dye-test antibody may be demonstrated from the sixth day after infection and the titre remains high for a long period.

Antibody titres are usually high at the time of abortion but the levels can vary over a wide range. Residual infection in the tissues, particularly in the brain, can result in the persistence of high levels of detectable antibody (Rawal, 1959; Jacobs and Moyle, 1963; Roever-Bonnet, 1963). These may, in fact, be as high in the year following abortion due to toxoplasmosis as at the time of abortion (Watson and Beverley, 1971a). Care must therefore be taken in the interpretation of the dye test in the diagnosis of toxoplasma abortion. Rising titres in paired serum samples are a more reliable indication of recent infections than the results on single samples.

It has been demonstrated experimentally that ewes infected before pregnancy do not produce congenitally infected lambs and the serum-antibody levels reflect their immunity to challenge. Ewes which abort with toxoplasmosis have normal pregnancies subsequently (Beverley and Watson, 1971; Watson and Beverley, 1971a). As far as is known, congenitally infected lambs do not pass infection to their offspring.

Diagnosis

1. *Histological.*—The rather characteristic necrotic lesions in a placenta may suggest toxoplasmosis as the cause of abortion and histological examination will provide confirmatory evidence. Occasionally, however, bacterial infections may result in colliquative necrosis with lesions not unlike those of toxoplasmosis.

2. *Isolation of the Parasite.*—Toxoplasma may be isolated from the foetal brain or placenta by mouse inoculation (*Plate VII, Fig. D*). Mice of a known toxoplasma-free strain are inoculated subcutaneously with 1 ml. of brain or cotyledon emulsion, with added penicillin and streptomycin. Six to 8 weeks later the mice are killed and the brain ground and suspended in 1 ml. *N* saline. Toxoplasma cysts appear as rounded forms 5–50 μ in diameter, consisting of aggregates of crescent forms. The isolation rate in mice is reduced by the decomposition or the mummification of the material.

3. *Fluorescent Antibody Techniques.*—The development of the immunofluorescent method for the diagnosis of toxoplasmosis has been described by Archer and others (1966). A high-titre human anti-toxoplasma serum and an anti-human fluorescent conjugate were used. The initial trials were done on material from experimentally infected ewes but the technique has been successfully used on a wide range of experimental and field material (Archer and others, 1971; Archer, Beverley, and Watson, 1971). The fluorescent antibody test has been found to be as sensitive as conventional histological examination, except when tissue degeneration is very advanced. It is quicker and easier and avoids the need for the critical evaluation of the varying types of histological changes. There is no reason to doubt the specificity of the method.

4. *Serological Tests.*—Serological tests, other than on paired sera, are mainly of value in establishing the immune status of a flock and cannot be used effectively to demonstrate that toxoplasmosis is the cause of an abortion outbreak. Other infectious agents responsible for ovine abortion may be present with toxoplasma in a flock. A sufficient number of specimens should be examined to demonstrate other pathogens.

Prevention and Control

Toxoplasmosis is often seen in closed flocks. Infection appears to be transmitted at all times of the year and not only at lambing time (Hartley, 1966; Beverley and Watson, 1971). Newly purchased ewes should be mixed with the resident flock on a farm where toxoplasmosis exists so that these may become infected before pregnancy.

When toxoplasma abortions occur, the live lambs, and ewes which do not abort, should be mixed with the affected group so that they may acquire an immunity.

There is scope for the development and application of an effective dead vaccine for this disease, but experimental work to date has not proved encouraging. A killed toxoplasma vaccine gave only partial protection from foetal death in challenged ewes and it did not prevent foetal or placental infection (Beverley, Archer, and others, 1971).

REFERENCES

Archer, J. F., Beverley, J. K. A., Fry, B. A., and Watson, W. A. (1966), *Vet. Rec.*, **78**, 369.

— — — — and Watson, W. A. (1971), *Ibid.*, **88**, 206.

— — — — — — — and Hunter, D. (1971), *Ibid.*, **88**, 178.

Beverley, J. K. A., Archer, J. F., Watson, W. A., and Fawcett, A. R. (1971), *Br. vet. J.*, in the press.

— — and Mackay, R. R. (1962), *Vet. Rec.*, **74**, 499.

— — and Watson, W. A. (1959), *Nature, Lond.*, 184, Suppl. No. 26, 2041.

— — — — (1961), *Vet. Rec.*, **73**, 6.

— — — — (1962), *Ibid.*, **74**, 548.

— — — — (1971), *Ibid.*, **88**, 39.

— — — — and Payne, J. M. (1971), *Ibid.*, **88**, 124.

— — — — and Spence, J. B. (1971), *Ibid.*, **88**, 174.

Cole, C. R., Sangar, V. L., Farrell, R. L., and Kornder, J. D. (1954), *N. Am. Vet.*, **35**, 265.

Crowley, J. P. (1964), *Ir. J. agric. Res.*, **3**, 159.

Galuzo, I. G. (1965), *Toxoplasmosis of Animals*, p. 553, Alma—Ata. Izdatel' Stvo Nauka, 33 pp. (Russ.). Reviewed *Vet. Bull.* (1966), **36**, 463, abstr. 2887.

HARTLEY, W. J. (1961), *N.Z. vet. J.*, **9**, 1.
— — (1966), *Ibid.*, **14**, 106.
— — JEBSON, J. L., and MCFARLANE, D. (1954), *Aust. vet. J.*, **30**, 216.
— — and MARSHALL, S. C. (1957), *N.Z. vet. J.*, **5**, 119.
HULLAND, T. J., and TOBE, S. B. (1961), *Can. vet. J.*, **2**, 45.
HUTCHINSON, W. M. (1965), *Nature, Lond.*, **206**, 961.
— — DUNACHIE, J. F., SIIM, J. CHR., and WORK, K. (1970), *Br. med. J.*, **1**, 5689.
JACOBS, L. (1961), *N.Z. vet. J.*, **9**, 85.
— — and MOYLE, G. G. (1963), *Am. J. vet. Res.*, **24**, 673.
NICOLLE, C., and MANCEAU, L. (1908), *C. r. Acad. Sci.*, **147**, 763.
OLAFSON, P., and MONLUX, W. S. (1942), *Cornell Vet.*, **32**, 176.
OSBORNE, H. G. (1959), *Aust. vet. J.*, **35**, 424.
RAWAL, B. D. (1959), *Lancet*, **1**, 881.
ROEVER-BONNET, H. DE (1963), *Tijdschr. Diergeneesk.*, **88**, 940.
SABIN, A. B., and FELDMAN, H. A. (1948), *Science, N.Y.*, **108**, 660.
WATSON, W. A., and BEVERLEY, J. K. A. (1963), *Int. vet. Congr.*, **1**, 775.
— — and BEVERLEY, J. K. A. (1971a), *Vet. Rec.*, **88**, 42.
— — — — (1971b), *Ibid.*, **88**, 120.
WOLFE, A., COWEN, D., and PAGE, B. H. (1939), *Science, N.Y.*, **89**, 26.
WORK, K., and HUTCHINSON, W. M. (1969a), *Acta path. microbiol. scand.*, **75**, 191.
— — — — (1969b), *Ibid.*, **77**, 414.
ZLOTNIK, I. (1959), *Lancet*, **2**, 295.

PLATE VI

TOXOPLASMA ABORTION IN SHEEP

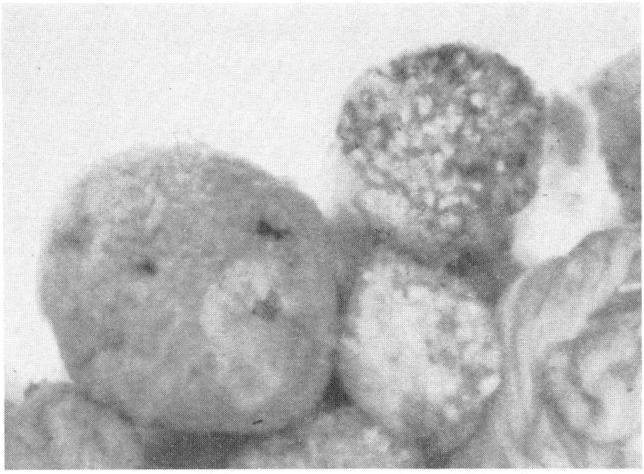

Fig. A.—Placenta of ewe aborting from toxoplasmosis.

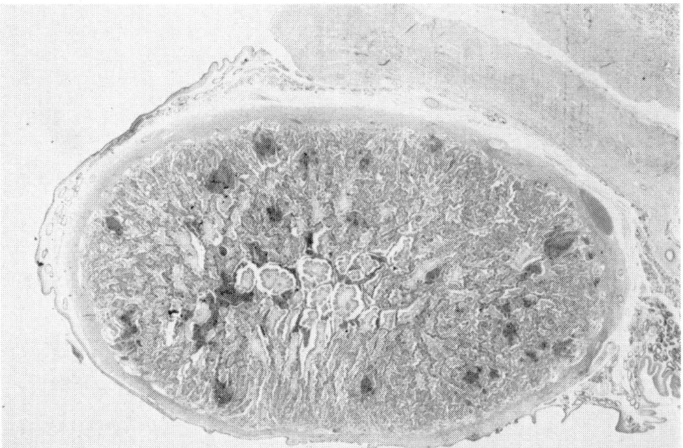

Fig. B.—Low power view of section of cotyledons still attached to uterus—experimental infection.

PLATE VII

TOXOPLASMA ABORTION IN SHEEP—*continued*

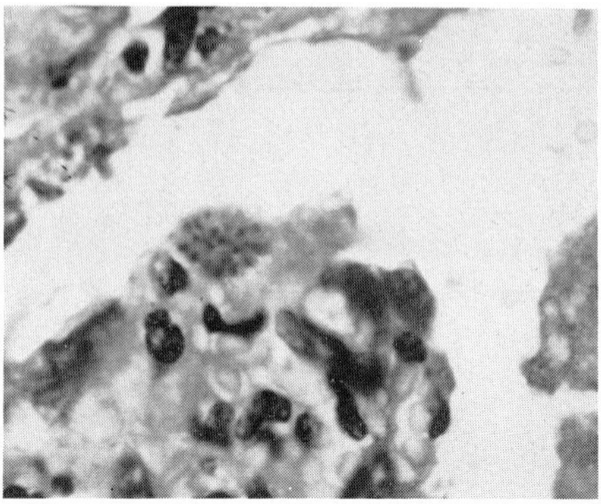

Fig. C.—Pseudocyst (terminal colony) of toxoplasma in section of placenta.

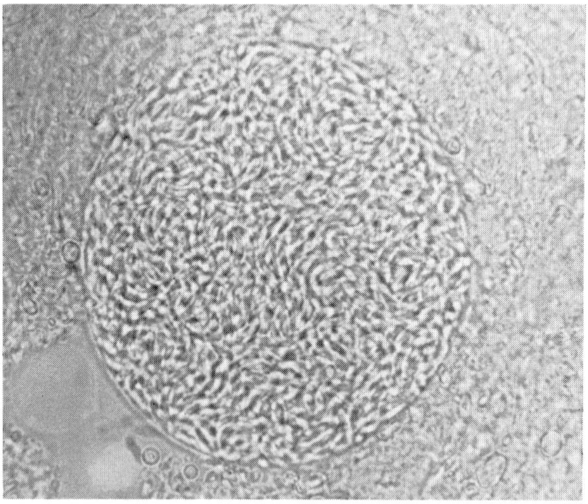

Fig. D.—Toxoplasma cyst in mouse brain emulsion.

SALMONELLA ABORTION IN SHEEP

E. J. Jack, M.R.C.V.S.

Introduction

Salmonella abortus ovis was first associated with abortion in sheep in Germany in 1920 (Zeh, 1920) and since then has been recorded from many other parts of the world including France, Russia, the Balkans, Italy, Israel, South America, and the British Isles. In Britain the disease was once common in East Anglia (Bosworth and Glover, 1925) but is now localized in Devon and Cornwall where it is the major cause of ovine abortion (Jack, 1968). Odd outbreaks have occurred in various parts of England and Wales during the past 15 years (Hunter, Sinclair, and Williams, 1969), but there has been no tendency for it to become established or to spread to neighbouring flocks.

Other salmonellae have been recognized as causing disease in sheep since 1919 (Fricklinger), but the symptoms described were those of general malaise, sometimes with diarrhoea, and death rather than abortion. In some areas of Australia and New Zealand *S. typhimurium* was endemic and caused severe losses (Walker, 1939). It was not until 1957 that Shearer gave his report on abortion in sheep associated with *S. dublin* in Britain and not until 1965 that *S. typhimurium* was described as causing abortion in Australian sheep (Dennis and Armstrong, 1965).

Fig. 12, compiled from data presented by Sojka and Field (1970) and Sojka (1971), represents the total number of incidents of ovine salmonellosis diagnosed at laboratories of the Ministry of Agriculture, Fisheries, and Food for the years 1958–70. The 1960s not only saw the continuance of *S. abortus ovis* in the West Country but the emergence of *S. dublin* infection as a cause of severe abortion throughout England and Wales and there was a tenfold increase in the number of reported incidents of this disease in that decade. Over the same period the incidence of *S. typhimurium* infection and disease associated with other salmonellae remained constant and in the main was not associated with abortion.

Further aspects of abortion caused by *S. dublin* in Britain are described by Watson (1960), Gitter and Sojka (1970), and Baker, Faull, and Rankin (1971). Examples of other salmonellae causing outbreaks of abortion are *S. reading* (Yucel, 1961) and *S. ruiru* (Gitter and Sojka, 1964).

The Disease

Natural infection is probably acquired by mouth. Both *S. dublin* and *S. abortus ovis* may be made to produce abortion when administered by this route (Bosworth and Glover, 1925; Jack, 1968; Arsov and Dhawedkar, 1969; Minershagen, Waldhalm, and Frank, 1970). Venereal transmission has been postulated for *S. abortus ovis* infection (Mura and Contini, 1954; Wojtek, 1959) and the organism may be isolated from the male's genital tract on rare occasions (Bartmann, 1957; Stanoev and Milev, 1967), but Jack (1968) was unable to produce evidence of coital transmission. Because of high blood titres in rams from aborting flocks Mura, Altieri, and Contini (1952) and Jack (1968) concluded that male infection was common, but

Watson (1960) examining blood samples from 6 rams in a flock infected with *S. dublin* could not demonstrate antibodies although 1 was a faecal excretor. Gitter and Sojka (1964) found 1 ram with a positive blood reaction and 1 with a negative reaction in an outbreak of abortion associated with *S. ruiru*. Conjunctival infection seems unlikely (Jack, 1968).

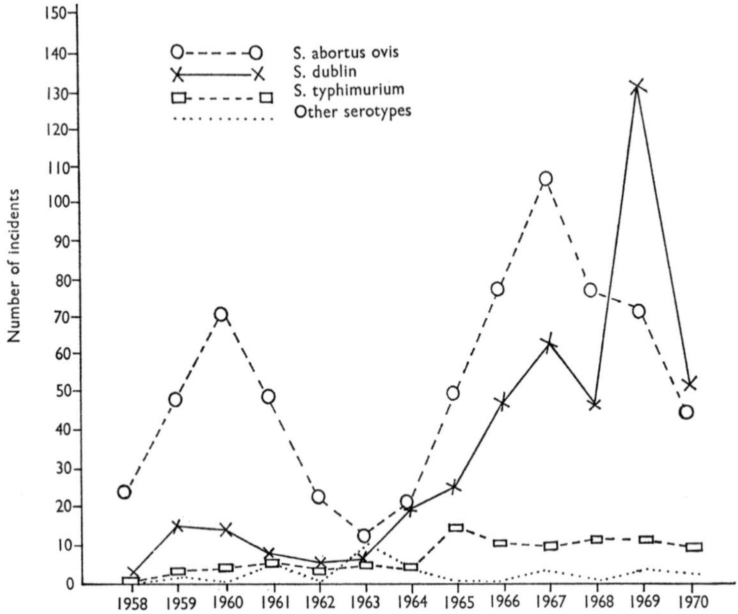

Fig. 12.—Incidents of salmonella infection in sheep in England and Wales, diagnosed at the Ministry of Agriculture's laboratories during the period 1958–70. (From Sojka and Field (1970) and Sojka (1971).)

Stress factors precipitating abortion are mentioned by several authors. In particular, *S. typhimurium* outbreaks in Australia are associated with exercise and lack of food, particularly at 'mobbing' (Salisbury, 1957). Baker and others (1971) associated the same factors with an outbreak of *S. dublin* abortion. Jack (1971) was unable to demonstrate stress factors precipitating *S. abortus ovis* outbreaks in 25 flocks.

Ovine abortion due to salmonellosis is normally uncomplicated by other disease although Nevjestic and Forsek (1968) and Popovichi (1966) commented on *S. abortus ovis* and enzootic abortion occurring concurrently.

In outbreaks caused by any of the serotypes more sheep may be infected than actually abort. Gitter and Sojka (1964) in investigating *S. ruiru* infection carried out serum-agglutination tests and reported an infection rate of about 72 per cent with an abortion rate of approximately 40 per cent. Similarly, Shearer (1957) estimated a minimum of 20 per cent of sheep to be affected with *S. dublin* although only 11 per cent aborted.

Baker and others (1971) found many more sheep excreting *S. dublin* in the faeces than actually aborted. With *S. abortus ovis* infection it is assumed that most susceptible sheep become infected within a flock in the course of an outbreak.

In *S. abortus ovis* infection disease occurs in the last 6 weeks of pregnancy. The average abortion rate is 10 per cent but this may vary from a single animal to 60 per cent of the flock. The majority of sheep in a group become affected but show mild, transient symptoms which are rarely observed by the shepherd. Arsov and Dhawedkar (1969) infected 8 pregnant ewes by mouth and on the second day all developed pyrexia and nasal discharge. By the third and fourth days the vaginal mucosa was hyperaemic and oedematous. *S. abortus ovis* was isolated from the vagina of all sheep but 1 week after infection symptoms had disappeared and only 1 sheep subsequently aborted. With 31 experimentally infected ewes that aborted Jack (1968) found that abortions occurred from the 6th to the 38th day. Although Zhelev and Pavlov (1962) described lesions in foetuses from which *S. abortus ovis* was isolated, they have not been described by other workers and would not appear to be diagnostic of the condition. Foetuses expelled early show no abnormalities. As the interval between infection and abortion lengthens so foetuses remain dead in the womb longer and when aborted are mascerated and putrefied. There are no pathognomonic placental changes as have been described for enzootic abortion, vibriosis, or toxoplasmosis.

After abortion the vaginal discharge persists for about a week and ewes generally show no other ill effects. However, on rare occasions some flocks have a high mortality associated with metritis caused by secondary organisms (Fincham, 1956).

Mortality in lambs is a feature of some outbreaks. Newborn lambs may be born weak and die quickly or healthy lambs, less than a fortnight old, may suddenly become ill and die showing lesions of a typical pneumonia.

The clinical picture resulting from *S. dublin* infection is similar to that described for *S. abortus ovis.* The differences are that the organism is more pathogenic for the ewe, putrefaction of foetuses is a more common finding, and disease in lambs is not identical. Ewes which abort commonly show malaise sometimes with diarrhoea. After abortion there is a purulent vaginal discharge associated with a metritis caused by *S. dublin.* Anorexia, loss of condition, and loss of wool are features of most outbreaks. The abortion rate is the same as that experienced with *S. abortus ovis* infection, varying from the single animal (Jack, 1971) to 60 per cent of the flock (Minershagen and others, 1970), but the majority of references (Watson, 1960; Gitter and Sojka, 1970; Baker and others, 1971) give the abortion rate as varying between 5 and 12 per cent with from a third to three-quarters of affected ewes dying subsequently. However, ewe mortality is not a constant finding (Shearer, 1957). Mortality in lambs varies from about 1·5 to 7 per cent of lambs born. This again is not constant and some outbreaks may occur in which no lambs die. In affected flocks lambs may be born weak and die quickly or after a normal birth become ill and die in the first few days of life. Baker and others (1971) found that less than half of the lambs which died yielded salmonellae and about a third of lamb carcasses showed no lesions. Most of the remainder were affected with gastro-enteritis with marked prominence of the serosal vessels of the small intestines. There was also a tendency for there to be subcutaneous haemorrhage and oedema of the ventral thoracic and abdominal walls. Less commonly there was peritonitis, joint ill, or liver abscesses. The typical pneumonia associated with *S. abortus ovis* has not been described for *S. dublin* infection in young lambs.

In the *S. ruiru* outbreak described by Gitter and Sojka (1964) all the ewes aborted without signs of malaise. Vaginal discharges were so sparse that it was not always possible to say which animals had aborted and the abortion rate was assessed on aborted foetuses instead of on aborting ewes.

Diagnosis

Isolation of the Causal Organism

Salmonellae may be isolated from the products of the abortion and from vaginal discharges before and after abortion. However, the bacteriological examination of discharge cannot be relied upon as a method of diagnosis for *S. abortus ovis* infection, and particularly when this serotype is suspected it is advisable to examine several fresh foetuses together with their placentae. There should be no difficulty in identifying the causal organisms by normal laboratory examinations, although Gitter and Sojka (1964) experienced initial difficulty in identifying *S. ruiru* because the diagnostic polyvalent 'O' sera they were using did not contain antibodies to *S. ruiru.*

Serological Reaction

The serum agglutination test may be used for diagnosis but in low dilutions positive reactions may occur in non-infected sheep particularly to phase I 'H' antibody. It is advisable, therefore, to sample several sheep and to test in dilutions of 1 in 40 and above when positive reactions to 'O' and phase II 'H' antibodies will indicate infection.

In *S. abortus ovis* infection the highest concentration of antibodies is during the first 8 weeks after abortion (Kotsche and Jerichow, 1967) and there is normally a return to 'negative' during the next 4–6 weeks. Therefore several samples must be taken soon after abortion and if most have titres to 'O' and 'H' 1·6 ('H' phase II) antibodies a reasonably sure positive diagnosis of disease may be given (Jack, 1968). With *S. dublin*, however, possibly because of a higher carrier rate, antibodies fluctuate and persist much longer, sometimes reaching their highest titres months or even years after abortion (Gitter and Sojka, 1970). Because of this, high titres to *S. dublin* may not necessarily be associated with recent abortion but may be due to a previous infection.

Prevention

Natural Immunity

With *S. abortus ovis* there is a general assumption that immunity follows infection. In the years following an abortion storm few abortions occur in affected flocks and then only in new arrivals. In flocks in endemic areas abortion may be confined to a group of sheep of particular origin, suggesting that the remainder of the flock is immune. Thus the advice that is normally given is that non-pregnant females should be mixed with the aborting flock so that they may gain an immunity. This practice may produce more carriers of the disease but that is thought to be of little consequence in an area of the country in which the disease is already endemic. It is perhaps worth noting that there is no experimental proof that immunity to *S. abortus ovis* actually exists. Certainly individual sheep have been known to abort twice in a lifetime due to that infection.

Mixing non-pregnant and infected sheep following *S. dublin* abortion might be valuable but at the moment there is too little clinical experience of the disease to be dogmatic. The high carrier rate that might result could be unacceptable.

Vaccination

A dead vaccine against *S. abortus ovis* was produced soon after the causal organism was first isolated (Schermer and Ehrlich, 1931) and similar vaccines have been reported by Tavelskij (1930), Manley (1932), Suchaci and Isopescu (1937), Mura (1948), and Selivanov (1959).

The testing of any vaccine against *S. abortus ovis* infection is exceedingly difficult. Sheep are the only satisfactory experimental animals, but numbers used tend to be limited, because of expense, and results of trials are not, therefore, always reliable. There is also a problem in selecting the method of challenge. Intravenous inoculation of the organisms is overpowering and will produce abortions whatever the immune status (Draganov, 1968; Jack, 1968) and oral administration will often fail to produce abortions even in susceptible animals; thus results of vaccine tests have too often been based upon experiments with mice and guinea-pigs, the comparison of blood titres in sheep, or on observations on poorly controlled field trials. There are no clear-cut, experimental results on the prevention by vaccination of salmonella abortion in sheep under controlled laboratory conditions. Some of the vaccines described by the various European workers may well prevent abortion, but generally speaking a serviceable immunity is not produced against salmonellosis from dead vaccines. The apparent exception to this is the *S. typhimurium* vaccine used in Australia where protection is described both in field and experimental cases (Cooper, 1967; Wallace and Murch, 1967). Theoretically live, rough vaccines such as the ones used by Smith (1956, 1965) in calves, pigs, and poultry would appear to offer the best hope of protection, but there is always a difficulty in ensuring that they are non-pathogenic as well as immunogenic and extensive laboratory testing would need to be undertaken before they could be put on the market. Such vaccines which are now available would appear to be unsuitable. Baker and others (1971) vaccinated 102 ewes with a live *S. dublin* vaccine prepared for use in calves. Not only did 8 ewes abort subsequently but from 3 of these a rough *S. dublin* was isolated which could have been the vaccinal strain. When Jack (1967) vaccinated 5 ewes with the same vaccine 1 aborted and 1 non-pregnant animal died. The vaccinal strain of *S. dublin* was isolated from various organs of the dead ewe and from the products of the abortion of the other. Experiments with live vaccines are described by Draganov (1968) and with anatoxins by Nikolaenko and Nefedev (1950) and Popov (1955), all with inconclusive results.

Treatment

British experience is that administration of antibodies will neither prevent abortion nor bring about bacterial cure in field cases. Streptomycin, chloramphenicol, furazolidone, and synthetic penicillin have all been used without success (Watson, 1960; Gitter and Sojka, 1964, 1970; Jack, 1968; Baker and others, 1971). White and Withnell (1971) state that trimethoprin and sulphonamides in combination are effective in experimental ovine salmonellosis, but there is no evidence of the use of these drugs in natural disease.

Discussion

S. abortus ovis is unusual, first because it is associated almost entirely with abortion rather than with enteric disease, and secondly because it is host-specific. Under field conditions British workers have rarely isolated it except in strict relation to clinical disease, namely from the uterus of the aborting ewe, the products of the abortion, or the diseased lamb. They have not recovered it from the vagina after the first week following abortion. There is no record of faecal isolation and carriers are rarely found (Jack, 1968). The organism differs culturally from other salmonellae and is much less robust. Many strains either fail to grow or grow very slowly on such selective media as desoxycholate-citrate agar, MacConkey agar, and brilliant green agar. They will not grow in competition with heavy contamination by other organisms such as *Escherichia coli* and growth on nutritive media like blood-agar is never as profuse as with other salmonellae. This means that the organisms may well be present in tissues but cannot always be demonstrated.

Foreign workers have had a much greater success in isolation of the organism from sites and in circumstances not relating to abortion. Thus Tamarin, Shamir, and Landau (1962), Arsov and Dhawedkar (1969), and Zakhariev and Kaloyanov (1970) reported isolation from blood, faeces, milk, and vaginal excretions and were able to find carriers of the disease with apparent ease. Their results may have been due to different cultural methods or to the fact that they were in the main working with ewes which had been infected experimentally.

S. dublin is an organism that grows well on all selective media. It is not host-specific, can be isolated from many sites in the sick ewe, and may be carried in a variety of sites for an indeterminate time after active infection. Baker and others (1971) cultured ewes which died in an outbreak of *S. dublin* abortion and found 86 per cent yielded the organism from the reproductive tract, 83 per cent from the rumen, 78 per cent from the faeces, and 30 per cent from the gall-bladder. Most of the survivors ceased faecal excretion 4–5 months after abortion. Gitter and Sojka (1970) retained 7 ewes from an *S. dublin* abortion outbreak. From 1 animal they recovered the organism in the faeces intermittently for 4 months, from another on a single occasion at 4 months, and from a final animal intermittently for over 2 years. At post-mortem examination 32 months after the outbreak *S. dublin* was isolated from the tonsils and mammary glands of this last animal.

Epidemiologically both *S. abortus ovis* and *S. dublin* pose interesting questions. Why has *S. abortus ovis* disappeared from East Anglia and become localized to cause severe disease in one small area of the British Isles only? Why has disease caused by *S. dublin* increased so alarmingly in recent years? If salmonella infection is thought to be associated with intensification of livestock, why has there been an increase in salmonellosis in sheep when sheep husbandry has been intensified least of all? Why is there no difference in incidence between housed and unhoused sheep?

The increase in *S. dublin* abortion in the 1960s appears to be associated with the great increase of disease in cattle caused by the same organism during that period, but the relationship is not always a direct one. Outbreaks are not necessarily related to overt disease in cattle, the disease sometimes occurring on farms where no cattle are kept. In Devon where the disease in cattle is rife, *S. dublin* infection in sheep is comparatively rare (Fincham, 1971). Although Watson (1960) found a calf, geese, and bitches infected in association with an outbreak of *S. dublin* and Gitter and Sojka (1970) found an infected calf in similar circumstances, there was no evidence that these had been the source of infection in the sheep and the reverse may well have been the case.

REFERENCES

ARSOV, R., and DHAWEDKAR, R. G. (1969), *Indian vet. J.*, **46**, 1.
BAKER, J. R., FAULL, W. B., and RANKIN, J. E. F. (1971), *Vet. Rec.*, **88**, 270.
BARTMANN, E. (1957), *Occurrence of* Salmonella abortus ovis *in the Male and Female Genital Organs of Sheep*. Inaugural Dissertation, Munich University.
BOSWORTH, T. J., and GLOVER, R. E. (1925), *Br. vet. J.*, **81**, 319.
COOPER, B. S. (1967), *N.Z. vet. J.*, **15**, 215.
DENNIS, S. M., and ARMSTRONG, J. M. (1965), *Aust. vet. J.*, **41**, 178.
DRAGANOV, M. (1968), *Archs exp. vet. Med.*, **22**, 7.
FINCHAM, I. H. (1956), personal communication.
— — (1971), personal communication.
FRICKLINGER, H. (1919), *Z. Fleisch- u. Milchhyg.*, **29**, 346.
GITTER, M., and SOJKA, W. J. (1964), *J. comp. Path. Ther.*, **74**, 322.
— — — — (1970), *Vet. Rec.*, **87**, 775.
HUNTER, D., SINCLAIR, W. B. V., and WILLIAMS, D. R. (1969), *Ibid.*, **84**, 350.
JACK, E. J. (1967), *Ibid.*, **80**, 78.
— — (1968), *Ibid.*, **82**, 558.
— — (1971), unpublished data.
KOTSCHE, W., and JERICHOW, A. (1967), *Mh. VetMed.*, **22**, 296.
MANLEY, F. (1932), *J. comp. Path. Ther.*, **45**, 239.
MINERSHAGEN, W. A., WALDHALM, D. G., and FRANK, F. W. (1970), *Am. J. vet. Res.*, **31** (10), 1769.
MURA, D. (1948), *Atti Soc. ital. Sci. vet.*, **2**, 100.
— — ALTIERI, M., and CONTINI, A. (1952), *Zooprofilassi*, **7**, 210.
— — and CONTINI, A. (1954), *Vet. ital.*, **5**, 787.
NEVJESTIC, A., and FORSEK, Z. (1968), *Veterinaria, Saraj.*, **16**, 545.
NIKOLAENKO, N. P., and NEFEDEV, A. P. (1950), quoted by DRAGANOV, M. (1968).
POPOV, B. W. (1955), quoted by DRAGANOV, M. (1968).
POPOVICHI, V. (1966), *Archiv. Vet.*, **1**, 29.
SALISBURY, R. M. (1957), *N.Z. vet. J.*, **6**, 76.
SCHERMER and EHRLICH (1931), *Berl. Munch. tierärztl. Wschr.*, **37**, 469.
SELIVANOV, A. W. (1959), quoted by DRAGANOV, M. (1968).
SHEARER, G. C. (1957), *Vet. Rec.*, **69**, 693.
SMITH, H. WILLIAMS (1956), *J. Hyg., Camb.*, **50**, 21.
— — (1965), *Ibid.*, **63**, 117.
SOJKA, W. J. (1971), personal communication.
— — and FIELD, H. I. (1970), *Vet. Bull., Weybridge*, **40**, 515.
STANOEV, S., and MILEV, M. (1967), *Vet. Sbir., Sof.*, **64**, No. 1, p. 12(B).
SUCHACI, I., and ISOPESCU, I. (1937), *Arhiva vet.*, **29**, 17.
TAMARIN, R., SHAMIR, A., and LANDAU, M. (1962), *Refuah Vet.*, **19**, 240.
TAVELSKIJ, P. W. (1930), quoted by DRAGANOV, M. (1968).
WALKER, D. J. (1939), *Yb. Inst. Insp. Stk. N.S.W.*, p. 27.
WALLACE, G. V., and MURCH, O. (1967), *N.Z. vet. J.*, **15**, 62.
WATSON, W. A. (1960), *Vet. Rec.*, **72**, 62.
WHITE, G., and WITHRELL, C. G. (1971), *Ibid.*, **88**, 371.
WOJTEK, H. (1959), *Tierärztl. Umsch.*, **14**, 129.
YUCEL, A. (1961), *Bull. Soc. Pat. exot.*, **54**, 939.
ZAKHARIEV, Ts., and KALOYANOV, I. (1970), *Vet. Bull., Weybridge*, **41**, 1609.
ZEH, O. (1920), *Berl. Münch. tierärztl. Wschr.*, **36**, 257.
ZHELEV, V., and PAVLOV, N. (1962), *Nauchni Trud. vissh. vet.-med. Inst. Prof. G. Pavlov*, **10**, 109.

PIGLET SURVIVAL

A REVIEW OF SOME PHYSIOLOGICAL CONSIDERATIONS

D. B. Stephens, B.V.Sc., Ph.D., F.R.C.V.S.

Introduction

The environmental conditions under which piglets are born and reared can vary enormously. Bond, Heitman, and Kelly (1964) defined environment as 'all conditions, circumstances and influences surrounding and affecting the development of an organism or group . . . often contrasted with heredity'. Clearly, the total environment in which the animal survives is multivariate and probably equals the complexity of the physiological responses induced in the animal by changes in the nature of the environment. Mount (1968) suggested that it might be simpler to divide the environmental parameters into two groups: those which have primarily a thermal relationship with the animal, and those which do not. The rate of energy exchange between the pig and its environment is particularly suitable for quantitative analysis and has been extensively investigated in the laboratory and reported by Mount (1968). In the main, it is intended here to seek evidence from the literature to substantiate the hypothesis that excessive cold exposure in piglets can lead to a lowering of viability, disease resistance, and growth rate.

Energy Exchange with the Environment

It may be useful initially to review the physical processes which govern the rate of heat exchange between the animal and its environment. Heat energy is generated and released centrally as a by-product of metabolic processes in the tissues and is distributed by the blood-stream to all parts of the organism including the surface skin areas. At birth, the pig has a core temperature in the region of 39° C. (Mount, 1959) so that normally it is exposed to ambient temperatures well below that of its own body. The resulting temperature gradient at the skin–air boundary causes an outward flow of heat and this is illustrated diagrammatically in *Fig*. 13. If the body is regarded as a simple physical homogeneous mass the heat loss would proceed according to Newton's law of cooling, which states that the cooling rate varies with the temperature gradient. However, Büttner (1932) and Kleiber (1961) more correctly regard animal heat loss as the flow of heat through an insulating surface layer according to Fourier's law, which states that the rate of heat flow is proportional to the thermal gradient and the conductance.

From this, the conductance of a given material is a measure of the ease with which heat flows through it. Its reciprocal value corresponds to the resistance, R, of an electrical circuit, and can be looked upon as a measure of the degree of impedance to the flow of heat which a material shows. In the case of an animal, R can thus be defined as the animal's total 'specific insulation' (Kleiber, 1961) and comprises two components ($r_1 + r_2$) both resisting heat flow from the core of the animal to the environment where r_1 is the internal thermal insulation between core and skin and r_2 is the external thermal insulation between skin and environment.

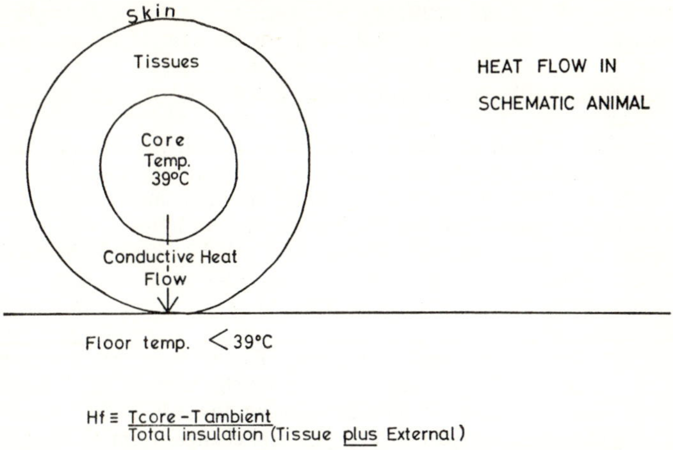

Fig. 13.—Diagrammatic representation of outward heat flow (hf) from an animal lying in contact with a solid floor at an ambient temperature below 39° C.

The heat flow from the animal can therefore be expressed by the equation

$$Q_h = \frac{T_c - T_a}{R},$$

where Q_h is the quantity of heat flowing per unit of time from the animal (this represents its total heat production); R is the total insulation between the core and environment (this comprises both the *internal* and *external* components of insulation); and $T_c - T_a$ is the temperature gradient between the body core and the environment.

Effective distribution of excess tissue heat is ensured by the circulatory system since all body tissues if unperfused are poor conductors of heat, and a purely conductive heat loss from the core to the environment would require an extremely large temperature gradient.

A complete partition of the various channels of heat flow from the newborn pig when it is lying on a concrete floor at 20° C. indicates that 39 per cent is accounted for by radiation, 39 per cent by convection, 15 per cent by conduction, and the remainder (7 per cent) by evaporation (Mount, 1967).

Thermoregulation

Homeothermic animals are able to maintain deep-body or core temperature within relatively narrow limits. The newborn pig is a homeothermic animal (Mount, 1959), which means that the body will respond to any thermal stimulus in such a way as to attempt to keep the core temperature constant, near to 39° C. in the case of the newborn pig, so that total heat production is balanced by the total heat loss to the environment through all channels. Within the relatively narrow zone of thermal neutrality, the rate of heat production (known also as the 'basal metabolic rate') equals the total heat loss, thus allowing the core temperature to remain constant. The lower end of this zone of thermal neutrality is known as the 'critical temperature' and has been shown to be around 34° C. in the case of the newborn pig (Mount, 1959). The rate of heat production must increase in order to maintain homeothermy if ambient temperature becomes lower than this.

If for any reason, such as a further lowering of ambient temperature, the thermal demand from the environment is increased, the animal is able to maintain a constant deep-body temperature in several ways:—

1. Increase its rate of heat production by raising its metabolic rate.

2. Reduce its rate of heat loss to the environment by:—

a. Decreased peripheral blood-flow. This will be relatively ineffective in the newborn because it has very little insulative fat under the skin.

b. Pilo-erection of the hair. This traps the air near the skin to form an insulative layer.

c. Behavioural activity and adaptation. The physiological processes can be greatly extended by the newborn pig by the behavioural activities of huddling with its mates or mother, moving towards a heat source, or modifying its conductive heat loss by postural changes to minimize the area in contact with the floor or wall, as shown by Mount (1960, 1963, 1967).

The above considerations allow a consideration of the effect of a changing thermal environment on the young piglet. As ambient temperature becomes cooler, the gradient between the animal and its environment is progressively increased, thereby raising the rate of heat loss, which in turn can only be offset by an increasingly vigorous metabolic response on the part of the animal. If ambient temperature is further progressively lowered the intensity of the cold stress increases rapidly so that for a small, relatively hairless animal such as the newborn piglet, the situation becomes critical and finally one of survival. The increasing rate of oxygen consumption accelerates rapidly to a maximum and an example is illustrated in *Fig*. 14. At this point of summit metabolism total heat loss from the animal equals the piglet's maximum capacity for heat production. When this heat loss exceeds the animal's maximum rate of heat production and as ambient temperature becomes still lower, the body cools, since the animal can no longer maintain homeothermy by metabolic and behavioural adaptations. Finally, the animal's metabolic rate falls rapidly and, if the cold is prolonged sufficiently, the animal lapses into a coma and dies.

Conversely, the reverse process occurs if the ambient temperature is gradually elevated up to and beyond the animal's critical temperature. Heat energy is released as an obligatory by-product of metabolic activity and must therefore be dissipated in order to maintain homeothermy. Above the critical temperature, the total rate of heat production exceeds total heat loss, so that eventually body temperature rises. This, together with the panting effort to increase evaporative heat loss, tends to elevate metabolism, so leading to hyperthermia and death in convulsions.

Energy Reserves and their Utilization

Several workers have shown that important changes occur in the chemical composition of the body of the pig during its growth and development. Chemical analyses of the whole body have been carried out by Widdowson (1950), Berge and Indrebø (1954), Manners and McCrea (1963), Brooks and others (1964), and Elsley (1964). The anatomical distribution in terms of fat, bone, and muscle tissue was analysed by gross dissection by McMeekan (1940) and Cuthbertson and Hosie (1963).

Pig embryos contain subcutaneous lipoid cells (Alexandrowicz, 1949), and Curtis and Rogler (1970) showed that at 12 hours postpartum fat tissues could be identified histologically in the interscapular skin region. At birth, fat accounts for under 1 per cent of the wet weight and increases to 10 per cent

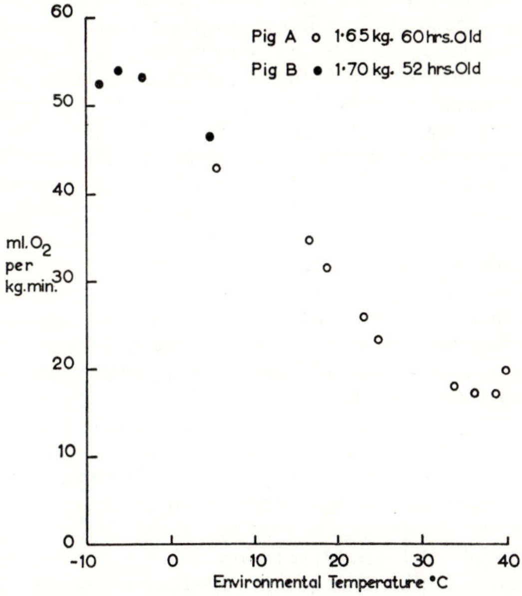

Fig. 14.—Maximum and minimum metabolic rates in the newborn pig. One pig, 52 hours of age and weighing 1·70 kg. (filled circles), was exposed to a decreasing environmental temperature for the detection of the maximum rate. Another pig, 60 hours of age and weighing 1·65 kg. (open circles), was exposed to a rising environmental temperature for the measurement of minimum metabolic rate. (*From Mount and Stephens*, 1970, *by kind permission of* '*Journal of Physiology*', *London.*)

by 1 week of age. However, the glycogen content of the skeletal muscles is relatively high at birth, therefore suggesting that glucose is an important source of energy in the immediate postpartum period. The hypoglycaemic syndrome in the piglet was first reported by Graham, Sampson, and Hester (1941), and later Goodwin (1957) showed that the lowered blood-sugar level is associated with a decreased heart-rate and a gradual decline of body temperature leading eventually to convulsions, coma, and death (Mount and Stephens, 1970).

During the first week of life the hypoglycaemic syndrome can be induced by fasting and its onset speeded by the lowering of ambient temperature (Morrill, 1952; McCance and Widdowson, 1959). After the first week of age this is not so (Hanawalt and Sampson, 1947), although the reasons for this are not quite clear. Recent studies on the respiratory quotient in the newborn piglet (Mount, 1969a, b; Curtis and Rogler, 1970; Curtis, Christison, and Robertson, 1970) suggest that fat can be catabolized at an early age to supplement energy derived from glucose catabolism.

Effects of Modifying the Physical Environment

The newborn piglet has a relatively large ratio or surface area to body-weight. Its capacity for heat conservation is further limited by having only a sparse covering of hair and a poorly developed subcutaneous adipose layer which minimizes the insulating effect of peripheral vasoconstriction.

Further studies are required to determine precisely at what age the piglet's hair and adipose tissues are able to form effective insulative coverings, and very little information exists about the ontogeny of thermoregulatory mechanisms in young piglets (Curtis, 1970). It has been shown (Mount, 1959) that the pig's metabolic rate is lower during the first day of life, so that any environmental factors which affect heat loss can influence the degree of chilling to which the animal is exposed. Very interesting results have recently been reported by Foley and others (1971) of experiments designed to compare the thermoregulatory responses to cold environment of neonatal wild and domestic piglets. The wild-strain piglets were more cold-resistant than the Large Whites at both 6 and 54 hours after birth. They concluded that the wild piglets were better able to resist cold exposure than the domestic animals due to their extra hair covering and also an ability to generate a more vigorous metabolic response to cold.

Since the baby pig normally spends a large proportion of time lying in direct contact with the floor, it is clear that conductive heat loss could have an effect large enough to effect growth and to be a potential hazard to its survival. McLagan and Thompson (1950) reared piglets on different types of floors and concluded that piglets could be successfully reared in a farrowing house with an ambient temperature as low as 7° C. provided that the floor was well insulated. Furthermore, pigs provided with electrically warmed beds have been shown to weigh considerably more at 8 weeks of age than piglets reared in pens with solid concrete floors (Lucas and Thompson, 1953). Floors have also been shown to conduct less heat when dry (Inglis and Robertson, 1953).

Some information on conductive heat loss has been provided by MacHardy (1960), who used an analytical approach to relate transient heat flows from adult pigs to the floor in an attempt to explain physiological phenomena in engineering terms, and Kelly, Bond, and Garrett (1964) measured heat loss from the skins of fattening pigs with a heat-flow transducer, and showed that the rate of heat loss to the floor rose slightly with an increase in floor temperature, suggesting an increase in peripheral blood-flow due to vasodilatation.

The insulative properties of floors in livestock buildings were studied by Haartsen (1967) using a plastic bag containing thermostatically warmed water placed on the floor. Such experiments, however, do not take into account thermoregulatory changes in behaviour by the live animal and the particular importance of postural adaptations was emphasized by Grommers, Christison, and Curtis (1970) when they demonstrated photographically that floor-contact area in the pig was nearly halved on changing from a relaxed to a tensed posture. Direct measurements of conductive heat loss from newborn pigs to the floor showed that conduction varied with both the type of floor material and the animal's posture (Mount, 1967).

Supplementary radiant heat is often supplied from a hover suspended over the creep area and is a conveniently simple and rapid method of reducing the thermal stress imposed by the environment on the young piglet during the first week of its life. Taylor and others (1952) concluded that such heating should be supplied during the first week of life when the ambient temperature falls below 7° C. Ambient temperatures below 7° C. constitute a cold stress for newborn piglets resulting in a gradual fall of body temperature (Curtis, Heidenreich, and Foley, 1966). The same authors also found that blood-glucose levels of the cold-stressed pigs remained high suggesting that newborn pigs are incapable of utilizing carbohydrate in adequate quantity to prevent a drop in body temperature.

While these attributes of the physical environment can combine to affect markedly the viability of newborn pigs, they can also be modified artificially to reduce significantly the effects of rapid changes in environmental temperature. Possible deleterious effects due to transient disturbances in the thermal environment are absorbed and their direct effects thereby limited. Such modification is clearly most important for the young piglet with its small body size.

Although physiological thermoregulatory mechanisms such as vasoconstriction have been shown to operate in the adult pig (Stephens and Fox, 1969) and also in the newborn (Mount, 1964a), they are relatively ineffective at an early age due to the paucity of the subcutaneous fat layer. Chiefly for this reason and also on account of its small body size, the piglet has to rely on its ability to vigorously increase metabolic rate in order to maintain homeothermy in the face of an increased thermal demand from the environment.

In view of the importance of thermogenesis in the piglet's resistance to cold exposure a series of experiments has recently been carried out (Stephens, 1969, 1970a, b, 1971; Stephens and Start, 1970) designed to compare the effects of the nature and temperature of the floor, supplementary radiant heating, and ambient temperature on the oxygen consumption of piglets during the early neonatal period.

The open-circuit system used to measure the rate of oxygen consumption is illustrated in *Fig.* 15. The test chamber containing the animal was situated in a controlled-temperature room and the rate of oxygen uptake measured for 30 minutes under each test situation. The total period of observation varied from 1 to 3 hours. It was shown that radiant heat alone, or moving the piglets on to straw from a concrete floor, reduced the rate of heat production by around 20 per cent. Using a wooden or rubber floor produced only a slight effect on metabolic rate, whereas a straw floor and radiant heat combined reduced metabolic rate by 46 per cent.

Further experiments showed that the rate of oxygen consumption was increased from 19·7 ml. per kg. per minute to 31·5 ($P < 0{\cdot}01$) by lowering the mean floor temperature from 33·5 to 6·8° C. while the chamber air temperature changed from 37·1 to 34·3° C. The reverse procedure of raising the floor temperature from 6·7 to 31·2° C. while the chamber temperature changed from 7·7 to 11·8° C. significantly reduced metabolic rate from 41·8 ml. per kg. per minute to 31·5 ($P < 0{\cdot}01$).

As these experiments were performed at temperatures below the critical level, the relative humidity was unlikely to be very important due to the pig's low rate of evaporative heat loss (Mount, 1962; Ingram, 1964a, b).

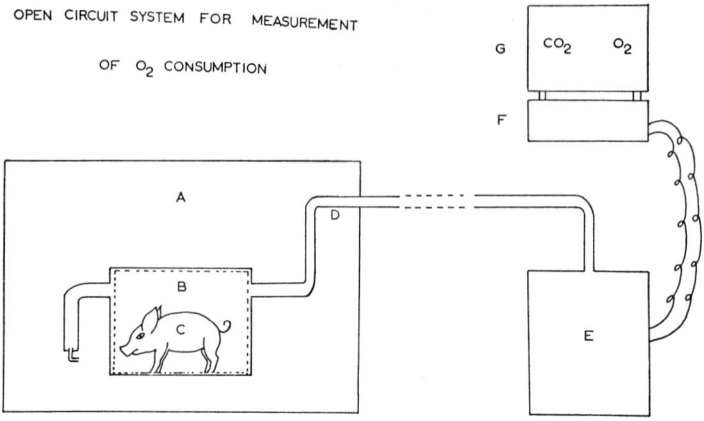

Fig. 15.—Open-circuit system for measurement of oxygen consumption. A, Temperature-controlled room. B, Metabolism chamber. C, Animal under investigation. D, Pipe connecting chamber to diaferometer. E, Diaferometer (Kipp and Zonen). F, Preamplifier. G, Chart recorder.

Suckling Behaviour in the Piglet

The piglet normally doubles its body-weight during the first week of life so that one of the critical factors which bears on its viability is the rate at which milk is ingested. Birth-weight has been shown to be particularly important. A heavier birth-weight increases the probability of a piglet choosing to feed from the pectoral teats (Allen and Lasley, 1958; McBride, James, and Wyeth, 1965) which have been shown to yield more milk than the inguinal teats (Donald, 1937; Gill and Thompson, 1956) and which are also in a safer position away from the sow's hind-legs.

In the lamb, the suckling drive is abolished if the core temperature is experimentally lowered from 37 to 32° C. (Alexander, 1964), and under cold conditions piglets normally tend to lie in a stiff, tensed posture (Mount, 1967; Stephens, 1971) suggesting a lowered probability of an effective response to stimuli which initiate suckling.

Practical Implications

Recent laboratory studies (Mount and Stephens, 1970) have shown that cold conditions can lead to hypothermia and eventually death in the piglet. However, such severe climatic conditions are not commonly observed in the field, although cold and exposure can cause a severe strain on the newborn animal's energy reserves, particularly in animals of low birth-weight with a lowered summit metabolism capability.

In a detailed study of factors contributing to preweaning mortality in pigs, Hutchinson and others (1954), Bauman, Kadlec, and Powlen (1966), and Sharpe (1966) found that the death-rate was highest during the first 24 hours of life. Pomeroy (1960) and Sharpe (1966) further showed that low birth-weight was the most important single contributing factor to death losses; this follows from the observation of Newland, McMillan, and Reineke (1952) that smaller baby pigs have lower energy reserves than heavier litter mates. A lowering of energy reserves reduces locomotive vigour and reduces the probability of successful suckling. The effect of floor insulative properties on energy expenditure, reported by Stephens (1971), shows that the mean reduction in oxygen consumption on going on to a straw floor was 18 per cent for pigs of the 2–9-day age-group at 10° C., and 12 per cent for the pigs exposed at an ambient temperature of 30° C. Mount (1969a, b) has shown that for similar piglets from 1 to 3 days of age, the respiratory quotient (R.Q.) had a mean value of 0·79, and concludes that for piglets over 24 hours of age the R.Q. is between 0·75 and 0·85 during their first week of life. Assuming that the R.Q. is near to 0·80 for pigs of this age (Mount, 1969a, b) and with a caloric equivalent of oxygen of 4·801 kcal. per litre (Weir, 1949), the daily saving on a straw floor would be 44·35 kcal. per kg. body-weight. At 30° C. the equivalent saving would be reduced threefold to 14·5 kcal. per kg. body-weight.

The practical importance of floor insulation can be expressed in terms of the total thermal demand of the environment as measured in these experiments (Stephens, 1970a, b). Mount (1959) showed that the critical temperature of piglets over 12 hours of age was 34° C. with an oxygen consumption of nearly 17 ml. per kg. per minute. Using these values combined with mean figures for O_2 consumption on concrete flooring at 10° C., it is possible to derive a relation between oxygen consumption and ambient temperature for the newborn pig (Stephens, 1971). The mean oxygen consumption for piglets when moved from concrete on to a straw floor was reduced from 35·1 to 28·7 ml. per kg. per minute. Using the relation derived above between O_2 consumption and ambient temperature, for a consumption rate of 28·7 ml. per kg. per minute, the equivalent ambient temperature was 18° C. This means that in terms of thermal demand for a week-old piglet, a straw floor at 10° C. is equivalent to a smooth concrete slab at 18° C. However, a similar calculation for piglets at 30° C. raises the equivalent temperature by approximately 2° C. Therefore as the ambient temperature falls, so the benefit derived from placing the piglets on a floor with a high insulative value markedly increases.

The Possible Role of Cold in Death-losses and Disease

In a general investigation of bacterial content and disease incidence in piggeries in Northern Ireland Gordon (1963) showed that the incidence of pneumonia was lower in pigs housed at high temperature. It is also well recognized that the susceptibility of piglets to infectious diseases is greatly increased under conditions where thermal demand from the environment is enough to constitute a cold stress. In the present context, cold stress has been taken to mean an environmental temperature which is low enough to stimulate marked physiological and metabolic responses by the animal.

Recent studies of the micro-environment in man (Lewis and others, 1969) and piglets (Stephens and Start, 1971) provide clear evidence of the dynamic nature of the transitional zone bridging the integument and the free air. This layer of air which is in direct contact with an animal's skin usually differs in temperature and density from the free air beyond its limits. These small differences in air density can be visualized and photographed using Schlieren techniques. When applied to the piglet, such techniques revealed that the boundary layer of air surrounding the animal, which forms part of the piglet's micro-environment, is in a constant upward movement with the displaced air, then being continually replaced by ambient air.

Any movement or disturbance of the ambient air, as found under draughty conditions, obviously affects this boundary layer around the animal. Ingram (1971) states that even small changes in wind speed in the rage 0–100 cm. per second have a marked effect on heat loss in pigs due to their sparse hair coat. In piglets this can be serious under cold conditions as it leads to shivering, which in turn disturbs the boundary layer and increases convective heat loss (Mount, 1968). This leads to even more vigorous shivering and an elevation of the rate of oxygen consumption. The piglet also becomes tensed and immobile in order to maximize heat conservation and the motivation to suckle is greatly reduced or extinguished.

Of considerable interest is the fact that this boundary layer has been shown in man to contain a significantly greater number of micro-organisms than the ambient air (Lewis and others, 1969), probably because the boundary layer picks up infected particles from either the skin and/or the ambient air. If this should be the case with the young pig it could explain the possible deleterious effect of a cold stress on the piglet's resistance to bacterial invasion. It could be postulated that airborne and droplet infectious agents descend on to the floor and piglet skin. If ambient temperature is lowered, the piglet shows a vigorous metabolic response and thereby greatly increases its rate of heat loss with a concomitant increase in surface air movement. In the cold, piglets also huddle closely to minimize the surface area available for heat loss (Mount, 1960) and therefore share a common portion of boundary layer. Clearly these factors greatly increase the possibility of the entry of bacteria via the nasal and oral routes on to the serous body surfaces and also cross-infection between animals in the litter. Although this area of epidemiology deserves further study, its relative importance should be assessed in relation to other factors which are known to be concerned with the epidemiology of cross-infections such as the design of creeps and the tendency of piglets to investigate their surroundings.

REFERENCES

ALEXANDER, G. (1964), *Proc. Aust. Soc. anim. Prod.*, **5**, 113.
ALEXANDROWICZ, S. (1949), *Bull. int. Acad. pol. Sci. Lett., Cl. Sci. math. nat., Sér. B, Sc. Nat.*, **4**, 261.
ALLEN, A. D., and LASLEY, J. F. (1958), *J. Anim. Sci.*, **17**, 1223.
BAUMAN, R. H., KADLEC, J. E., and POWLEN, P. A. (1966), *Purdue Univ. Agric. exp. Sta. Bull.*, p. 810.
BERGE, S., and INDREBØ, T. (1954), *Meld. Norg. LandbrHøisk*, **34**, 481.
BOND, T. E., HEITMAN, H., jun., and KELLY, C. F. (1964), *Int. Congr. agr. Engrg*, **1**, 356.
BROOKS, C. C., FONTENOT, J. P., VIPPERMAN, P. E., THOMAS, H. R., and GRAHAM, P. P. (1964), *J. Anim. Sci.*, **23**, 1022.
BÜTTNER, K. (1932), *Klin. Wschr.*, **17**, 1508.
CURTIS, S. E. (1970), *J. Anim. Sci.*, **31**, 576.
— — CHRISTISON, G. I., and ROBERTSON, W. F. (1970), *Proc. Soc. exp. Biol. Med.*, **134**, 188.
— — HEIDENREICH, C. J., and FOLEY, C. W. (1966), *J. Anim. Sci.*, **25**, 655.
— — and ROGLER, J. C. (1970), *Am. J. Physiol.*, **218**, 249.

CUTHBERTSON, A., and HOSIE, K. F. (1963), *Anim. Prod.*, **5**, 220.
DONALD, H. P. (1937), *Emp. J. exp. Agric.*, **5**, 361.
ELSLEY, F. W. H. (1964), *Sémin. Int. Inst. nat. Rech. agron., Paris*, p. 75.
FOLEY, C. W., SEERLEY, R. W., HANSEN, W. J., and CURTIS, S. E. (1971), *J. Anim. Sci.*, **32**, 926.
GILL, J. C., and THOMPSON, W. (1956), *Br. J. Anim. Behav.*, **4**, 46.
GOODWIN, R. F. W. (1957), *J. Physiol., Lond.*, **135**, 208.
GORDON, W. A. M. (1963), *Br. vet. J.*, **119**, 263.
GRAHAM, R., SAMPSON, J., and HESTER, H. R. (1941), *Proc. Soc. exp. Biol. Med.*, **47**, 338.
GROMMERS, F. J., CHRISTISON, G. I., and CURTIS, S. E. (1970), *J. Anim. Sci.*, **304**, 552.
HAARTSEN, P. I. (1967), *De Isolatie van Stalvloeren* ('The Insulation of Floors in Livestock Buildings'). Publ. 35, I.L.B. (Institute of Farm Building Research), Wageningen, The Netherlands.
HANAWALT, V. M., and SAMPSON, J. (1947), *Am. J. vet. Res.*, **8**, 235.
HUTCHINSON, H. D., TERRILL, S. W., MORRILL, C. C., NORTON, H. W., MEADE, R. J., JENSEN, A. H., and BECKER, D. E. (1954), *J. Anim. Sci.*, **13**, 1023.
INGLIS, J. S. S., and ROBERTSON, A. (1953), *Vet. Rec.*, **65**, 875.
INGRAM, D. L. (1964a), *Res. vet. Sci.*, **5**, 348.
— — (1964b), *Ibid.*, **5**, 357.
— — (1971), *Progress in Biometeorology*, Section A. *Progress in Human Biometeorology*, Vol. 1 (ed. TROMP, S. W.). Amsterdam: Swets & Zeitlinger.
KELLY, C. F., BOND, T. E., and GARRETT, W. (1964), *Trans. Am. Soc. agric. Engrs*, **7**, 34.
KLEIBER, M. (1961), *The Fire of Life*. New York: Wiley.
LEWIS, H. E., FOSTER, A. R., MULLAN, B. J., COX, R. N., and CLARK, R. P. (1969), *Lancet*, **2**, 1273.
LUCAS, I. A. M., and THOMPSON, W. (1953), *J. agric. Sci., Camb.*, **43**, 192.
MCBRIDE, G., JAMES, J. W., and WYETH, G. S. F. (1965), *Anim. Prod.*, **7**, 67.
MCCANCE, R. A., and WIDDOWSON, E. M. (1959), *J. Physiol., Lond.*, **147**, 124.
MACHARDY, F. W. (1960), *Can. agric. Engng*, **2**, 13.
MCLAGAN, J. R., and THOMPSON, W. (1950), *J. agric. Sci., Camb.*, **40**, 367.
MCMEEKAN, C. P. (1940), *Ibid.*, **30**, 276.
MANNERS, M. J., and MCCREA, M. R. (1963), *Br. J. Nutr.*, **17**, 495.
MORRILL, C. C. (1952), *Am. J. vet. Res.*, **13**, 164.
MOUNT, L. E. (1959), *J. Physiol., Lond.*, **147**, 333.
— — (1960), *J. agric. Sci., Camb.*, **55**, 101.
— — (1962), *J. Physiol., Lond.*, **164**, 274.
— — (1963), *Nature, Lond.*, **199**, 122.
— — (1964a), *J. Physiol., Lond.*, **170**, 286.
— — (1964b), *Ibid.*, **173**, 96.
— — (1967), *Res. vet. Sci.*, **8**, 175.
— — (1968), *The Climatic Physiology of the Pig*. Monograph of the Physiological Society. London: Arnold.
— — (1969a), *Proc. Nutr. Soc.*, **28**, 52.
— — (1969b), *Br. J. Nutr.*, **23**, 407.
— — and STEPHENS, D. B. (1970), *J. Physiol., Lond.*, **207**, 417.
NEWLAND, H. W., MCMILLAN, W. N., and REINEKE, E. P. (1952), *J. Anim. Sci.*, **11**, 118.
POMEROY, R. W. (1960), *J. agric. Sci., Camb.*, **54**, 31.
SHARPE, H. B. A. (1966), *Br. vet. J.*, **122**, 99.
STEPHENS, D. B. (1969), *Anim. Prod.*, **11**, 289.
— — (1970a), *Int. J. Biomet.*, **14**, 186.
— — (1970b), Fellowship Thesis, Royal College of Veterinary Surgeons, London.
— — (1971), *Anim. Prod.*, **13**, 303.
— — and FOX, R. H. (1969), *Res. vet. Sci.*, **10**, 305.
— — and START, I. B. (1970), *Int. J. Biomet.*, **14**, 275.
— — — — (1971), *Cornell Vet.*, in the press.
TAYLOR, J. G., OREM, M. T., DOYLE, L. P., and VESTAL, C. M. (1952), *Agric. Enging, St. Joseph, Mich.*, **33**, 213.
WEIR, J. B. DE V. (1949), *J. Physiol., Lond.*, **109**, 1.
WIDDOWSON, E. M. (1950), *Nature, Lond.*, **166**, 626.

PORCINE IMMUNOGLOBULINS

F. J. Bourne, B.Vet.Med., Ph.D., M.R.C.V.S.

General Structure of the Immunoglobulins

Antibodies are members of a group of related proteins called the 'immunoglobulins'. Immunoglobulins are multi-chain proteins made up of four polypeptide chains linked by non-covalent and by disulphide bonds in a fashion similar to that proposed by Porter (1962). Different classes of immunoglobulins can be separated from serum by physical and chemical techniques and five classes of immunoglobulins have been defined according to their general properties and the class of their heavy chains. They are designated (World Health Organization, 1964): IgG, IgA, IgM, IgD, and (World Health Organization, 1968) IgE.

Each four-chain unit consists of two polypeptide chains of low molecular weight (light chains) and two polypeptide chains of high molecular weight (heavy chains), as shown in *Fig.* 16. The chains are linked by interchain

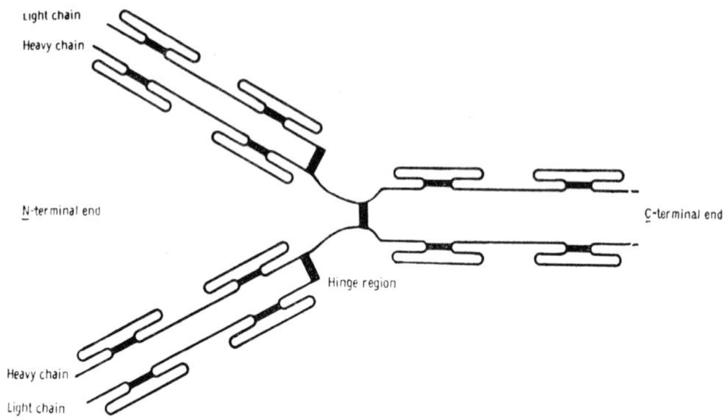

Fig. 16.—Basic immunoglobulin four-chain structure.

disulphide bonds and there are intrachain disulphide loops on each chain. The light chains have a molecular weight of about 23,000 and are of two types, kappa (K) and lambda (L), which are found in all the immunoglobulin classes. An individual immunoglobulin molecule contains either two kappa chains or two lambda chains, never one of each. The heavy chains are specific to and determine the class to which the immunoglobulin belongs and are designated gamma, alpha, mu, delta, and epsilon according to their class. Within a given class of heavy chains subclasses have been distinguished by their antigenic determinants. Four closely related human IgG subclasses are known—IgG_1, IgG_2, IgG_3, and IgG_4. Two subclasses of IgA also occur and IgM exists in more than one form. Differences in the subclasses are reflected in variations in the amino-acid sequences of the carboxyl-terminal parts of the heavy chains.

Although they share the same overall structure, immunoglobulins within a single class and subclass are a heterogeneous mixture of chemically different molecules produced by differing cell lines; even purified antibodies directed against a simple hapten antigen are a population of diverse molecules. This heterogeneity makes structural studies on normal immunoglobulins difficult, but in some pathological conditions great quantities of homogeneous immunoglobulin molecules are produced.

Malignancies of plasma cells may produce IgG or IgA myeloma globulins, whereas malignancies of the lymphocyte series of cells may produce IgM. In about half the cases of plasma-cell tumour, but less frequently in lymphocyte malignancies, there is a urinary excretion of a homogeneous light chain which is known as a 'Bence Jones protein'. Bence Jones proteins are identical with the light chain of the corresponding myeloma globulin and are related to the light chains of normal immunoglobulins. There are two types corresponding to the light chains of type K and L. Myeloma proteins have not been shown to be antibodies in the sense that they have been electively induced by stimulation with known antigens. However, although they do not meet this biological criterion, they have the same structure as normal immunoglobulins and each myeloma protein appears to be a unique example of one of the many different immunoglobulin molecules in the normal heterogeneous

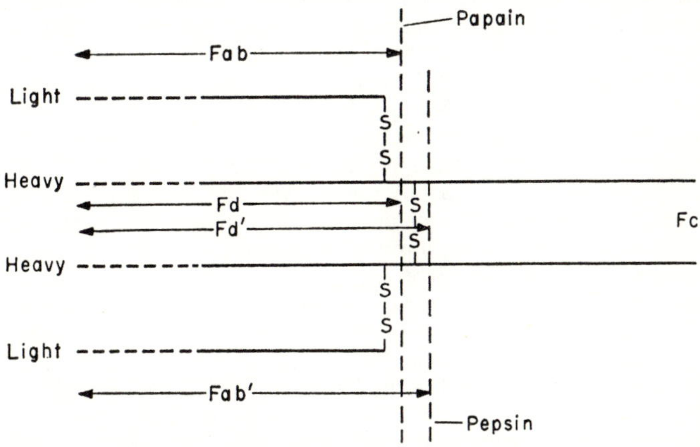

Fig. 17.—Schematic representation of IgG immunoglobulin structure showing the sites of papain and pepsin cleavage. The broken lines indicate regions of marked viability in primary amino-acid sequence.

population. These monoclonal immunoglobulins are ideal for study because of their uniform biosynthetic origin, presence in large amounts, and relative ease of isolation. Multiple myelomas occur in man and some strains of mice but have not been recognized in any of the domesticated species.

A model for IgG immunoglobulin has been proposed having three compact regions (the Fab and Fc regions) (*Fig.* 17) linked by highly extended flexible portions. This allows free rotation of the three compact portions with the angle between the arms varying from 0° to 180°.

Immunoglobulin IgM molecules are made up of five monomeric units each of 180,000 molecular weight held together in the form of a ring, each unit consisting of two light chains and two mu chains. Electron micrographs support the idea that 19S IgM is a flexible pentameric structure.

IgA immunoglobulin molecules like IgG are made up of light (kappa and lambda) and heavy chains (alpha). These immunoglobulins exist both in serum and in external secretions. Serum IgA immunoglobulins exist both as monomeric proteins, containing two light and two heavy chains, and as polymers of two or more of the monomeric units.

It is now established that two subclasses of human IgA globulins are present in serum and certain external secretions and that the antigenic differences between IgA_1 and IgA_2 are associated with the heavy polypeptide chains. Structural differences between these molecules also occur (Grey and others, 1968).

Tomasi and Zigelbaum (1963) first demonstrated that normal serum immunoglobulin ratios do not occur in mucous surface secretions and that IgA, which is only a minor component of the serum immunoglobulins, is the major antibody component of saliva, colostrum, urine, tears, bile, and small intestinal secretions. These findings have been extended to other body fluids and it is now generally accepted that IgA is the major antibody system of the mucous surfaces which open to the exterior. It is also recognized that IgA in human external secretion has physico-chemical and antigenic properties that differentiate it from its counterpart in serum. Human-serum IgA exists mainly in the form of a 6·9S monomer but secretory IgA is found mainly in an 11·5S form, although high polymers exist (Tomasi and others, 1965). The antigenic determinants of secretory IgA that are not present in serum IgA are due to an additional fragment termed the 'transport piece', 'T-piece', 'secretory piece', 'secretory component', or 'S-component'.

The human secretory 11S IgA immunoglobulin contains subunits of 7S IgA and the glycoprotein S-component. The number of subunits is not definitely established, but most available evidence indicates two molecules of 7S IgA and one of S-component.

Electron-microscopy studies have postulated a molecular model in which two IgA monomers are superimposed on each other in a close-packed state with the S-component inserted in the C-terminal part of the alpha chains.

The constituents of the IgA molecule are very probably synthesized in different cells, the IgA light and heavy chains being synthesized in local plasma cells, whereas the S-component polypeptide chain is formed in the epithelial cells of the exocrine glands. The extent of synthesis of both constituents of the exocrine IgA molecule need not necessarily run parallel. If a relative over-production exists, free S-component or free IgA molecules can be expected in the excreta. It is a well-known fact that in persons lacking IgA in their plasma, free S-component can be demonstrated in their secretions. In normal human colostrum free S-component is not present (van Munster, Stoelinga, and Poels-Zanders, 1969), but it can be found in milk, where a relative over-production of S-component occurs.

Halpern and Koshland (1970) have recently described a further polypeptide unit in secretory IgA molecules of 23,000 molecular weight which they designate J-chain. This polypeptide has been found in rabbit and human secretory IgA molecules and is disulphide linked to the alpha chain. The suggested role of J-chain is to provide a binding site for secretory component either directly through the contribution of groups to the site or indirectly through an induced conformational change in the alpha chains. It was further suggested that J-chain was synthesized in the same plasma cell as the heavy and light chains and may provide the recognition signal for the interaction between the plasma cell synthesizing the J-dimer complex and the epithelial cell synthesizing the S-component. J-chains have been found in the dimer but not the monomer form of human IgA and seem to be responsible for the dimer structure, characteristic of secretory IgA molecules. This observation would also agree with the findings that rabbit colostral IgA is secreted from plasma cells as a dimer and not formed by the joining together of monomers outside of the cell by secretory component.

A fourth class of human immunoglobulin, IgD, has been described (Rowe and Fahey, 1965a, b). Each IgD molecule is made up of two light and two heavy chains (delta). The high frequency of lambda chains in IgD molecules is unusual and unexplained. No special function of IgD is known.

Immunoglobulin IgE is associated with skin-sensitizing activity and has been distinguished from the other classes of immunoglobulin (Ishizaka, Ishizaka, and Hornbrook, 1966). IgE has a molecular weight of 200,000 and is made up of two light (kappa or lambda) and two heavy chains (epsilon).

Porcine Immunoglobulins

Very few studies have determined the physico-chemical data of pig gamma-globulins. Tiselius and Kabat (1939) found an isoelectric point of *p*H 5·86 in respect of gamma-globulins and one of *p*H 5·1 in respect of isolated pig pneumococcal antibody. The molecular weight of the antibody was determined to be 990,000 with a sedimentation constant of 19·8. Later Koenig (1949) found for isolated pig gamma-globulin a sedimentation constant of 7·25–7·28. Cammarata and Deutsch (1950), using free electrophoresis, divided the gamma area into $gamma_1$ and $gamma_2$, which were separated by alcohol fractionation. A sedimentation constant of 7·1 was found in respect of both fractions and a molecular weight of 168,000. The isoelectric point was 6·1 for $gamma_1$ and 7·2 for $gamma_2$. No component was found with a higher sedimentation constant. However, this was achieved by Franek, Riha, and Sterzl (1961), who in respect of gamma-globulin in mature pigs found sedimentation constants of 6·7 and 18S.

Many direct comparisons have been made between porcine and human immuno-electrophoretic patterns and on this basis porcine IgG, IgA, and IgM precipitin arcs have been described. Karlsson (1966) identified such precipitin arcs in porcine serum, colostrum, and milk, and Kim, Bradley, and Watson (1966) recognized similar immunoglobulins in serum. In neither case, however, was the protein isolated or a relationship with the immunoglobulins established. Brummerstedt-Hansen (1967) also observed immuno-electrophoretic precipitin arcs which he suggested could be comparable to the precipitin arcs of human immunoglobulins, but emphasized that there was little justification for this comparison until the porcine immunoglobulins had been isolated and characterized.

The isolation of a porcine immunoglobulin was first described by Metzger and Fougereau (1967). These authors isolated two IgG immunoglobulins, IgG_1 and IgG_2, which differed in electrophoretic mobility. The latter protein was isolated in a pure form but the former protein was always contaminated with IgG_2. An antigenic relationship between the two proteins was not established because of this contamination.

Franek and others (1961) described a gamma-globulin in mature pigs with a sedimentation constant of 18, and antibody activity in 19S molecules of pig serum has been demonstrated by several authors. Porter (1969a) isolated an IgM-rich fraction from porcine serum which was contaminated with $alpha_2$ macroglobulin and later showed it to possess antibody activity. The protein, however, was not obtained in a pure form and characterized, nor was its relationship to the other immunoglobulins established.

The isolation of porcine IgA immunoglobulin was first reported by Bourne (1969a) from milk and colostrum. Its presence was also demonstrated in saliva, urine, and serum. The isolation of IgA from serum was later described by the same author (Bourne, 1969b), who showed that secretory IgA possessed antigenic determinants that were not present on the isolated protein. Porter (1969a) also described the isolation of an IgA immunoglobulin from porcine colostrum, but the isolated protein was not characterized and its relationship to other immunoglobulins was not established.

Four pig immunoglobulins are now recognized and have been isolated and characterized in this laboratory (Bourne, 1971). They are designated IgG_1, IgG_2, IgM, and IgA. Physico-chemical and antigenic studies on these proteins have demonstrated their analogy to the three major classes of human immunoglobulins—IgG, IgA, and IgM. (*See Table I.*)

Table I.—Some Properties of Porcine Immunoglobulins

	Sedimentation Coefficient	Nitrogen	Carbohydrate (μmoles per mg.)							Extinction Coefficient (*E*)
			Fuc	Man	Gal	Glc	GlcNAc	GalNAc	SA	
Serum IgG_1	7S	14·6	9	65	17	13	56	6	6	13·7
Serum IgG_2	7S	14·5	6	53	17	11	51	—	4	—
Serum IgM	19S	13·4	25	178	76	21	146	—	75	12·5
Serum IgA	7S; 89·55	—	—	—	—	—	—	—	—	—
Milk IgA	9·55; 11·65	14·0	27	102	75	33	110	17	43	13·9

Fuc: Fucose. Gal: Galactose. GlcNAc: *N*-acetyl glucosamine. SA: Sialic acid. Man Mannose. Glc: Glucose. GalNAc: *N*-acetyl galactosamine. $E^{1\%}_{282\ nm.}$ 1 cm. 0·1*N* NaOH

Porcine immunoglobulin IgG is the main immunoglobulin of serum, and the presence of two subclasses, an electrophoretically fast IgG_1 and a slow IgG_2, has been demonstrated. Both subclasses possess a sedimentation coefficient of 7 and a nitrogen content of 14·6 per cent and 14·5 per cent for IgG_1 and IgG_2 respectively. This is slightly lower than the value for human IgG of 16 per cent but the extinction coefficients for these proteins are very similar. Antigenic differences occur between the subclasses, as do differences in their susceptibility to the proteolytic action of papain in the presence of cysteine. Although porcine IgG immunoglobulins are more resistant than the corresponding human proteins, the same features of resistance to papain hydrolysis do occur.

Only small amounts of porcine immunoglobulin IgM were recoverable as a euglobilin precipitate; in this respect it is similar to rabbit IgM but contrasts with the precipitating behaviour of human IgM. Like the corresponding immunoglobulin in other species it possesses an S value of 19. The nitrogen content of 13·4 per cent compares with a value of 14·3 per cent for rabbit IgM.

Immunoglobulin IgA of porcine external secretions is composed principally of two molecular types—a 9·5S and 11·6S molecule. Colostrum and milk during the first week of lactation is made up of about 60 per cent of the smaller molecule and 35–40 per cent of the 11·6S molecule; smaller amounts of 7, 15, and 18S molecules also occur. After the first week of lactation the proportion of 9·5S molecules increases.

A similar molecular make-up has been shown for porcine urine IgA and the elution position on G200 Sephadex of pig intestinal juice IgA and salivary IgA also indicates a similar size for these proteins. Vaerman (1970) has also demonstrated two molecular types of porcine milk IgA, of 8·9 and 11·2S.

Serum IgA has been shown to occur in approximately equal proportions of a 7S and 9·5S molecule, which differs markedly from the situation found in man but is similar to the situation described in the dog (Vaerman, 1970). The latter author has also shown that the intestinal mucosa is a major source of serum IgA in the dog, forming 60–90 per cent of this protein. The predominance of IgA-containing lymphoid cells in the pig intestinal tract and the scarcity of them elsewhere, plus the presence of an IgA dimer in serum, suggests that this may also be the case in the pig.

Pig secretory IgA possesses antigenic determinants in addition to those possessed by the serum 7S IgA molecule; they are associated with secretory component. This polypeptide chain has been isolated and shown to have a sedimentation value of 4·3S and a suggested molecular weight of 80,000–90,000. Secretory component is bonded covalently to the parent IgA molecule and has been demonstrated in epithelial cells of gastric mucosa but not in plasma cells; it is found free in milk.

Antigenic differences between secretory IgA and serum IgA could only be shown when 7S serum IgA was used in the immunodiffusion. When whole serum was used, or serum IgA containing molecules larger than the 7S form, no antigenic differences could be shown.

This is probably due to the presence in serum of secretory IgA, the pig being similar to the human, bovine, ovine, and caprine species in this respect.

On the basis of dissociation and reduction studies two structural types of IgA molecule are recognized in the pig equivalent to IgA_1 and IgA_2 of man. The IgA_1 and IgA_2 molecules occur in equal proportions in colostrum and milk but IgA_1 predominates in serum (4 : 1).

A shared antigenic relationship exists between human and porcine IgA molecules, emphasizing their homology, and the carbohydrate contents of human and porcine immunoglobulins are similar, showing a close analogy between the species.

Immunoglobulin Quantitation

Mean immunoglobulin concentration in serum from pork pigs and sow serum, colostral whey and milk whey are shown in *Table II* (Curtis and Bourne, 1971).

Table II.—IMMUNOGLOBULIN LEVELS IN SERUM, COLOSTRUM, AND MILK

	MEAN IMMUNOGLOBULIN CONCENTRATION (mg. per ml.)±S.E.				TOTAL SERUM AND WHEY PROTEIN (mg. per ml.)
	IgG	IgG_2	IgA	IgM	
Serum from pork pigs	18·31±0·67	12·41±0·48	1·44±0·12	3·15±0·19	70
Sow serum	24·33±0·94	14·08±0·49	2·37±0·20	2·92±0·18	70
Colostrum (0 hour)	61·80±2·44	40·29±1·66	9·66±0·59	3·19±0·21	196
Milk (24 hours)	11·83±4·82	8·04±3·21	3·76±0·99	1·79±0·31	41
Milk (2 days)	8·16±3·17	5·02±1·80	2·72±0·67	1·81±0·41	35
Milk (3–7 days)	1·91±0·64	1·31±0·32	3·41±1·01	1·17±0·23	33
Milk (8–35 days)	1·37±0·62	0·99±0·45	3·04±0·74	0·89±0·25	33

Immunoglobulin IgG constitutes over 80 per cent of the total immunoglobulin content of colostrum which contains two and a half to three times more IgG than serum. A fivefold drop in colostral IgG concentration occurs in the first 24 hours of lactation and a thirtyfold drop in the first week; IgG accounts for 20–30 per cent of milk immunoglobulin. The IgA concentration in colostrum is four times higher than in serum. A threefold drop in concentration occurs in the first 24 hours of lactation, after which milk IgA levels remain at 3 mg. per ml., IgA accounting for 50–60 per cent of milk immunoglobulin. IgM is the minor component of both colostrum (4 per cent) and milk (18 per cent) immunoglobulin.

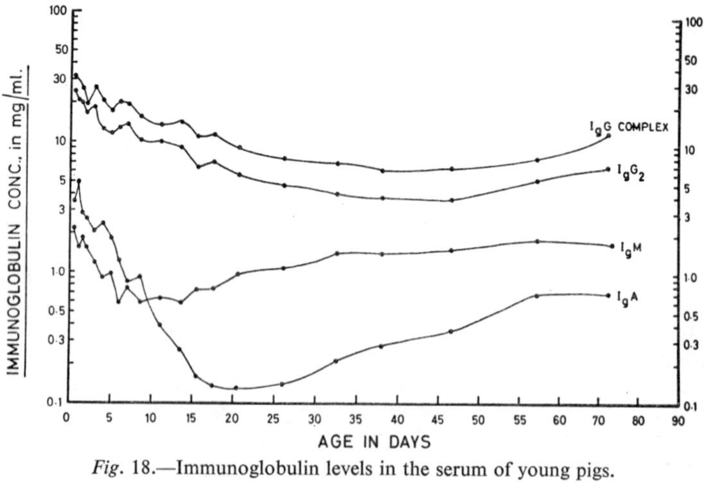

Fig. 18.—Immunoglobulin levels in the serum of young pigs.

Immunoglobulin levels in the serum of young pigs is shown in *Fig.* 18. Immunoglobulins IgG, IgM, and IgA are all absorbed from colostrum by the newborn piglet. Peak serum levels are obtained at about 24 hours of age with a great deal of variation in levels between litters.

At 24 hours the litter means of IgG concentrations ranged from 18·7 to 39·0 mg. per ml.; levels then fell slowly to reach a minimum (6·3 mg. per ml.) at 36–40 days of age. Immunoglobulin IgA levels varied from 2·1 to 8·6 mg. per ml. and fell rapidly after 24 hours, reaching a trough at 17–22 days of age. IgM levels varied from 1·1 to 2·0 mg. per ml. at 24 hours and then fell rapidly to their lowest level (0·6 mg. per ml.) at 8–14 days of age.

The half-lives of absorbed IgM, IgA, and IgG are 4·5, 3·5, and 14·2 days respectively in piglet serum. IgG_2 was on average two-thirds of the total IgG concentration throughout the period studied and had a half-life of 12 days.

From our studies it is clear that in general IgM levels in the young suckled piglet are lower than those in the adult throughout the first 12 weeks of life. Absorbed IgA reaches a maximum concentration which is double adult levels, but falls rapidly to a minimum at 3 weeks and is only half adult levels at 12 weeks. The concentration of absorbed IgG at 24 hours is about 20 per cent higher than that of mature animals but falls below adult levels in 4 days. A mature serum profile has not been attained in pigs of 16 weeks of age since the IgA and IgG concentrations are only three-fifths and three-quarters respectively of those in the adult.

If the adult immunoglobulin profile represents the optimum for efficient systemic immunity, then throughout the growing period systemic immunity is far from optimum. Three age-groups of pig are most commonly affected by enteritis due to *Escherichia coli* infection. These are at 12–48 hours after birth, 3 weeks of age, and during the first 1–2 weeks after weaning (Stevens, 1963). Susceptibility to infection in the first few days of life may be due to low levels of passive immunity. There is a great deal of variation between pigs and between litters in the amount of immunoglobulin absorbed. At 3 weeks of age the levels of all three classes of immunoglobulins are very low. At weaning (5–6 weeks) IgM and IgA levels are low, the serum concentration of IgG reaches its lowest level, and the protection afforded by copro-antibody in milk is removed. It must be appreciated that although systemic immunoglobulin levels may give an indication of the general immune status of the animal, they give no indication of the specificity of immunity that may be present and little indication of the development of the intestinal-tract immune system, which must be vitally important in relation to gut infections.

It has been demonstrated that the newborn piglet is capable of absorbing colostral IgG, IgM, and IgA from the intestinal tract as whole protein molecules. A study of the molecular characteristics of colostrum, milk, and piglet serum IgA at 1 day and 3 days after birth using gel-filtration and preparative and analytical ultracentrifugation has confirmed that this absorption is non-selective. The proportion of 11·6S to 9·5S molecules in 1-day piglet serum IgA was only slightly different to that found in colostral IgA. However, in milk and particularly in 3-day piglet serum IgA, there was a markedly reduced proportion of the larger molecule. When the proportion of secretory IgA in these IgA preparations was quantitated using a colostral IgA preparation as an arbitrary standard it showed a reduced proportion of the secretory molecule in milk IgA and particularly in 3-day piglet serum IgA. This study indicates that the 11·6S molecule of colostral IgA is absorbed by the newborn piglet but it possesses a shorter half-life than the 9·5S molecule. The findings of a half-life of 24 hours for human 11S secretory

IgA compared with a 5·6-day half-life of monomer serum IgA (Butler, Rossen and Waldmann, 1967) would lend support to this observation. A further implication of this study is that only the 11·6S molecule is secretory in type, the 9·5S being non-secretory and similar to the 9·5S molecule found in serum.

These findings disagree with the observation of Porter (1969b) that secretory IgA is not absorbed by newborn piglets and that antibody activity against *E. coli* antigens present in colostrum IgA is not transferred to the serum of newborn pigs. Porter (1969b) suggests that absorption recognition sites on the Fc part of the molecule are blocked by secretory component. However, the age of pig studied was not given; if the piglet was 3 days or older one would expect to find only low levels of secretory IgA, also the haemagglutination and antiglobulin haemagglutination test results described by Porter could not be repeated by Knop (1971).

Intestinal Immunoglobulins

Studies on the immunoglobulin components of the intestinal tract of adult pigs revealed that IgA was the main immunoglobulin in intestinal juice and gut mucosa, the IgA : IgG ratios being 12 : 1 and 5 : 1 respectively (*Table III*). The IgA immunoglobulins isolated from these two sites were immuno-electrophoretically and antigenically similar to each other and also to other

Table III.—Immunoglobulin Levels (mg. per ml.)

	IgG	IgA	IgM	IgA/IgG
Serum	24·3	2·4	2·9	0·1/1
Colostrum (0 hour)	61·8	9·7	3·2	0·16/1
Milk	1·4	3·0	0·9	2·1/1
Intestinal juice (relative levels)	0·2	2·6	Trace	12/1

secretory IgA molecules. Elution positions on Sephadex G200 suggest that these immunoglobulins have the same molecular size as milk IgA and in common with other secretory IgA molecules possess an additional heavy-chain antigenic determinant analogous to secretory component in man (Bourne, Pickup, and Honour, 1971).

There are no previous reports of intestinal immunoglobulin levels in domestic animals, but Vaerman and Heremans (1969) have shown that the dog possesses a gut IgA secretory system similar to that known to occur in the mouse and in man. Chodirker and Tomasi (1963) reported that the IgG : IgA ratio in adult human intestinal fluid was 3·8 : 1 and although it was later suggested that the concentration of IgG was over-estimated their findings are not in agreement with those of Plaut and Keonil (1969), who showed that IgA is the major immunoglobulin of upper small-intestinal juice and that it predominated over IgG by 5 : 1.

Immunofluorescent studies on the pig intestinal tract have confirmed that IgA-containing lymphoid cells predominate. In the adult pig IgA cells occurred in a 5 : 1 ratio compared to IgM, whereas IgG were only present in low numbers. In the spleen the position was reversed: IgG predominated and were about twenty times more prevalent than IgM cells; IgA cells only occurred in small numbers. In the gut of the pig there are relatively larger numbers of IgM and IgG cells than in the intestinal tract of man where the ratio of IgA to IgM and IgG cells is 20 : 1.

The immunofluorescent findings of a significant number of IgM-containing cells in the lamina propria is in contrast to the quantitation of only small amounts of this immunoglobulin in intestinal juice and gut mucosa. The reason for this is not clear. However, the absolute levels of immunoglobulin quantitated were not very high due to difficulties in handling highly concentrated intestinal juice; consequently IgM may have lost some of its significance due to this factor. Both IgA and IgM staining was present on crypt epithelium and the suggestion by Brandtzaeg (1968) that both of these immunoglobulins have secretory mechanisms would appear to gain support from these studies. Immunoglobulin IgG staining was observed in the connective-tissue ground substance of the gut, but no crypt fluorescence was seen and it would appear that this immunoglobulin has no secretory mechanism equivalent to that of IgA and IgM.

Examination of the intestinal tract of pigs slaughtered for bacon (16–20 weeks of age) showed that the number of IgM containing cells equalled those of IgA. Further studies are necessary on the development of the immune system of the gastro-intestinal tract of the pig, but it would appear that a mature profile is obtained at a relatively late stage of growth, certainly beyond the normal life span of animals killed for food production. The immunoglobulin-containing cell picture in the spleen of the immature animal mirrored to some degree that seen in the gut, since although IgG cells were predominant IgM cells occurred in relatively greater numbers than in the adult sow spleen.

In mesenteric lymph-nodes of the adult pig IgA and IgM cells were present in equal numbers and were relatively more numerous than IgG-staining cells. In the 16–20-week-old pig relatively fewer IgG-staining cells were present but IgM and IgA-containing cells were equal in number.

The Site of Formation of Immunoglobulins

The site of formation of colostral and milk immunoglobulins is very pertinent to any discussion on their protective value in the alimentary tract of the young pig. In the mammary gland of the cow and sheep there is evidence that the secretory immunoglobulins are derived from serum by a highly selective transport mechanism (Tomasi and Bienenstock, 1968). Whether the human mammary gland also shows selective transport rather than local synthesis remains to be determined. Adinolfi and others (1966) could find little relationship between the antibody activity of serum and colostral IgA against *E. coli* and concluded that colostral IgA was formed locally in mammary tissue. Genco and Taubmann (1969), by comparing local and systemic immunoglobulin activity in response to parenteral and local vaccination of mammary tissue, have demonstrated that most colostral IgA is also produced locally in the rabbit, and Lawton, Asofsky, and Mage (1970) have suggested that local synthesis can account for all the IgA found in rabbit colostrum. Our studies in the pig on the transfer of I^{125}-tagged immunoglobulins IgG, IgA, and IgM from serum into mammary secretions suggest that virtually all colostral IgG and half of colostral IgA and IgM are derived from serum, so colostrum must be regarded more as a transudate than as a secretion. In milk, however, a different situation exists; about one-third to one-half of IgG and IgM are derived from serum, but only a minor amount of IgA (2–17 per cent), suggesting that the bulk of these immunoglobulins and certainly IgA is formed locally in mammary lymphoid tissue. This situation would thus appear to be similar to that occurring in the rabbit.

It is reasonable to expect that local immunization at a mucosal surface induces secretory IgA antibody with protective effects at that surface. Parenteral immunization would not be as likely to provide comparable levels of local protection. Work is at present under way at Langford to determine the class and antibody activity of locally and systemically produced immunoglobulins following local and systemic immunization.

The development of the immune system in piglets is also being studied. We have shown that the piglet in utero is capable of eliciting an immune response, following intra-uterine stimulation, after the 55th day of gestation. This lends support to the findings of Binns (1967) and Fennestad, Borg-Petersen, and Brummerstedt-Hansen (1968). The immune response is principally macroglobulin in character, which suggests that this could be a useful parameter in the study of pig intra-uterine disease.

REFERENCES

ADINOLFI, M., GLYNN, A. A., LINDSAY, M., and MILNE, C. M. (1966), *Immunology*, **10**, 517.

BINNS, R. M. (1967), *Nature, Lond.*, **214**, 179.

BOURNE, F. J. (1969a), *Biochim. biophys. Acta*, **181**, 485.

— — (1969b), *Biochem. biophys. Res. Commun.*, **36**, 138.

— — (1971), Ph.D. Thesis, University of Bristol.

— — PICKUP, J., and HONOUR, J. W. (1971), *Biochim. biophys. Acta*, **229**, 18.

BRANDTZAEG, P. (1968), *Acta path. microbiol. Scand.*, **74**, 624.

BRUMMERSTEDT-HANSEN, E. (1967), *The Serum Proteins of the Pig. An Immunoelectrophoretic Study*. Copenhagen: Munksgaard.

BUTLER, W. T., ROSSEN, R. D., and WALDMANN, T. A. (1967), *J. clin. Invest.*, **46**, 1883.

CAMMARATA, P. D., and DEUTSCH, H. F. (1950), *Archs Biochim.*, **25**, 354.

CHODIRKER, W. B., and TOMASI, T. B. (1963), *Science, N.Y.*, **142**, 1080.

CURTIS, J., and BOURNE, F. J. (1971), *Biochim. biophys. Acta*, **236**, 319.

FENNESTAD, K. L., BORG-PETERSEN, C., and BRUMMERSTEDT-HANSEN, E. (1968), *Res. vet. Sci.*, **9**, 378.

FRANEK, F., RIHA, I., and STERZL, J. (1961), *Nature, Lond.*, **189**, 1020.

GENCO, R. J., and TAUBMANN, M. A. (1969), *Ibid.*, **221**, 679.

GREY, H. M., ABEL, C. A., YOUNT, W. J., and KUNKEL, H. G. (1968), *J. exp. Med.*, **128**, 1223.

HALPERN, M. S., and KOSHLAND, M. E. (1970), *Nature, Lond.*, **228**, 1276.

ISHIZAKA, K., ISHIZAKA, T., and HORNBROOK, M. M. (1966), *J. Immun.*, **97**, 840.

KARLSSON, B. W. (1966), *Acta path. microbiol. scand.*, **67**, 237.

KIM, Y. B., BRADLEY, S. G., and WATSON, D. W. (1966), *J. Immun.*, **97**, 189.

KNOP, J. (1971), personal communication.

KOENIG, V. L. (1949), *Archs Biochim.*, **23**, 229.

LAWTON, A. R., ASOFSKY, R., and MAGE, R. G. (1970), *J. Immun.*, **104**, 388.

METZGER, J. J., and FOUGEREAU, M. (1967), *C. r. hebd. Séanc. Acad. Sci., Paris*, **265**, 724.

PLAUT, A. G., and KEONIL, P. (1969), *Gastroenterology*, **56**, 522.

PORTER, P. (1969a), *Biochim. biophys. Acta*, **181**, 381.

— — (1969b), *Immunology*, **17**, 617.

PORTER, R. R. (1962), in *Basic Problems in Neoplastic Disease* (ed. GELLHORN, A., and HIRSCHBERG, E.). New York: Columbia University Press.

ROWE, D. S., and FAHEY, J. L. (1965a), *J. exp. Med.*, **121**, 171.

— — and FAHEY, J. L. (1965b), *Ibid.*, **121**, 185.

STEVENS, A. J. (1963), *Br. vet. J.*, **119**, 520.

TISELIUS, A., and KABAT, E. A. (1939), *J. exp. Med.*, **69**, 119.

TOMASI, T. B., and BIENSTOCK, J. (1968), in *Advances in Immunology* (ed. DIXON, F. J., and KUNKEL, H. G.), Vol. 9, p. 1. New York: Academic.
— — TAN, M. M., SOLOMON, A., and PRENDERGAST, R. A. (1965), *J. exp. Med.*, **121**, 101.
— — and ZIGELBAUM, S. (1963), *J. clin. Invest.*, **42**, 1552.
VAERMAN, J. P. (1970), *Studies on IgA Immunoglobulins in Man and Animals.* Catholic University of Louvain.
— — and HEREMANS, J. F. (1969), *Immunochemistry*, **6**, 779.
VAN MUNSTER, P. J. J., STOELINGA, G. B. A., and POELS-ZANDERS, S. (1969), *Immunology*, **17**, 165.

ALLERGIC SKIN CONDITIONS IN THE DOG

G. S. Walton, B.V.Sc., M.R.C.V.S.

Many agents that come into either direct contact with the skin or enter the body by other routes are capable of inducing changes in immunologic reactivity.

Such changes may be protective and benefit the individual, or they may be detrimental and result in a state of allergic hypersensitivity (von Pirquet, 1906; Coombs and Gell, 1968). In the latter case, subsequent antigenic challenge results in mobilization of one or more allergic mechanisms (Coombs and Gell, 1968) which may then produce either localized tissue damage and inflammatory changes within one organ, such as the skin, or may evoke a more generalized systemic response in which the skin may become involved.

Cutaneous allergic hypersensitivity responses occur sporadically in the dog and they never follow a first exposure to a given allergen. They have been found in association with certain arthropods, food and food-products, pollens and inhaled agents, therapeutic agents, infections, and foreign agents residing within the body. They may also be associated with certain agents that come into direct contact with the skin.

Responses to Arthropods

Insects and ectoparasites may produce changes within the skin by causing mechanical damage, introducing cytotoxic or pharmacologically active substances, introducing infection, inducing a foreign-body response, or stimulating an allergic hypersensitivity response. The relative importance of each of these mechanisms in the ensuing cutaneous response will depend on the potentialities of the arthropod and the responsiveness of the host.

Allergic hypersensitivity plays a decisive role in certain ecto-parasitic infestations of the dog. It is very important, for instance, in the cutaneous responses noted in individual animals during flea infestation. The salivary secretions of the dog, cat, and human flea contain no cytotoxic or pharmacologically active substances and the cutaneous responses found in animals result from mobilization of allergic mechanisms which had been induced at the time of previous challenge. The clinical features of flea hypersensitivity responses in the dog are well known. They comprise severe pruritus, followed by varying degrees of self-inflicted skin damage, exfoliation, and thinning of the coat, which is most pronounced along the spine and dorsum of the body. Circumscribed areas of exfoliation, sometimes described as ‘wet eczema’, are occasionally seen in individual animals. In cases of long duration the skin may become grossly thickened and heavily pigmented.

Kissileff (1938) observed in the flea-hypersensitive dog that artificial challenge resulted in an immediate response at the test site, with recurrence of irritation several hours later. Subsequent challenge produced a similar response at a second site 3 days later, and also recurrence of irritation over the original area. It has been shown subsequently that artificial challenge may produce an immediate and/or delayed response within the skin of hypersensitive dogs (Walton, 1965). Hypersensitivity may develop in dogs of any age, but is rare in animals under the age of 6 months. How and why sensitivity develops is not known. Many animals infested sporadically or continually over many years never develop a hypersensitivity.

The salivary secretions of the cat flea contain several antigenic constituents (Young and others, 1963) which are haptenic in nature (Benjamini and others, 1963) and require to be linked to a skin collagen fraction before they reach full antigenicity (Feingold, Benjamini, and Michaeli, 1968).

Diagnosis may be confirmed by isolation of the parasite, or by finding evidence of flea debris in brushings, associated with remission of symptoms following parasiticidal therapy.

Intradermal testing using flea extracts is of limited value (Muller and Kirk, 1969).

Desensitization using whole flea extracts has been investigated in the dog (Owen, 1941; Collins, 1966; Keep and Taylor, 1967; Michaeli and Goldfarb, 1968), but although improvement has been noted with this form of therapy, it is usually of very short duration, lasting on average only 5–6 weeks (Michaeli and Goldfarb, 1968).

Natural desensitization appears to be rare; sensitized animals show recurrence of symptoms following further challenge in subsequent years.

At the present time reliance has still to be placed on empirical treatment of lesions and the use of parasiticidal baths and dressings or the use of collars impregnated with organophosphorus compounds, together with thorough treatment of the bedding and premises, and in-contact animals.

Responses in the dog to the venom of the bee and other members of the order Hymenoptera are complex. The venom contains numerous toxic and pharmacologically active substances which can produce local irritation, inflammation, and pain (Mueller, 1959), or if injected in sufficient amounts can produce systemic anaphylactic-like effects (Torsney, 1968).

Bee, wasp, hornet, and yellow-jacket extracts contain at least four to six antigenic fractions, some of which are species-specific, while others show cross-reactivity with other members of the order Hymenoptera (Langlois, Shulman, and Arbesman, 1965; Arbesman, Langlois, and Shulman, 1965; Arbesman and others, 1966). Thus an animal may become sensitized when attacked by one member of this order and subsequent challenge by another member of the same group may produce a severe anaphylactic response (Johnson and Halperm, 1966).

Fatalities have been recorded in the dog (Antin, 1963) and man (Parrish, 1963) following bee stings.

Desensitization of individuals suffering from severe general reactions to bee stings, using allpyral antigens, has given encouraging results in man (Fox, 1968) but has yet to be evaluated in the dog.

Although mechanical damage plays an important role in clinical demodex infestation of the dog, histological investigations suggest that hypersensitivity responses may be an added complication in a small percentage of animals (Walton, 1966; Gaafar, 1967), where cutaneous changes are accompanied by massive infiltrations of monocytic cells and severe pruritus.

The precise role of allergic mechanisms in Sarcoptes, Otodectes, and forage-mite infestations of the dog has not yet been elucidated.

Responses have been suspected in the dog to black fly (Schwartzman and Orkin, 1962) but require further investigation, and it is known that the saliva of this group of insects contains histamine and an anticoagulant (Hutcheon and Chivers-Wilson, 1953). Reactions have also been recorded in the dog to mosquitoes (Schwartzman and Orkin, 1962).

Responses to Food and Food Products

Responses to ingested allergens probably account for 1 per cent of cutaneous disease in the dog and cat (Walton, 1968). They were first described in the dog by Phillips (1922) and subsequently observed by a number of other workers (Collins, 1966).

Sensitization may occur suddenly at any age, often after many months or years of repeated or continuous challenge.

Once established, exacerbation of lesions will follow each subsequent challenge. Natural desensitization appears to be rare. Lesions may be confined to the skin or may involve also the alimentary or respiratory tracts.

Alimentary involvement may result in vomiting or abdominal discomfort within 2 hours of feeding and/or voiding of fluid or haemorrhagic faeces several hours later.

Unlike the alimentary changes noted in individual animals showing an intolerance to a given food, symptoms never follow the initial challenge and can only be prevented by complete elimination of the substance from the diet and not by merely reducing its amount.

Respiratory involvement is usually manifested by asthmatic seizures several hours after ingestion of the allergen.

Cutaneous changes follow within 12–24 hours of challenge and persist for 12–18 hours, unless further challenge occurs or self-inflicted damage is marked, in which case cutaneous changes may last longer. The most frequent manifestation of cutaneous hypersensitivity to ingested allergens in the dog is generalized pruritus accompanied by self-inflicted skin damage (Walton, 1968). The pattern of self-infliction shows marked individual variation. Such lesions may be confined to a relatively small body area or be widely distributed over the body surface; the remaining areas of the skin appear macroscopically normal.

Less frequently, there may be evidence of papular urticaria, plaque formation, or generalized hyperaemia, which can be accompanied by cutaneous oedema leading to swelling of the eyelids and entropion, and bilateral otitis.

Occasionally exfoliative lesions may be seen. In cases of long duration, the skin may become thickened, pigmentation may increase, and hair growth become sparse. The skin may also develop a greasy texture and a rancid odour.

Investigations have shown (Walton, 1968) that, although multiple sensitivities can occur, they are rare; most patients develop a very precise response to a single antigen. The antigen concerned may be a major constituent of the diet or it may be ingested infrequently and in very small amounts.

Sensitivity may be produced to any one of a very large number of dietary constituents. In many cases antigenicity can be lost or enhanced by cooking or processing the substance concerned. Certain animals have been shown to react to cooked, as opposed to raw, meat from a given species. Cross-reactivity between the meats from different species has not been encountered, although it can occur between cow beef and cow milk. Sensitivities may also be encountered to cereals, and these, too, are precise; thus an animal reacting to wheatmeal will not react to oats, maize, or barley.

Reactions to shellfish and to some fruits may not be allergic, since certain of these foods contain substances which act as histamine releasers when they gain entry to the body (Champion, 1968).

No precise knowledge is available of the mechanisms responsible for certain papular urticarial responses occurring in the younger dog, which appear suddenly, on a single occasion, and cannot be reproduced either naturally or artificially at a later date.

Diagnosis of food allergy in the dog rests on a thorough clinical examination, elimination of possible parasitic infestations and other causes of pruritus, and the carrying out of test-meal investigations as follows.

Animals are placed on a defined diet, such as beef and vegetables, or mutton and maize, etc., for a week. If no improvement occurs this suggests that the trial diet contains the causative agent. If improvement does occur, the diet is enlarged by one constituent a week until a response is observed and the food containing the allergen is detected.

Serological tests are at present of little practical value. Similarly, results of intradermal scratch or prick test procedures are extremely disappointing, probably because the allergen concerned has been altered by digestion or by the forming of serum complexes so that it bears no resemblance to the presently available commercial test antigens.

Responses to Pollens and Other Inhaled Agents

Allergic hypersensitivities have been recorded in the dog to plant and tree pollen (Wittich, 1941; Joshua, 1956; Ripps, 1958; Patterson, 1959). They show a distinct seasonal incidence, related directly to the flowering season of the plant concerned.

Sensitization may result in rhinitis, conjunctivitis, and other forms of respiratory involvement and may in turn lead directly to the production of self-inflicted lesions on the face and corresponding lesions on the inner aspects of the forelimbs.

Alternatively, skin changes identical to those described with ingested allergens may accompany sensitization to inhaled allergens (Schwartzman and Rockey, 1967) and sometimes even in the absence of upper-respiratory involvement (Muller and Kirk, 1969).

Hypersensitivity to the pollens of ragweed presents a serious problem in certain areas of the world, but not in the British Isles. Ragweed pollinosis has a marked familial predisposition in the dog (Patterson, 1959). It causes an immediate anaphylactic response, induced by reaginic antibodies (Patterson, Pruzansky, and Janis, 1963, 1964; Patterson, Chang, and Pruzansky, 1964; Patterson, Roberts, and Pruzansky, 1969) and the sensitivity may be passively transferred by serum to the skin of normal dogs (Patterson, 1959).

Generalized cutaneous responses to inhaled plant and tree pollens are also occasionally noted in the United Kingdom but their relative importance has not been fully elucidated. Allergic responses have also been noted to animal and poultry danders.

Intradermal testing using pollen extracts is of diagnostic value (Patterson, 1959; Baker, 1970) provided that steroid therapy has not been given recently.

Desensitization using pollen antigens has also proved successful (Schwartzman and Rockey, 1967; Halliwell and Schwartzman, 1971).

The blocking activity of antiserum against ragweed has been demonstrated in the dog (Patterson and others, 1965).

Responses to Therapeutic Agents

The adverse responses that may follow injection, ingestion, inhalation, or cutaneous application of a therapeutic dose of a given drug may result from mobilization of either allergic or non-allergic mechanisms within the body.

Individual animals may develop symptoms of overdosage when given minute amounts of a drug to which they possess an intolerance. Other animals may exhibit potentiation of certain adverse side-effects associated with a drug. Occasionally, individual species, strains, or individual animals may possess an idiosyncrasy to a particular drug by virtue of their intrinsic biochemical make-up. In all the above cases no allergic mechanisms are involved.

Unfortunately the true allergic hypersensitivity responses to therapeutic agents are poorly documented in the dog. They may be produced to (1) the drug itself, (2) a drug–protein complex, the drug acting as a hapten, (3) a degradation product of the drug, and (4) a complex composed of a drug-degradation product and a protein (Simon and Rantz, 1961). Similar responses may also be produced to the base or vehicle in which the agent is transported or to a protein complex associated with these. On rare occasions allergic hypersensitivity responses may be produced to an impurity in a drug.

Injected, ingested, and inhaled agents may produce cutaneous symptoms in the sensitized animal identical to those described in association with ingested food allergens. The rapidity of onset of such symptoms varies with the mode of administration of the drug. The duration of symptoms varies with the rapidity of drug breakdown or excretion. Responses to drugs may be prolonged, with symptoms recurring spontaneously over a variable period of time, e.g., if the drugs were given in depot form.

In some cases subsequent administration of a drug may produce more profound systemic effects. General anaphylaxis, characterized by salivation, shivering, vomiting, and collapse, has been observed in the dog. It has been found in individual animals, following repeated administration of a number of different therapeutic agents by veterinary surgeons taking part in a survey at present being carried out in the north-west of England. Previously, Clarke (1960) recorded salivation, shivering, vomiting, hyperaemia, and urticaria in a dog following the injection of procaine penicillin G. Walton (1971a) recorded a similar case in an animal receiving a course of framomycin injections. The dog became unconscious and showed profound circulatory collapse following the seventh daily injection of framomycin. The subject required intubation, artificial ventilation, and the administration of intra-cardiac adrenaline followed subsequently by intravenous injections of adrenaline and cortisone before recovering consciousness several hours later. Anaphylactic responses and serum sickness reactions have been reported in the dog following the use of certain vaccines and antisera (Kral and Schwartzman, 1964; Collins, 1966).

Responses to Infective Agents

During the course of many bacterial, viral, fungal, and parasitic infections changes in immunological reactivity may occur. Certain of these may be beneficial by leading to direct destruction of the infective organism or by countering the toxic side-effects associated with such infections.

During the course of certain infectious diseases the body produces allergic hypersensitivity responses to the invading organism with such regularity that such responses may be used by the clinician as a valuable diagnostic tool, e.g., in tuberculosis, glanders, and certain deep mycoses and parasitic diseases.

In many cases the value of allergic hypersensitivity to the host is open to conjecture, however.

It is probable that this type of response plays a profound role in the invasiveness and subsequent inflammatory responses associated with many cutaneous infections.

Observations on the course of cutaneous staphylococcal infections in the rabbit suggest that hypersensitivity responses can be detrimental to the host by increasing the susceptibility of the skin to subsequent infection by the original or by other antigenically related organisms (Johnson and others, 1961).

To what extent allergic hypersensitivity responses influence the course of streptococcal, *Proteus*, and *Pseudomonas* infections of the canine skin is not known.

Endotoxin production by many Gram-negative organisms is often of much importance in the disease picture (Braude, 1964). It has been suggested, however, that in some cases tissue damage is enhanced further by superimposition of an arthus-type response.

Delayed hypersensitivity responses associated with tuberculosis may also prove to be detrimental in that tubercular masses may mechanically interfere with the normal functioning of organs and cushion the bacillus against destruction by chemotherapeutic agents. Conversely, it has been contended that tubercle formation is beneficial by localizing further spread of the organism (Gresham and Jennings, 1962).

It has also been suggested that hypersensitivity responses may be beneficial to the host during vaccinia virus invasions by marshalling humoral defences at the site of invasion by the virus and by destroying the virus together with the host cells, so making the latter unusable by any further virus particles—a sort of 'scorched earth' policy (Beveridge, 1967).

It has been shown that anaphylactic and delayed hypersensitivity responses can be induced in experimental animals to water-soluble extracts of ringworm mycelium (Jillson and Huppert, 1949; Wood and Cruickshank, 1962), but the role of such responses in canine ringworm infection has not been fully investigated.

On rare occasions cutaneous responses similar to those found in association with ingested food allergens may be produced in the dog and cat by enteric tapeworm infections or encapsulated round-worms. Diagnosis is often difficult, but in the former the response to taeniacidal therapy is spectacular. Treatment of encapsulated ascarids is difficult since treatment with diethylcarbamazine may produce a generalized anaphylactic reaction.

The occurrence of cutaneous autosensitization resulting in skin disease has not been established.

The role of immunological changes noted in a condition identical to human systemic lupus erythematosus, which has been recorded in the dog (Lewis and others, 1963; Lewis, 1965; Lewis, Schwartz, and Gilmore, 1965; Lewis, Schwartz, and Henry, 1965; Lewis and Hathaway, 1967) is still, as in man (Rowell, 1968), open to conjecture.

In the dog a normocytic, haemolytic anaemia is a constant finding. Phagocytosing polymorphonuclear leucocytes containing nuclear inclusion bodies (L.E. cells) may be demonstrated in blood samples, together with a non-species-specific antinuclear factor.

Changes in vascular and connective tissues are widespread, frequently giving rise to symptoms of nephritis and a progressive crippling arthritis.

Thrombocytopaenia may give rise to epistaxis petechiation and purpuric reactions within body tissues including the skin.

Alopecia and facial skin eruptions have also been noted in individual cases, but still require further investigation.

Responses to Contact Agents

Contact hypersensitivity in the dog may be induced by close and repeated contact with the skin. In contrast to physical or chemical contact reactions it is rare for other animals in the same environment to be similarly affected. Lesions are usually confined to the more hairless areas of the body, since the coat provides a sufficient barrier over the other areas (unless the allergen is in fluid form and present in large quantities).

Most contact allergens are haptenic in nature (Landsteiner and Jacobs, 1935) and require to be linked to a skin fraction before they reach full antigenicity (Eisen and Tabachnick, 1958). Many are single ions such as cobalt and nickel. Others are relatively simple compounds such as formaldehyde. Yet others are more complex, including higher alcohols or sterols. Most of such agents possess either chemical lability or a high reaction constant (Calnan, 1968).

Allergic contact hypersensitivities to pollen are found in individual animals during the summer months. The onset and duration of the individual cutaneous response coincide with the flowering period of the plant concerned and the effects disappear spontaneously in the autumn.

Most affected dogs show a regional distribution of lesions. Inflammation and irritation of the skin between the foot pads are usually present. Lesions also often involve the abdomen, axilla, anterior aspects of the face, periorbital skin, inside the ear flaps, and occasionally the perineum. The back is usually spared unless the animal has been closely clipped.

Sensitivity in pollen dermatitis is produced to the oleoresin fractions of pollen, in contrast to the immediate response which follows inhalation of pollen and is due to sensitization to the protein fractions.

Patch testing using the oleoresins is yielding valuable information on the common allergens responsible for this type of reaction in the dog, but they are not yet available commercially in the United Kingdom.

Contact hypersensitivities are also found in the dog to many household items. The pattern of response varies slightly, depending on whether the animal lies and walks on, or only walks on, the object concerned.

Responses may occur to the dyes used in carpeting and fabrics. Responses to cotton, wool, and man-made fibres themselves are rare and the responses are most frequently produced by acid and azo dyes or by mordants used in the dyeing process. Responses have not been seen to vegetable dyes (Walton, 1971a).

Less frequently, responses may be noted to antioxidants and accelerators used in the production of rubber matting, or to wood resins and polishes or detergents.

Although patch testing may yield valuable information as to the precise contact allergen involved, it rarely gives sufficient information as to which object within the environment is directly responsible for the reaction. Diagnosis is best achieved by making a detailed inventory of all potential agents within the environment and systematically excluding certain of these from contact with the subject for at least 7 days and looking for any remission of symptoms. Once a potential cause has been isolated, the animal should be subjected to provocative exposure to confirm diagnosis, but it must be remembered that, since this is a delayed response, symptoms may not appear until 2–5 days after initial exposure.

Desensitization techniques are not available for this condition and efforts must rest on prevention of further contact with the causative agent.

REFERENCES

ANTIN, I. P. (1963), *J. Am. vet. med. Ass.*, **142**, 775.

ARBESMAN, C. E., LANGLOIS, C., BROWNSON, P., and SCHICKMAN, S. (1966), *J. Allergy*, **38**, 1.

— — — — and SHULMAN, S. (1965), *Ibid.*, **36**, 147.

BAKER, E. (1970), *J. Am. vet. Med. Ass.*, **157**, 1607.

BENJAMINI, E., FEINGOLD, B. F., YOUNG, J. D., KARTMAN, L., and SHIMIZU, M. (1963), *Expl. Parasit.*, **13**, 143.

BEVERIDGE, W. I. B. (1967), 'Immunity to Viruses', in *Viral and Rickettsial Infections of Animals* (ed. BETTS, A. O., and YORK, C. J.), vol. 1, p. 313. New York: Academic.

BRAUDE, A. I. (1964), *Scient. Am.*, **210**, 36.

CALNAN, C. D. (1968), 'Allergic Contact Dermatitis', in *Clinical Aspects of Immunology* (ed. GELL, P. G. H., and COOMBS, R. R. A.), 2nd ed., p. 756. Oxford: Blackwell.

CHAMPION, R. H. (1968), 'Urticaria', in *Textbook of Dermatology* (ed. ROOK, A. J., WILKINSON, D. S., and EBLING, F. J. G.), p. 412. Oxford: Blackwell.

CLARKE, P. B. (1960), *Vet. Rec.*, **72**, 1054.

COLLINS, D. (1966), *Vet. Med. small Anim. Clin.*, **61**, 679, 761, 871.

COOMBS, R. R. A., and GELL, P. G. H. (1968), 'Classification of Allergic Reactions responsible for Clinical Hypersensitivity and Disease', in *Clinical Aspects of Immunology* (ed. GELL, P. G. H., and COOMBS, R. R. A.), 2nd ed., p. 575. Oxford: Blackwell.

EISEN, H. N., and TABACHNICK, M. (1958), *J. exp. Med.*, **108**, 773.

FEINGOLD, B. F., BENJAMINI, E., and MICHAELI, D. (1968), *Ann. Rev. Entomol.*, **13**, 137.

FOX, L. A. (1968), *Ann. Allergy*, **26**, 639.

GAAFAR, S. M. (1967), 'Pathogenesis of Canine Demodicosis', in *Veterinary Medical Review: The Reaction of the Host to Parasitism* (ed. SOULSBY, E. J. L.), p. 59. Proceedings of 3rd International Conference of World Association for the Advancement of Veterinary Parasitology, Lyons, France.

GRESHAM, G. A., and JENNINGS, A. R. (1962), *An Introduction to Comparative Pathology*. New York: Academic.

HALLIWELL, R. E. W., and SCHWARTZMAN, R. M. (1971), *Vet. Rec.*, **89**, 209.

HUTCHEON, D. E., and CHIVERS-WILSON, V. S. (1953), *Rev. Can. Biol.*, **12**, 77.

JILLSON, O. F., and HUPPERT, M. (1949), *J. invest. Derm.*, **12**, 179.

JOHNSON, J. E., CLUFF, L. E., III, and GOSHI, K. (1961), *J. exp. Med.*, **11**, 235.

JOHNSON, R. B., and HALPERN, S. R. (1966), *Cutis*, **2**, 311.

JOSHUA, J. O. (1956), *Vet. Rec.*, **68**, 682.

KEEP, J. M., and TAYLOR, J. H. (1967), *Aust. vet. J.*, **43**, 425.

KISSILEFF, A. (1938), *J. Am. vet. Med. Ass.*, **93**, 21.

KRAL, F., and SCHWARTZMAN, R. M. (1964), *Veterinary and Comparative Dermatology*. Philadelphia: Lippincott.
LANDSTEINER, K., and JACOBS, J. (1935), *J. exp. Med.*, **61**, 643.
LANGLOIS, C., SHULMAN, S., and ARBESMAN, C. E. (1965), *J. Allergy*, **36**, 109.
LEWIS, R. M. (1965), *J. Am. vet. Med. Ass.*, **147**, 939.,
— — and HATHAWAY, J. E. (1967), *J. small. Anim. Pract.*, **8**, 273.
— — HENRY, W. B., THORNTON, G. W., and GILMORE, C. E. (1963), *Scient. Proc. Am. vet. Med. Ass.*, p. 140.
— — SCHWARTZ, R. S., and GILMORE, C. E. (1965), *Ann. N.Y. Acad. Sci.*, **124**, 178.
— — — — and HENRY, W. B. (1965), *Blood*, **25**, 143.
MICHAELI, D., and GOLDFARB, S. (1968), *Aust. vet. J.*, **44**, 161.
MUELLER, H. L. (1959), *Ped. Clin. N. Am.*, **6**, 917.
MULLER, G. H., and KIRK, R. W. (1969), *Small Animal Dermatology*. Philadelphia: Saunders.
OWEN, F. H. (1941), *N. J. vet. med. Ass.*, 1.
PARRISH, H. M. (1963), *Am. J. med. Sci.*, **245**, 129.
PATTERSON, R. (1959), *J. Am. med. vet. Ass.*, **135**, 178.
— — CHANG, W. W. J., and PRUZANSKY, J. J. (1964), *Immunology*, **7**, 150.
— — PRUZANSKY, J. J., and JANIS, B. (1963), *J. Immunol.*, **90**, 35.
— — — — (1964), *Ibid.*, **93**, 51.
— — ROBERTS, M., and PRUZANSKY, J. J. (1969), *J. Immunol.*, **102**, 466.
— — TENNENBAUM, J. I., PRUZANSKY, J. J., and NELSON, V. L. (1965), *J. Allergy*, **36**, 138.
PHILLIPS, J. McL. (1922), *J. Am. vet. med. Ass.*, **78**, 497.
VON PIRQUET, C. (1906), *Munch. med. Wschr.*, **30**, 1457.
RIPPS, J. H. (1958), *J. Am. vet. Med. Ass.*, **133**, 479.
ROWELL, N. R. (1968), 'Lupus Erythematosus, Schleroderma, Dermatomyositis, Polyarteritis. The Collagen or Connective Tissue Diseases', in *Textbook of Dermatology* (ed. ROOK, A., WILKINSON, D. S., and EBLING, F. J. G.), p. 511. Oxford: Blackwell.
SCHWARTZMAN, R. M., and ROCKEY, J. M. (1967), *Archs Derm.*, **96**, 418.
— — and ORKIN, M. (1962), *A Comparative Study of Skin Diseases of Dog and Man*. Springfield, Ill.: Thomas.
SIMON, H. J., and RANTZ, L. A. (1961), *Ann. Rev. Med.*, **12**, 111.
TORSNEY, P. J. (1968), *N.Y. St. J. Med.*, **68**, 2765.
WALTON, G. S. (1965), 'Reactions to Arthropods in Domestic Animals', in *Comparative Physiology and Pathology of the Skin* (ed. ROOK, A. J., and WALTON, G. S.), p. 561. Oxford: Blackwell.
— — (1966), *J. small anim. Pract.*, **7**, 749.
— — (1967), *Vet. Rec.*, **81**, 704.
— — (1968), *Ibid.*, **82**, 204.
— — (1971a), 'Allergic Responses involving the Skin of Domestic Animals', in *Advances in Veterinary Science and Comparative Medicine* (ed. BRANDLY, C. A., and CORNELIUS, C. E.), vol. 15, 201. New York: Academic.
— — (1971b), in preparation.
WITTICH, F. W. (1941), *J. Allergy*, **12**, 247.
WOOD, S. R., and CRUICKSHANK, C. N. D. (1962), *Br. J. Derm.*, **74**, 329.
YOUNG, J. D., BENJAMINI, E., FEINGOLD, B. F., and NOLLER, H. (1963), *Expl Parasit.*, **13**, 155.

AVIAN SALMONELLOSIS

R. F. Gordon, D.Sc., D.V.Sc., F.R.C.V.S.

'Salmonellosis' is a collective term used to describe infections with any organism of the salmonella group other than *Salmonella pullorum* (pullorum disease) or *S. gallinarum* (fowl typhoid). In some countries salmonella infections are referred to as 'avian paratyphoid' whilst in other instances the name of the serotype concerned is used, e.g., 'typhimurium infection', 'thompson infection', etc. In ducklings infection with *S. anatum* was at one time referred to as 'keel disease'.

Of the more than 1000 serotypes in the salmonella group some 200 have been isolated from poultry and the number of new types isolated is continually increasing. Certain types, particularly *S. typhimurium* and *S. thompson*, may be regarded as endemic in poultry and indeed *S. typhimurium* accounts for some 50 per cent of recorded outbreaks of salmonellosis in poultry in this country (Stevens, 1971; Williams Smith, 1971). Exotic serotypes occur from time to time, although certain serotypes sometimes appear to become established in an area, breeding flock, or hatchery, and give rise to a number of outbreaks of the disease, e.g., *S. thompson* (Buxton and Gordon, 1947) and *S. menston* (Gordon and Tucker, 1965). Stevens (1971) lists the individual serotypes isolated by the Veterinary Investigation Service of the Ministry of Agriculture during 1969–70.

The exact incidence of salmonellosis in poultry is difficult to ascertain since in many cases mortality is so low that specimens are not submitted for diagnosis. Although mortality from infection with endemic salmonellae such as *S. typhimurium* can be high, the exotic and rarer serotypes generally speaking result in only low mortality, often about 2 or 3 per cent, but once the environment becomes contaminated an increase in mortality can take place.

Surveys have shown that the incidence in chicks has varied from about 5 per cent of all batches of chicks examined (Blaxland, Sojka, and Smither, 1958) to about 0·1 per cent (Stevens, 1971). Although the latter figures might suggest at first sight that salmonellosis is of little importance economically, the public health hazards created by these infections should not be disregarded. Stevens (1971) states that the methods used at poultry-processing plants in general, and the spin chillers used for cooling carcasses in particular, allow a high degree of dissemination of any bacteria present. Preservation by freezing and the subsequent slow thawing and quick cooking methods create further hazards. The large retailers and the public are becoming increasingly aware of the risks involved and these are having some adverse effects on the sale of poultry products. There is therefore a great need for better methods of ensuring freedom from these less common salmonellae for reasons quite outside those of controlling clinical disease.

Two further dangers were well illustrated by the *S. virchow* incident described by Pennington and others (1968). Livestock other than poultry can become infected from poultry sources. For example, cattle grazing lands dressed with poultry manure have become seriously affected and such cases are now a regular if not common occurrence in the Liverpool area. Secondly, although in the first instance there was no evidence of any clinical disease in birds associated with *S. virchow*, it has since become associated with mortality in chicks. This may indicate a change in the virulence of the organism though it is more probably a consequence of heavier challenge doses.

The host-specific salmonella types (*S. pullorum* and *S. gallinarum*) have undoubtedly yielded to control measures and have been virtually eradicated, particularly from flocks participating in the Poultry Health Scheme (Stevens, 1971). However, although there has been an apparent decrease in the incidence of infections with the motile salmonellae, there has been an increase in the number of serotypes involved, and these infections have not responded in a comparable manner to control measures. This will be discussed later.

Salmonella infection rarely clinically affects chicks over 3 weeks of age and even then mortality may be high only when other disease conditions are present. Unfortunately, however, a high proportion of survivors are likely to remain carriers and symptomless excretors. If these birds are used as breeders the excretors will continue the cycle of infection; if they are broilers they will, at slaughter, serve to infect the packing-station environment.

Cycle of Infection

The classic cycle of ovarian infection as first described for pullorum disease can occur in rare instances, particularly in relation to *S. typhimurium*, and is the main route of infection in ducks. In most instances, however, infection is carried on rather than in the egg and is not a true trans-ovarian infection such as occurs when the carrier harbours the organism in the reproductive organs. Carriers are intermittent faecal excretors and the organism contaminates the outside of the shell either during the passage of the egg through the cloaca or after the egg is laid, by soiling with faeces in the nest box. The organism can then penetrate the pores of the shell and set up infection of the embryo, further infection being transmitted at hatching time or during brooding. Most outbreaks of salmonellosis arising from the commoner serotypes result from hatchery infections originating in eggs from infected breeding stock.

Although lateral infection does occur from other sources such as rats and mice and human excretors (sexers, hatchery attendants, etc.), Hobbs (1971) states that infected food handlers may be more often victims of the environment than initiators of infection. Williams Smith (1971) makes a similar comment regarding vermin. Most outbreaks due to the rarer serotypes probably originate from infected imported feedingstuffs, usually animal protein. This was first high-lighted by Walker (1957) and followed by a Report in the *Monthly Bulletin of the Ministry of Health and Public Health Laboratory Service* (1959). A more recent survey (Dawkins and Robertson, 1967) indicated the relative incidence in animal feedingstuffs to be as shown in *Table I.*

McCoy (1970), examining animal protein supplements in current use in this country, found the following incidence of contamination in 5250 samples examined between 1961 and 1969: meat-and-bone meal, 9·6 per cent; fish meal, 2·3 per cent; feather meal, 6 per cent; poultry-offal meal, 9·6 per cent; oil-seed meal, 0 per cent; steamed bone-flour, 80 per cent; protein-concentrate meal, 53 per cent. The addition of feather meal and poultry offal to the supplements shown in *Table I* is significant.

Table I.—SALMONELLA ISOLATED FROM ANIMAL AND VEGETABLE PROTEIN DERIVATIVES. (*From Dawkins and Robertson*, 1967.)

PRODUCER	IMPORTED			HOME PRODUCED		
	No. of Samples Examined	No. Contaminated with Salmonellae	Percentage Contamination	No. of Samples Examined	No. Contaminated with Salmonellae	Percentage Contamination
Animal protein						
Bone meal	14	12	85·7	4	2	50
Meat meal	2	1	50	11	0	0
Meat-and-bone meal	14	6	42·8	38	16	42·1
Blood meal	2	0	0	3	1	33·3
Fish meal	25	2	8	21	2	9·5
Total	57	21	36·8	77	21	27·2
Vegetable protein						
Cotton cake	13	1	7·6	—*	—	—
Soya meal	13	1	7·6	—	—	—
Groundnut cake	25	0	0	—	—	—
Copra	3	0	0	—	—	—
Others	2	0	0	8	0	0
Total	56	2	3·5	8	0	0

* Samples not examined.

Table II gives figures for the same period showing the results of the examination of both home-produced and imported products.

Infected feedingstuff may give rise to a number of outbreaks in breeding stock with subsequent infection via their eggs to chicks emanating from the same hatchery, or it may initiate outbreaks in individual broiler crops. That such a cycle of infection may occur was demonstrated by Gordon and Tucker (1965) who fed adult birds on food contaminated with *S. menston* at a level of one organism per gramme of food. Infection even at this low level established a carrier state in the fowls, who then laid *S. menston*-infected eggs which produced *S. menston*-infected chicks which at maturity laid *S. menston*-infected eggs. The rate of infection of stored eggs was 5·6 per cent and of incubated eggs 8·6 per cent. Since over 3000 stored eggs and more than 2000 incubated eggs were examined the potential spread of infection via the hatchery will be appreciated. Most of the isolations were from the outsides of the egg shells.

An excellent example of a self-perpetuating cycle of infection in the field is given by Kauffman and Feeley (1968) who isolated the same salmonella types from live birds, their food, and the offal meal incorporated in the food (the meal having been prepared from offal from the company's birds killed on their own processing plant).

Figs. 19 and 20 show the two cycles of infection: (1) via the egg (in the egg or on the shell) and (2) from the environment.

Table II.—Samples of Home-produced and Imported Products examined between 1961 and 1969
(*From McCoy, personal communication*, 1970)

	Examined	+	Per Cent	Most Probable Number of Salmonellae per 100 g. Sample														
				1	2	4	6	10	23	36	51	69	92	120	161	230	357	511
Fish meals	728	17	2·3	6	1	5	3		1	1								
Meat-and-bone meals	2640	265	10·0	105	50	23	26	26	8	5	4	3	3	1	2	7	1	1
Feather meals	961	77	8·0	49	8	4	4	6	4	1		1						
Poultry offal	355	34	9·6	20	8	1	2	2	1									
Steamed bone meal	5	4	80·0					2								1		1
Protein concentrate	509	268	52·6	95	52	32	27	33	9	4	5	3	2	3	3			

One of the best documented outbreaks of food poisoning in man attributable to infected poultry products is that caused by *S. virchow* in 1968 in Cheshire (Semple, Turner, and Lowry, 1968; Pennington and others, 1968). Severe illness occurred in some 50 out of 120 people who attended a tennis-club supper in the Merseyside area. *S. virchow* was found to be present in chicken portions supplied by a cooked-meat shop which had obtained frozen eviscerated chicken from a Cheshire packing station which received the live birds

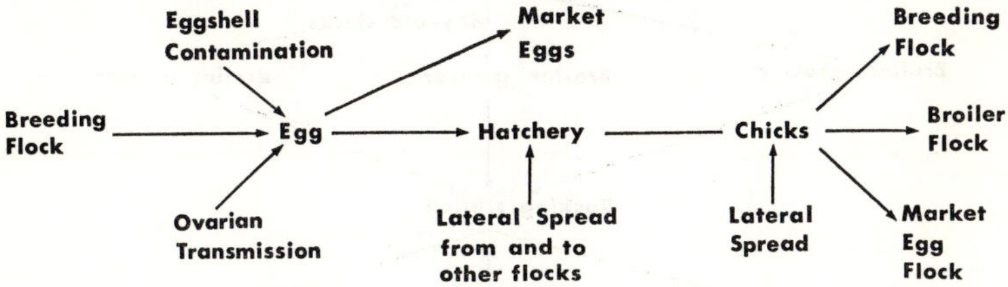

Fig. 19.—Transmission routes in poultry. (*From National Academy of Sciences,* 1969.)

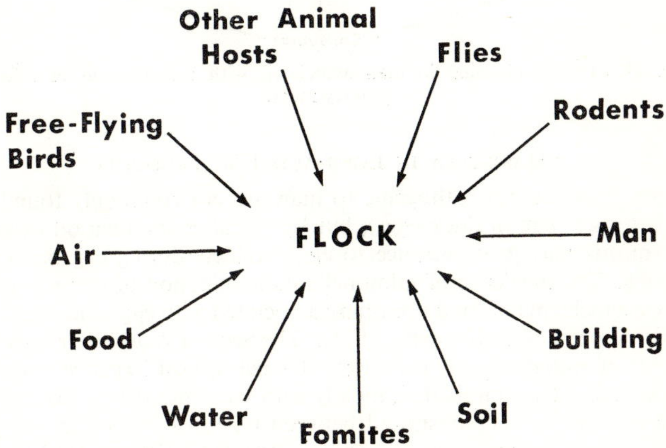

Fig. 20.—Methods whereby salmonellae gain entrance to poultry flocks. (*After Williams Smith,* 1971.)

from sixteen broiler farms in the area. *S. virchow* was isolated from the patients, the cooked chicken, the packing station, and the hatchery supplying the broiler units. The same organism was recovered from staff at the shop, the packing station, the broiler units, and the hatchery. Although no infection was found at the breeding farms supplying the hatchery, it seems likely that the original source of infection was contaminated food fed to the breeding stock. At the cooked-meat shop the chicken had been improperly thawed out before spit roasting and the general hygiene was poor.

A number of similar outbreaks in man have been recorded in which *S. agona* and *S.* 4.12:d:— have been involved (Hobbs, 1971), the origin of the latter having been shown to be imported fish-meal pellets. In *S. agona* outbreaks chicken and chicken giblets have been incriminated.

A typical cycle of infection is shown in *Fig.* 21.

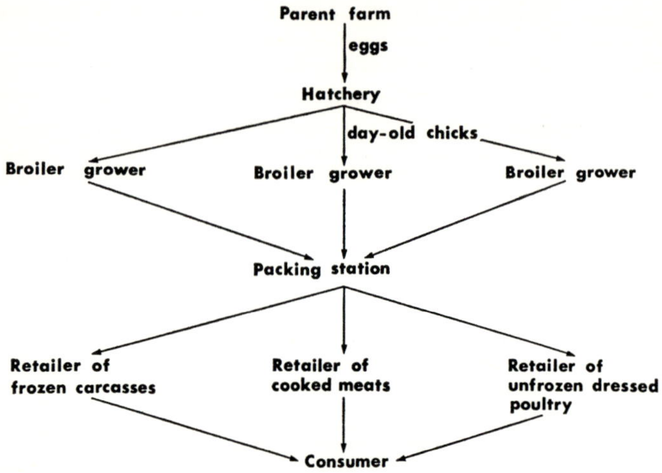

Fig. 21.—Food poisoning in man associated with consumption of infected poultry meat.

Salmonella in Eggs and Egg Products

Salmonella serotypes pathogenic to man are not commonly found in egg contents (other than in duck eggs), but by faecal contamination of the shell the organisms may gain entrance to egg products during egg breaking-out operations. The incidence of salmonella contamination of raw egg products and known incidents of food poisoning associated with eggs and egg products are well documented by Knowles (1971). The Second World War high-lighted the danger of imported spray-dried egg, of which almost 10 per cent of samples were known to be contaminated, mostly with serotypes new to Great Britain. A close parallel was demonstrated between type distribution in spray-dried egg and cases of human food poisoning. Between 1950 and 1963 a number of severe outbreaks of food poisoning were reported in Great Britain attributable to both English and imported liquid and frozen egg products, with subsequent environmental infection of premises such as bakeries.

Experimental work in the United Kingdom (Knowles, 1953; Heller and others, 1962) established satisfactory procedures for the heat treatment of liquid whole egg which led to the introduction in 1963 by the Ministries of Health and Agriculture of regulations enforcing the pasteurization of liquid egg. Briefly this requires that liquid whole egg to be used for food for human consumption must be pasteurized by being retained at a temperature not lower than 64·4° C. for at least 2·5 minutes and immediately cooled to 3·3° C. A control test, the alpha-amylase test, was developed, by which the accuracy of the heat-treatment process can be checked (Brooks, 1962; Shrimpton and others, 1962).

Since the introduction of the regulations for the pasteurization of liquid egg the British Egg Marketing Board has carried out continual monitoring of liquid and dried egg from processing plants in this country and no samples have been found to contain viable salmonella organisms. Knowles (1971) states that the overall improvement in the sanitary quality of pasteurized egg has made possible the development of chilled bulk liquid egg deliveries without any intervening process of freezing and defrosting. The dangers previously associated with raw whole liquid egg have now been eliminated and heat treatment methods have now been extended to other egg products such as liquid yolk and albumen.

Control

Serology

In view of the marked success achieved in controlling and, under the Poultry Health Scheme, virtually eradicating pullorum disease by the use of the agglutination test, it is difficult to explain to the poultry breeder why equally effective results cannot be achieved in the control of salmonellosis. To explain this it is necessary to recapitulate certain basic facts, as follows:—

1. *S. pullorum* and *S. gallinarum* are the only two non-motile members of the salmonella group. As such they have only somatic or O antigens of a relatively simple nature. All other serotypes are motile and contain both O antigens and flagellar or H antigens, the latter being of a highly complex nature. A vast number of serological permutations and combinations can therefore occur and it is unlikely that a polyvalent antigen which could cover the whole spectrum can ever be perfected. O antigens stimulate a more clear-cut and more consistent antibody response so that a bird once positive to the *S. pullorum*/*S. gallinarum* test is likely to remain so at subsequent tests. H antigens, however, produce poor agglutination responses which tend to fluctuate from test to test so that a bird positive at one test may be negative at a subsequent one, or conversely; furthermore, cross-agglutination between H antigens is common.

2. A further difference between *S. pullorum*/*S. gallinarum* and the other serotypes is that the former seldom colonize the alimentary tract and their presence in the tract is the consequence of an infection in other organs such as the spleen, gall-bladder, or gonads. It is this tissue infection which gives rise to consistent and detectable antibodies which are responsible for the higher reliability of blood testing in these two infections. The motile salmonellae are usually restricted to the intestinal tract and birds so infected react intermittently to the agglutination test. Organ-infected birds, e.g., *S. pullorum* carriers, seldom excrete the causal organism in their faeces, so that once carrier birds have been removed from a flock further infection is unlikely. Where motile salmonellae are involved, intestinal excretion is usual; thus the environment becomes contaminated and even when reactors are removed, further carriers become established as a result of contact with an infected environment. Under modern intensive housing conditions it is impracticable to move the flock to fresh quarters after removal of reactors.

3. *S. pullorum* and *S. gallinarum* are virtually host-specific and restricted to the avian species and once reactors have been removed it is reasonably simple to prevent the further introduction of infection. The motile salmonellae, conversely, are host-ubiquitous and thus reinfection can occur from a variety

of sources, such as vermin, man, other domestic animals, flies and other insects, fomites, etc.

Extensive field experiments using serology supplemented by rectal swabbing have given unreliable results and have led to continual depletion of the flocks and, by interference with long-term breeding programmes, have proved economically impracticable. Nevertheless, under certain circumstances, particularly in the case of endemic infection with *S. typhimurium*, control by elimination of carriers should be considered.

Pen Testing

Snoeyenbos (1967) reports promising results in the eradication of salmonellosis by the cultural examination of samples of pen litter. The flock status can be determined with some accuracy when chicks are 4–14 days of age. This method, however, necessitates the sacrifice of entire pens of future breeding stock and this means rearing chicks in relatively small groups. The test declines in accuracy as chicks and litter become older. Nest-box litter is often more reliable than floor litter. This method can be supported by regular monitoring of unhatched chicks, incubator dust and debris, the pots used by sexers to collect faeces, and brooder house and hatchery attendants. Work still requires to be carried out to evaluate different methods of sampling, e.g., sample size, location of samples in house, frequency of testing, different techniques of isolation, etc., in an attempt to establish reliable methods which are simple and cheap enough to be used routinely.

Hygiene

In view of the fact that transmission is mainly by shell contamination a considerable measure of control can be exercised by improved clean egg production and hatchery hygiene. It has been shown that an increase in the number of egg collections from nest boxes per day can effect a considerable measure of control in that eggs are removed from contact with contaminated faeces in the nest boxes before they have cooled. Collections of not less than three per day are recommended; eggs should be stored in a vermin-proof room kept solely for that purpose and maintained at a temperature between 9° C. and 13° C. and at a humidity of 75 per cent. Nest-box litter must be kept clean and dry and renewed frequently; wood shavings are preferable to straw or hay. Dirty, cracked, or 'floor' eggs should not be incubated.

The establishment of separate hatcheries for the hatching of eggs from infected breeding flocks is also of value. Routine fumigation for 20 minutes of eggs at the farm, using 3 oz. potassium permanganate to $4\frac{1}{2}$ oz. formaldehyde per 100 c. ft. air space or 1·4 oz. paraformaldehyde if the hot-plate method is used, in an efficient fumigation chamber (now commercially available), is often more effective than fumigation at the central hatchery when the organisms may already have penetrated to sites inaccessible to the gas. However, routine fumigation of incubators as outlined in the Poultry Health Scheme regulations should also be carried out.

Dipping of eggs in germicidal solutions has also been shown to be effective (Gordon, Harry, and Tucker, 1956). A number of effective egg dips are now commercially available. An essential point in egg dipping is that the dipping fluid must be at a temperature higher than that of the egg, i.e., at least 80° F.

---

* Obtainable from M.A.F.F., Animal Health Division, Hook Rise South, Tolworth, Surbiton, Surrey.

throughout the operation. Where large numbers of eggs are involved, thermostatically controlled heating devices are required to maintain the dip temperature. The eggs (usually in wire baskets) are immersed for 15 minutes and then hung up to 'drip dry' before setting.

Salmonellae are fairly easily destroyed by most disinfectants and by heat (60° C. for 15 minutes), but can remain viable in the environment for lengthy periods (up to 5 weeks in old litter and 20 weeks in new litter; Tucker, 1967). Broiler-house litter, after an outbreak, is best dealt with by incineration, although heaping of litter may be of some value.

Foodstuffs

The part played by infected foodstuff, already referred to, is well recognized by the food compounders who have done much to reduce the level of infection by monitoring consignments of imported animal protein and discontinuing supplies from the more seriously contaminated sources (Riley, 1969). The recently developed practice of recycling poultry-house litter, packing-station offal, and feathers is one which must be viewed with considerable suspicion; records of the isolation of salmonella organisms from such products are numerous (McCoy, 1970). Even if the method of treatment of the material is efficient, recontamination after processing is probably unavoidable. Attention has frequently been drawn to the effectiveness of pelleting of foodstuffs in reducing the incidence of salmonellae and an excellent description of the pelleting process, temperatures obtained, etc., is given by Riley (1969). Unfortunately, for a number of reasons, pelleted food is not favoured for breeding stock; apart from the fact that the cost of production is higher than that for mash, the latter is preferred for husbandry reasons. Some breeders have gone to the extent of recrushing pelleted food for breeding stock.

Treatment

There are numerous reports of the effective treatment of salmonellosis in chicks with furazolidone and it has been shown that this drug at a level of 0·04 per cent for 10 days was highly effective in reducing mortality in chicks if the treatment was initiated sufficiently early in the outbreak. Tucker (1963) tested some 28 different compounds in chickens artificially infected with *S. typhimurium* and found that only furazolidone and its soluble form, furaltadone, showed any real efficiency in the control of mortality. However, the majority of surviving chicks became carriers and as some carriers were still found when the chicks reached maturity, treatment cannot be recommended for birds intended for use as breeding stock. Prophylactic medication with furazolidone in the food at 0·01 or 0·02 per cent has been used successfully in broiler units with a recurrent history of salmonellosis.

Summary

The following extracts from the summary of the 1970 Association of American Avian Pathologists Salmonellosis Workshop serve as an excellent précis of avian salmonellosis:

1. It has been demonstrated that salmonellosis is a clinical problem in poultry; however, many birds may be intestinal carriers of salmonellae without clinical disease.

2. Salmonellosis continues to be a serious public health problem, and poultry are a common source of the organism for man.

3. The disease may be introduced into a flock through the food.

4. Also important in introducing the infection into clean flocks of both chickens and turkeys are the contaminated natural environment and infected eggs.

5. Nest and floor-litter sampling may offer a means of conducting an industry-wide surveillance to establish the incidence of salmonella carriers in poultry flocks and may be utilized as a means of monitoring breeding flocks.

6. There is a need for industry-wide application of effective methods for early reduction of the bacterial populations on the surface of egg shells for prevention of avian salmonellosis.

7. The use of wire-floored houses or cages considerably decreases the bacterial populations on eggs and offers great promise as an effective means of significantly reducing bacterial contaminants, including salmonellae, on the surface of eggs.

8. Improvement in diagnostic laboratory methods is needed for eventual effective control of avian salmonellosis.

9. Standard laboratory procedures are paramount for the successful operation of regulatory programmes which require recognition of products contaminated with salmonellae.

10. Pelleting greatly reduces the level of salmonellae in poultry foods.

11. Some progress has been made in eliminating salmonellae in poultry foods by the co-operation of industry.

12. Examination of poultry carcasses at various stages of processing has indicated points of processing at which decontamination and recontamination of carcasses occurred. Spray washes were very effective in the decontamination procedures. Recontamination of carcasses occurred during evisceration and during chilling.

13. The most effective means of controlling salmonella infections is the production of eggs free of shell contamination with salmonella organisms.

14. Early on-the-farm fumigation of hatching eggs with high levels of formaldehyde gas has been found very effective in preventing egg-borne infections with motile salmonellae.

15. Quaternary ammonium compounds at 200 p.p.m. have been reported as completely eliminating bacteria on the shells of eggs and providing a residual bactericidal film on the shell for at least 21 days.

BIBLIOGRAPHY

BLAXLAND, J. D., SOJKA, W. J., and SMITHER, A. M. (1958), *Vet. Rec.*, **70**, 374.

BROOKS, K. J. (1962), *J. Hyg., Camb.*, **60**, 145.

BUXTON, A., and GORDON, R. F. (1947), *Ibid.*, **45**, 265.

DAWKINS, H. C., and ROBERTSON, L. (1967), *Mon. Bull. Minist. Hlth*, **26**, 215.

GORDON, R. F., HARRY, E. G., and TUCKER, J. F. (1956), *Vet. Rec.*, **68**, 23.

— — and TUCKER, J. F. (1965), *Br. Poult. Sci.*, **6**, 251.

HELLER, C. L., ROBERTS, B. C., AMOS, A. J., SMITH, M. E., and HOBBS, B. C. (1962), *J. Hyg., Camb.*, **60**, 135.

HOBBS, B. C. (1971), in *Poultry Disease and World Economy* (ed. GORDON, R. F., and FREEMAN, B. M.), p. 65. Edinburgh: Longman for *British Poultry Science.*

KAUFFMAN, A. F., and FEELEY, J. C. (1968), *Pub. Hlth Rep., Wash.*, **83**, 417.

KNOWLES, N. R. (1953), *Proc. Soc. appl. Bact.*, **16**, 107.
— — (1971), in *Poultry Disease and World Economy* (ed. GORDON, R. F., and FREEMAN, B. M.), p. 81. Edinburgh: Longman for *British Poultry Science.*
McCOY, J. H. (1970), personal communication.
NATIONAL ACADEMY OF SCIENCES (1969), *An Evaluation of the Salmonella Problem.* Publication 1683, Committee on Salmonella. National Research Council: Washington, D.C.
PENNINGTON, J. H., BROOKSBANK, N. H., POOLE, P. M., and SEYMOUR, F. (1968), *Br. med. J.*, **4**, 804.,
REPORT (1959), *Mon. Bull. Minist. Hlth*, **18**, 26.
REPORT (1970), *Avian Dis.*, **14** (4), 817.
RILEY, P. B. (1969), in *Bacterial Food Poisoning* (ed. TAYLOR, J.), p. 101. Royal Society of Health.
SEMPLE, A. B., TURNER, G. C., and LOWRY, D. M. O. (1968), *Br. med. J.*, **4**, 801.
SHRIMPTON, D. H., MONSEY, J. B., HOBBS, B. C., and SMITH, M. E. (1962), *J. Hyg., Camb.*, **60**, 153.
SMITH, H. WILLIAMS (1971), in *Poultry Disease and World Economy* (ed. GORDON, R. F., and FREEMAN, B. M.), p. 37. Edinburgh: Longman for *British Poultry Science.*
SNOEYENBOS, G. H. (1967), *Proc. Poultry Hlth Conf.*, p. 30.
STEVENS, A. J. (1971), in *Poultry Disease and World Economy* (ed. GORDON, R. F., and FREEMAN, B. M.), p. 25. Edinburgh: Longman for *British Poultry Science.*
TUCKER, J. F. (1963), *Br. vet. J.*, **119**, 544.
— — (1967), *Ibid.*, **123**, 92.
WALKER, J. H. C. (1957), *Lancet*, **2**, 283.

THE NEWCASTLE DISEASE EPIDEMIC

'WHY' AND 'WHITHER'

J. I. Davies, M.R.C.V.S., D.V.S.M.

The hard facts of the 1970–1 epidemic of Newcastle disease in Great Britain have been recorded elsewhere (M.A.F.F., 1970) but there remain the two questions, 'Why did it happen?' and 'What does the future hold?'

The well-publicized fact that the general level of vaccination in the country had fallen progressively to a new low, which was very low indeed if only fully vaccinated flocks were counted, was undoubtedly a major reason why the epidemic was so disastrous. The whole history of disease outbreaks in Great Britain since 1963 is conclusive proof of the value of inactivated vaccines in limiting numbers of outbreaks and the severity of cases which do occur. The small series of outbreaks in Kent early in 1969 showed that the same is true when the virus involved is an acute variety, for in that series the mortality in unvaccinated flocks was 75 per cent whereas that in vaccinated flocks was only 2·6 per cent and recovery was very rapid. Yet the fact that that series only involved seven premises in a country with a fairly heavy poultry population suggests that all other factors involved were not similar. Furthermore, the Kent series occurred in February/March when weather conditions appear to favour development of epidemics of virus diseases whereas the 1970–1 epidemic began in the month of August, a time when weather conditions are normally unfavourable for virus survival.

Laboratory examination and trials have shown that whereas the virus of the epidemic (the 'Essex' virus) and the 'Kent' virus are very similar in virulence, as determined by a series of tests and expressed as the 'combined index', there are significant differences as far as their behaviour is concerned, the Essex virus having the properties of being particularly diffusible and markedly pneumotropic. These two factors would make it particularly suitable for wind-borne spread and this idea was in fact borne out by the progress of the epidemic. All too often a primary outbreak in an area gave rise to secondaries a few days later with no discoverable connexion other than that the secondary premises were located down-wind. This was to be expected perhaps when the initial case involved a large number of poultry, but it also happened following small and otherwise quite insignificant outbreaks. That the small flocks as a rule were not vaccinated at all or at any rate were not fully protected by vaccine did not help matters. But far more disturbing were cases that occurred down-wind from poultry-packing stations and even from motorways and highways with no apparent connexion with foci of infection, and one was left to speculate whether poultry in the incubative period had been slaughtered upwind or vehicles had merely passed by them during the night. Certainly tell-tale trails of feathers were occasionally reported.

However, the impression must not be given that all secondaries came with the wind. All the classic methods of spread, direct and indirect, were seen during the epidemic such as direct movement of poultry during the incubative stage, movement of poultry slaughterers' crates and other equipment, market contacts, movement of personnel, careless disposal of poultry offal, and inefficient boiling of swill. In fact the general level of safety precautions was deplorable. Some practices were almost unbelievable in their carelessness and disregard for danger and yet were continually repeated, even when the epidemic was at its worst, and no one could claim to be ignorant of the possibilities of acquiring infection. Some examples may be quoted:—

1. Flock supervisors, vaccinators, and egg collectors going from premises to premises within an organization without taking sufficient precautions regarding personal hygiene and disinfection.

2. Poultry slaughterers' dirty crates being taken into a shed for filling when only a proportion of the birds were being removed for slaughter.

3. Discarding raw offal from frozen carcasses without making certain that chickens could not gain access to it.

The actual appearance of the disease varied considerably from flock to flock dependent in particular on the vaccinal status. In general outbreaks were characterized by rapid onset, high mortality, marked dejection, pronounced respiratory symptoms, and early death. Fall in egg production was normally to zero and was protracted in unvaccinated flocks. Heavy mortality in unvaccinated or imperfectly protected flocks was the outstanding feature of the epidemic, as was also the high proportion of recovered birds exhibiting torticollis, especially in the case of turkeys. Turkeys seemed to be involved more frequently and more severely than ever before in Great Britain, as also were pheasants. There were numerous reports of infection with heavy mortality in pheasants, which being uncontrollable may also have been a factor in spread in the immediate vicinity.

Post-mortem findings were more striking than usual. Haemorrhages, which were often splashes rather than pin-point, were found in all the regular sites in large numbers, and, in the intestines, ulceration was a not unusual finding particularly in the early stages of the epidemic when vaccine usage was at its lowest. Diagnosis did not provide any difficulty, was normally made on clinical and post-mortem grounds, and in only a small percentage of cases was it necessary to resort to blood sampling and virus isolation in order to differentiate from other conditions.

This epidemic poses the question of future fowl-pest policy and what the prospects are for the poultry industry.

At the time of writing these thoughts, the incidence of the disease is still uncomfortably high and we must be prepared for it to continue through the summer and gather momentum again in the autumn. There are probably infected carcasses in cold stores throughout the country which will come out over the next few months and give rise to fresh cases, some of them in the most unlikely spots where even now people seem to be unaware of the dangers of unboiled swill and poultry scraps.

Have we any weapons in the armoury that we did not have in August, 1970? The approval of live vaccines of the Hitchner B_1 strain is now a matter of history and much has been said regarding their use. The principal arguments in the live/dead controversy were debated in an article by Davies (1971) and many veterinary surgeons, especially those from the Ministry's laboratory at Weybridge, have lectured to poultry-keepers up and down the country on the subject. Veterinary surgeons have a difficult and important part to play in advising on best methods and times for vaccination. Vaccines of the La Sota strain had not, at the time of writing, been licensed for general use, but present evidence suggests that they will be about as effective as inactivated vaccines for purposes of revaccination measured in terms of degree and longevity of protective effect achieved. As the vaccinal virus does spread fairly readily from bird to bird they are particularly suitable for mass administration in contradistinction to B_1 strains which hardly spread laterally at all. Fortunately this property of spread is not sufficiently great to cause a jump from one premises to another. However, the use of a La Sota vaccine would not solve all the problems as it is too virulent to be used safely in chicks under about 6 weeks of age especially where there is a likelihood of intercurrent infection. Thus it will not overcome the principal difficulty associated with the use of vaccines which is the attainment of a protective level of immunity in young birds. It is unfortunate that as the immunity level in breeding stock improves, this problem increases owing to the phenomenon of maternal immunity which has little or no protective property but precludes response to vaccines.

Last year the Minister asked persons with knowledge of the poultry industry to assist the State Veterinary Service in reviewing the course of the epidemic. Alterations to the control policy may have been introduced as a result of their inquiries, but in the final analysis there can be no doubt that the solution will rest collectively in the hands of the country's poultry-keepers.

Experience in this country from 1963 onwards showed that if a high level of vaccination is maintained throughout the country over a period there is a gradual damping down of disease incidence until it virtually disappears. In Great Britain this was achieved with inactivated vaccines. Experience in other countries has shown that the same is true with live vaccines though possibly more rapidly. But the fact that live, easy-to-apply vaccines have been available does not appear to have prevented falling off in usage as the disease situation improved with consequent resurgence of disease and one wonders whether this is to be the pattern of the future, a disease-incidence graph rising and falling with a periodicity of about 5 years and the peaks coinciding with the troughs in the vaccine-usage graph.

A high level of vaccination is, however, not sufficient by itself and the high standard of hygienic practices and isolation of premises that existed in earlier days must be re-established. There must be careful avoidance of any form of contact, direct or indirect, which might convey the disease unless full precautions of cleanliness and disinfection are taken. A particularly heavy responsibility will fall on small poultry-keepers who are the most likely to be handling carcasses and not disposing of offal in a safe manner, for they can be the cause of seeding otherwise clean areas and, if this diffusible virus persists, of setting up foci of infection.

The slogan 'Don't hesitate, vaccinate' is as true now in respect of Newcastle disease as it was when first coined in 1963, and if vaccines are applied properly and continually and are allied to general control measures both statutory and voluntary there is no reason why outbreaks of Newcastle disease should not once again fall to a very low level.

REFERENCES

Davies, J. I. (1971), *Agriculture*, **78**, No. 6, 236.

M.A.F.F. (1970), *Annual Report on the Animal Health Services in Great Britain.*

FISH DISEASES

W. E. Pearson, B.Sc., B.V.S., M.R.C.V.S., M.I.Biol.

In considering which way to tackle this article the Chinese proverb, 'Give a man a fish and you feed him for a day, teach him to fish and you feed him for life', comes to mind. This could today well be written with the addendum, 'Teach him to farm fish and you feed a whole community for life'. To achieve this end one must produce healthy fish so a knowledge of fish pathology, therapeutics, and hygiene is essential.

Ichthyopathology, the study of fish diseases, is assuming increasing importance as a result of the great increase in fish culture (fish farming) in recent times. Although fish have been cultured for about 4000 years, it is only comparatively recently that farming has assumed commercial importance. Another area in which fish keeping has developed is in the field of pets. In Britain, fish rank third in popularity as household pets. There are a large number of different species, coming from warm and cold, fresh or salt waters, that are kept in home aquaria.

A brief description of the main diseases will follow, to acquaint the veterinarian with the types of problem involved in this field. Fish live in water and hence depend on water for all their needs—oxygen, food, removal of waste-products, etc. Their metabolic rate depends on the ambient temperature of the water. One must accept these facts in order to understand fish pathology. However, the differences between the pathology of aquatic and terrestrial animals are minimal.

Fish are subject to viral, bacterial, and fungal diseases and to infestation by protozoal, helminth, and crustacean parasites. They also exhibit neoplasia and are sensitive to various toxic principles.

Viral Diseases

Infectious Pancreatic Necrosis

This acute viral disease affects the salmon family especially brown, brook, and rainbow trout, mainly in North America but it has been diagnosed in Britain and Europe. The virus can be cultured in fish-cell tissue culture, producing a cytopathogenic effect, and is pathogenic even after eight passages. In fish tissues the virus is infective after 4½ years at −20° C., 2½ years in 50 per cent glycerin at 4° C., but is inactivated at 60° C. after 1 hour. The incubation period is 7 days, and mortality 60–70 per cent.

Affected fish show intermittent spiral swimming movements and a darkening of the skin. There is an absence of food in the digestive tract but an abundance of mucus. Histological examination of the tissues reveals pancreatic necrosis and haemorrhages and necrosis in the muscles.

There is no specific treatment, in common with all viral diseases, and no effective vaccine as yet, although research along this line is proceeding. Hygiene and the removal of carriers are most important. A method has been developed for the detection of carriers.

Viral Haemorrhagic Septicaemia

This is an acute or subacute disease of salmonids affecting brook and rainbow trout, mainly those of 1–2 years of age. It occurs chiefly in the cold months at the end of winter and beginning of spring and when new fish are introduced on to the farm. The incubation period is from 5 to 20 days.

The virus can be grown in tissue culture and can survive for long periods in tissues frozen at $-20°$ C.

The non-specific symptoms are darkening of the skin, exophthalmos, anaemia, ascites, and atactic swimming. Specific lesions are haemorrhages scattered throughout the body—palate, fins, muscles, swim bladder, and the perivisceral fat. The liver may be very anaemic or show hyperaemic areas with microscopic necrotic foci.

There is no effective therapy so control is based on hygienic measures, e.g., isolation and destruction of affected fish, thorough disinfection of infected ponds, etc. Ensure that the feed is properly balanced and vitamin fortified. Present studies are being directed towards the development of a vaccine.

Lymphocystis

This viral disease, of world-wide incidence affecting many species of marine and fresh-water fish, is characterized by small verrucose nodules. It was originally thought to be a protozoan and was named *Lymphocystis johnsonei*, but this structure has been shown to be a massive hypertrophy of an epithelial cell (up to several mm. in diameter).

The disease has a chronic course and no mortality. Spontaneous recoveries have been described. Affected fish lose their market value.

The lesions have a greyish to yellowish colour, sometimes with haemorrhagic spots. They may run together and produce a mulberry appearance. Lesions are found most frequently on the fins and sides of the body and also internally.

No treatment is known.

Fish Pox

This disease was probably the first fish disease that was recognized, being described originally in 1563. It affects mainly carp, both wild and farmed. The virus involved is a typical pox virus, measuring 0·07–0·2 μ, which tends to group in masses in the affected cells. In tissue culture it shows a cytopathogenic effect.

The disease is characterized by cutaneous proliferations, especially on the fins and lips but also on the rest of the body. The lesions are milky in colour, firm, but easy to extirpate. When the lesions are extensive, the carp may show an osteomalacia. Again, in common with other viral diseases of fish, there is no known treatment so control is achieved by strict hygienic measures, disinfection of the ponds, and removal of affected fish.

Ulcerative Dermal Necrosis

This viral disease of salmon came into prominence in 1964 in Ireland. It would appear from the literature that this, or at least a very similar disease, has occurred at roughly 30-year intervals since 1830, each outbreak lasting some 4–5 years in any area. The aetiology is not yet clarified but it is safe to assume that the cause is a virus, since the agent passes a 200-μ filter.

The first lesion is a necrotic spot up to 1·5 mm. diameter, with a whitish appearance on the scaleless areas, e.g., the forehead, easily visible in water but difficult to see out of water. Later the ulcer deepens and usually becomes invaded by secondary fungi (*Saprolegnia* spp.) or bacteria (*Aeromonas liqueifaciens*, *Pseudomonas fluorescens*, etc.). The internal organs do not show changes. In a few cases degeneration of the liver due to secondary infection is seen. Treatment has not been studied to any extent, but dipping in malachite green or an injection of chloramphenicol is reputed to effect a cure.

Infectious Carp Dropsy

This acute or chronic viral disease affects carp and rarely tench. It was originally thought to be caused by *Pseudomonas punctata* but this is now shown to be a secondary invader to the virus that causes the disease. The disease occurs in the chronic form in the cold months and in the acute form in spring when the water temperature is rising. The acute form shows anaemia of the gills, haemorrhagic spots and ulcers on the skin, destruction of the fins, and ascites. The liver is pale and there is an enteritis. Mortality is high. In the chronic form, there is little mortality and one observes deep ulcers on the skin, frequently invaded by *Saprolegnia*, and necrosis of the fins.

The most successful treatment so far has been the injection intraperitoneally of chloramphenicol (10 μg. per kg. live-weight) or streptomycin (30 μg. per kg.). Chloromycetin can also be given in the feed—1 part per thousand for several days. Infected ponds should be disinfected with quick-lime (1·5–2·0 tons per hectare).

Work is proceeding to breed resistant strains of fish.

Bacterial Diseases

Furunculosis

Furunculosis is a very widespread bacterial disease of salmonids of all types from rivers, ponds etc., and farms. Salmon, brook and brown trout are most susceptible and rainbow trout less so. The grayling is also susceptible. The disease is caused by a Gram-negative non-motile bacterium, *Aeromonas salmonicida*. The incubation period is about a week.

Acute and chronic forms occur. In the acute form the lesions are not very specific being those of a septicaemia—congestion and haemorrhages in the viscera. Chronic cases show the typical 'furuncles', subcutaneously or in the muscles. These lesions are filled with a bloody fluid. They may rupture outwards leaving a deep and bloody ulcer.

Treatment is based on the administration of sulphonamides, antibiotics, or nitrofurans in the feed. Good results have been obtained with the following:—

Sulphamerazine	200–220 mg. per kg. live-weight per day for 10–15 days
Chloramphenicol, Chlortetracycline	50–75 mg. per kg. live-weight per day for 7 days
Furazolidone	90 mg. per kg. live-weight per day for 15 days

Hygienic measures such as the disinfection of ponds and equipment and of the eggs, and elimination of carriers are essential. Resistant strains should be reared on the farms, in preference to susceptible ones.

Kidney Disease

Kidney disease affects salmonids particularly the brook trout. It is caused by a Gram-positive non-motile *Corynebacterium* which has not been given a specific name. The disease has also been described under the name of 'Dee disease'.

Infection appears to be through the skin and the incubation period is from 1 to 3 months or even longer; the course is also chronic. Mortality is usually light, moderate to severe from fingerlings to adults. Affected fish often show exophthalmos and large cutaneous welts (especially on brook trout) or small unbroken pimples associated with small crater-like lesions along the sides of the fish (particularly in salmon and rainbow trout). The welts and pimples contain a red to creamy purulent fluid composed of red and white blood-cells and very many specific bacteria. These may rupture to give crateriform ulcers. The kidney is swollen and light and variegated in colour. The liver is pale. Both of these organs may show intact abscess-like lesions. The rest of the viscera and cavity walls are haemorrhagic and ascites is frequent.

The disease is difficult to treat. The best results have been obtained by the use of oral erythromycin (in the feed) at a dose of 4·5 g. per 100 lb. live-weight of fish for 3 weeks, but the control was not complete. Sulphamezathine at a dose of 2 g. per 100 lb. of fish per day controls mortality, but mortality recurs once the treatment is stopped.

Bacterial Gill Disease

Gill diseases are due to either bacteria or nutritional factors. The bacterial type is caused by what are inadequately described as 'aquatic myxobacteria', most likely associated with those causing Columnaris disease. Gill disease is characterized by swelling and fusing or clubbing of the gill filaments and lamellae.

The incubation period is 3–7 days. Affected fish lose their appetite and tend to swim against the current. The gill filaments thicken at the ends and fuse together. Microscopic examination shows them to be covered with long, thin bacteria. Often there is an abundant secretion of mucus. Chronic cases frequently show a secondary infection by *Saprolegnia.*

Treatment is by medicated baths of such as a 1 in 50,000 dilution of the 10 per cent commercial solution of Roccal (benzalkonium chloride), i.e., 20 p.p.m., pyridyl-mercuric acetate or Lignasan X at 2 or even 1 p.p.m. repeated for 2 or 3 days. Prophylaxis is by the use of the above once or twice a week.

Mycobacteriosis

Fish tuberculosis or mycobacteriosis was first described in France in 1898 in carp and has since been described in many other species, in fresh, brackish, and sea water. Six species of *Mycobacterium* are described but not all are recognized in *Bergey's Manual* (1957). These are *M. piscium*, *M. marinum*, *M. platypoecilus*, *M. anabanti*, *M. fortuitum*, and *M. salmoniphilum*, which are typical Gram-positive, non-motile, acid-resistant bacteria, which grow at low temperatures and are non-pathogenic for warm-blooded animals. There are five types of the disease, the *Macropodus* (*M. anabanti*) type, the ascitic type as in *Betta splendens*, the exophthalmos type as in *Brachydanio*, the caseous type as in the cyprinids, and the emaciation type as in poecilids.

The disease is chronic and the principal symptoms are loss of skin colour, anorexia, exophthalmos or sunken eyes, skeletal deformities, cutaneous ulcers or skin swellings, all or some of which are seen. Some fish only show internal lesions, e.g., numerous miliary tubercles or extensive yellowish adhesions or even pearl-like nodules in the viscera. Histopathologically the lesions resemble those in the mammal but generally the inflammatory reaction is less. There is much more fibrous tissue, typical giant cells may be absent, and there is much less caseation.

Isonicotinichydrazide and para-amino-salicylic acid have given good results in the treatment of tropical fish. Isonicotinichydrazide 3–5 μg. and streptomycin 10–20 μg. per g. of fish either injected or fed give good results. Kanamycin 20 μg. per g. of fish fed or injected has proved encouraging.

Nocardia asteroides has been incriminated in a similar disease of tropical aquarium fish, trout, and some other species.

Columnaris Disease

This disease of fish in warm waters is caused by myxobacteria, *Chondrococcus columnaris*, and *Cytophaga columnaris*, which may be isolated from the surface of the viscera. It affects many species, especially those without scales, e.g., the catfish but also trout, during the warm seasons of the year. Affected fish show whitish-grey spots and areas, resembling saprolegniosis, on the gills, head, fins, and the dorsolateral parts of the body. When examined fresh under the microscope the bacteria appear as thin, long filaments in wavy columns.

Medicated baths of copper sulphate (1 in 2000) for 1–2 minutes, malachite green (1 in 1500) for 10–30 seconds, pyridyl-mercuric acetate (1 in 500) for 1 hour, or chloramphenicol (5–10 in 1000) are advised for treatment of the external form, whereas for the internal form feeding with sulphamerazine in the feed at a rate of 200–220 g. per ton is recommended. Antibiotics can also be fed with success.

Ulcer Disease

Ulcer disease occurs widely in north-east America and affects salmonids, particularly the brook trout. Susceptibility decreases with age. The disease is caused by *Haemophilus piscium*, a non-motile Gram-negative bacterium which may be isolated from both the skin lesions and the internal organs. The incubation period is 10–15 days.

At first the affected fish show small, whitish lesions scattered over the body especially on the jaw and palate. Later these develop into open ulcers with a red surface. They may enlarge and run together to form large, irregular lesions.

Treatment is by the feeding of chloramphenicol and oxytetracycline at a dose of 5–7 g. per 100 kg. (approximately 55 mg. per lb.) of fish per day for 10–15 days. Prevention is best accomplished by regular disinfection of the tanks and equipment, elimination of carriers, and disinfection of the eggs.

Tail and Fin Rot

These two diseases have much in common so they are described together. In both cases various myxobacteria, not sufficiently identified, have been isolated. The disease affects young trout on farms. In the case of fin rot, the margins of the fins become opaque and thickened with necrosis of the soft tissues, leaving the hard rays exposed. Tail rot is shown as a swelling and inflammation, discoloration, and necrosis of the caudal peduncle.

Fin rot may be cured by the use of external disinfectants such as copper sulphate, formalin, malachite green, etc., along with disinfection and cleaning of the tanks. There is no satisfactory treatment for tail rot, however.

Red Pest of Eels

There are two forms of this disease, the first affecting eels in fresh water and the second those in salt or brackish water.

The first appears mainly from August to November and shows as a reddening of the ventral region, either as a diffuse, banded, or patchy reddening. Sometimes there are open bluish-white lesions, swellings, or ulcers particularly on the head. Blindness can also occur. This form is caused by *Pseudomonas punctata* var. *sacrowiensis.* Microscopical examination reveals inflammation of the terminal part of the intestine and haemorrhages in the liver.

The second form caused by *Vibrio anguillarum* occurs in eels in waters having a salinity greater than 2·5 parts per 1000 during the hot season. The affected eels show a patchy reddening on the borders of the fins and the skin and around the anus, swellings on the skin and reddish ulcers, muscular contractions, and a red swelling of the muscles in the cardiac region. Although the monotrichous Gram-negative *V. anguillarum* is a cause, it is very possible that other bacteria can produce similar symptoms.

Nothing is known of the therapy in these diseases.

Fungal Diseases

Several fungi have been shown to cause diseases in fish but only the three main ones will be discussed here.

Saprolegniosis

This can be regarded as a disease *per se* but generally it is a secondary condition to other concurrent disease. Several fungi of the genera *Saprolegnia* and *Achlya* are responsible for the condition. They attack diseased fish or even fish that are dead and have been left in water for some time. The fungi grow on wounds and other cutaneous lesions and are a complicating factor, for example, to ulcerative dermal necrosis. One observes lesions on the skin, gills, cornea, etc., that appear as greyish-white, cotton-wool-like tufts. Obviously the treatment should be directed against the primary condition, but treatment of the secondary fungal invasion with antimycotics is also indicated. The preferred treatment is with malachite green at a dilution of 1 in 180,000–200,000 in the water for 1 hour in the fish tanks. A bi-weekly treatment with this drug is used to maintain incubating eggs free from *Saprolegnia* (1 in 200,000 for 30–45 minutes).

Ichthyosporidiosis

Ichthyosporidiosis (ichthyophoniasis) affects farmed salmonids, marine, and tropical aquarium fish, and is caused by the fungus *Ichthiosporidium* (*Ichthiophonus*) *hoferi*, which grows slowly on special media at 10° C.

The disease is transmitted chiefly by feeding affected ground-up fish to farmed fish, but can be directly transmitted. Affected salmonids exhibit darkening of the skin, emaciation, exophthalmos sometimes followed by a panophthalmia, and loss of the eyes. Small translucent pin-point nodules appear especially on the ventral part of the body. In the case of the herring this latter is referred to as sand-paper skin. On opening the fish, one observes small, whitish nodules scattered throughout the organs affected, e.g., liver, kidneys, spleen, heart, etc.

No treatment is known so prophylactic measures must be adopted. Hygiene and disinfection are important, also avoid feeding of raw fish, etc. The development of balanced feeds will go a long way towards the prevention of transmission by feeding. In modern fish culture, such feeds are being used more and more so the disease should become rarer as time goes on.

Branchiomycosis

This disease is seen chiefly in carp, tench, and pike, having an acute course in the summer months in waters that have an excess of organic matter. It can cause a loss of from 30 to 50 per cent.

It is caused by *Branchiomyces sanguinis* in the carp and *B. demigrans* in the tench and pike. The fungi localize in the capillaries of the gills, thus causing necroses and severe respiratory distress and asphyxia. Affected gills are hyperaemic, with red and greyish spots and necrotic areas, which later become attacked by *Saprolegnia*. There is no satisfactory treatment. Hygienic measures aim towards the reduction of excess organic material by the application of 8–10 lb. copper sulphate per acre (according to the depth of the ponds) in the months of May, July, and August.

Protozoal Diseases

Protozoa exist on fish as external or internal parasites and in the blood-stream.

External

Wild fish usually harbour a small number of protozoa with no ill effects, but under farming conditions these become so numerous as to have detrimental effects, because of the facility with which they multiply. In general these parasites cause similar symptoms; thickening of the skin, increase in mucus (slime) on the gills and skin, emaciation, and anaemia. The main species involved are *Costia*, *Chilodonella*, *Trichodina*, and *Ichthyophthirius*, and the diagnosis is made by microscopic examination of smears of the slime. Treatment, where indicated, is done by adding disinfectants such as formalin diluted to 1 in 4000 in the tanks for 1 hour or less, depending on the reaction of the fish. With *Ichthyophthirius* the treatment should be repeated for 7–14 days consecutively. Malachite green at a dilution of 0·15 mg. per litre of water in the tank for 10 days is also useful in this case.

Internal

The *Myxosporidia* are the most important of these.

Lentosporiasis or Whirling Disease.—This is a chronic disease with an incubation period of 1–2 months affecting young salmonids during their first summer. The causal organism *Lentospora cerebralis* localizes in the cranium and vertebrae, and in the cartilage of young fish, causing foci of colliquation. This results in disturbances of ossification and exostoses which press on the spinal and peripheral nerves causing atactic swimming and skeletal deformities. The dark coloration is the result of a partial paralysis of the nerves supplying the chromatophores. Transmission is not known but is related to the feeding of infected fish tissues.

The symptoms are disturbed swimming seen especially at feeding time, etc., dark coloration of the tail, scoliosis, lordosis, deformities of the mandibles, and gill covers.

No treatment is known. On affected farms the tanks should be disinfected with calcium cyanamide at the rate of 1½–2 lb. per square yard, during the autumn and spring in dry tanks.

Myxoboliasis.—*Myxobolus pfeifferi* causes parasitic tumours in the barbel, and it is suspected that the parasite can also affect humans. The disease occurs in many European rivers in the summer months. The tumours are of various sizes and are localized on the dorsal area in the muscles. They are firm, pasty to fluid in consistency, and may be ulcerated or show scar tissue. In the muscles the lesions are yellowish and gelatinous, filled with a creamy, dense material. Lesions occur in the internal organs too. Again there is no treatment and the affected fish should be destroyed.

Octomitiasis or Hexamitiasis.—The correct name of the disease should be 'hexamitiasis' but the other name is still used to some extent in the literature. The parasite *Hexamita salmonis*, previously named *Octomitis trutta*, localizes in the lower part of the intestine and gall-bladder of young salmonids especially in the summer months. The course is chronic and losses of 50–75 per cent can occur.

The affected fish are very emaciated with sunken abdomens. Their heads appear large in comparison to the rest of the body as a result. The acute form is rarely seen and in this case the main symptom is a disturbed swimming movement.

It appears that fish can harbour small numbers of the parasites without ill effects for long periods, but various conditions such as infectious diseases, errors in feeding (nutrition), etc., can precipitate a rapid multiplication of the parasites with the resultant appearance of the disease.

Calomel at the rate of 0·2 per cent or carbazone 0·2 per cent for 2 or 4 days respectively in the feed has been used for treatment, but better results are given by aureomycin 0·1 per cent, fumigillin 0·2 per cent, or carbazone oxide 0·2 per cent which are more recent treatments.

Helminth Infestations

Trematodes

There are two groups of trematodes—the Monogenea and the Digenea—that affect fish. The Monogenea have a direct life cycle and are essentially parasitic on the gills and skin. In general, they are egg-layers, but one family the Gyrodactylidea (genus *Gyrodactylus*) is viviparous and is of particular interest in that the unusual condition of polyembryonia occurs. In the developing embryo a second embryo forms and in this a third can be seen and sometimes a fourth inside the third. Another genus *Diplozoon* has the unusual feature that the male and female fuse together completely in an X shape in which they remain for the rest of their life.

Whereas the Monogenea are almost without exception parasites of fish, the Digenea, having a complex life cycle, affect many species of animals. Their life cycles somewhat resemble that of the liver fluke *Fasciola hepatica*, well known in the veterinary field.

Monogenea.—As already mentioned, these parasitize the gills, when the main phenomena are those of asphyxia (in severe cases), or the skin, where the symptoms are similar to the external protozoal infestations already described. There are a large number of families and genera affecting all species of fish ranging from fresh-water to salt-water types, but the genera and species are very host specific. The most important genera found under fish farming conditions are *Dactylogyrus*, *Diplozoon*, *Monocoelium*, and *Gyrodactylus*.

Treatment consists of medicating the water in the tanks with 1 : 4000 formalin for 1 hour, combined with general hygienic measures.

Digenea.—The important infestations are by the larval stages of these parasites, the adult stages of which occur in fish-eating birds. Two groups are important, those that encyst in the eye and those in the skin, etc. Those that encyst in the eye cause the so-called 'verminous' cataract. *Diplostomum spathaceum* larvae up to 500 in an eye can cause complete blindness with the result that feeding and growth suffer and economic loss occurs. The life cycle is as follows: bird—egg—miracidium—snail (first intermediate host)—cercaria—fish (second intermediate host)—bird (final host). *Neascus brevicaudatus* is another Digenea that encysts in the eye.

Clinostomum complanatum carcariae encyst in the musculature and subcutis of fish and are referred to by fishermen as 'yellow grub'. The life cycle is similar to that of *Diplostomum* with the final host as fish-eating birds, e.g., herons, pelicans, and cormorants.

Obviously there is no treatment in the fish so the control is by breaking the cycle—keeping birds away from the fish tanks and the destruction of snails. The first can be achieved by stringing nylon threads across the tanks and the second by the use of molluscicides in the water.

Cestodes

Some cestodes occur in the adult stage in the fish, e.g., *Caryophyllaeus*, *Trieanophorus*, and *Protocephalus*. If the infestation is heavy, they retard the growth of the fish causing economic loss. Treatment is by the administration of taeniacides. Kamala at the rate of 1·5–2 per cent in the feed for 1–2 weeks has given good results. Other drugs should be considered.

The second group of cestodes that infest fish are those that employ the fish as an intermediate host. The most frequently encountered of these are those which cause ligulosis schistocephalosis, and Plerocercosis.

Ligulosis.—Here the adult parasite occurs in the intestine of birds and the plerocercoid larvae infest the body cavity of cyprinid fish, notably the tench and the roach. Affected fish show an enlargement of the abdomen, along with emaciation and anaemia. On opening the fish, a ribbon-like, yellowish-white worm, measuring from 10 to 100 cm. by 0·6–1·5 cm. is found in between the convolutions of the intestines. The parasite is *Ligula intestinalis* whose life cycle is: bird—coracidia—crustacean—fish—bird.

Schistocephalosis.—Another tapeworm, *Schistocephalus solidus*, has a similar life cycle to that of the previous cestode, but the size of the plerocercoids is much smaller, 2–4 cm. by 0·6 cm.

Plerocercosis.—Strictly speaking all forms of infestation with plerocercoids can be called 'plerocercosis' but this term is mostly reserved for the infestation with the plerocercoids of *Diphyllobothrium latum*, the human tape-worm. This is of great importance from a public health point of view. The larvae encyst in the muscles and viscera, appearing as milk-white cysts 2–20 mm. long, transversely striated and showing a retractable scolex with two bothria. The life cycle is: human—egg—coracidium—crustacean—fish—second fish—man or other host (dog, cat, etc.).

Nematodes

There are numerous nematodes which infest fish in both the larval and adult stages. Space does not permit a description in detail. In the intestine one finds various species of *Ascaris*, *Capillaria*, *Cucullanus*, *Camallanus*; in the swim bladder, *Ancyracanthus cystidicola*, and in the liver, *Capillaria eupomotis*—all in the adult stage. The liver parasite is common in trout, where affected fish show whitish, pin-point nodules in the liver that later increase in size and become brown to blackish.

The only treatment that has been investigated is against the nematode *Contracaecum bidentatum* in the sturgeon in Russia. They have had success with the use of santonin there.

Acanthocephalae

The thorny-headed worms are common in fish. They are provided with a head armoured with rows of hooks by which they anchor themselves to the intestinal wall. These worms do not possess a mouth or gut but absorb their food by osmosis from the intestinal contents. The intermediate host in their life cycle is generally an isopod such as *Gammarus*, or other aquatic insect larvae, and the final host a fish.

The most frequently encountered acanthocephalans are *Echinorynchus truttae*, *E. gadi*, *Neoechinorynchus rutilis*, *Pomphorynchus laevis*, *Acanthocephalus anguillae*, and *A. lucii*.

Treatment has not been studied to any extent, and the method of control advocated is to remove thin and sick fish and to disinfect the ponds with quick-lime.

Crustaceae

A large number of crustaceans parasitize fish, being localized on the skin, gills, and subcutis. The types most commonly encountered belong to the genera *Lernea*, *Ergasilus*, *Argulus*, and *Salmincola*. Some of these can transmit diseases, e.g., *Argulus foliaceus* can transmit fish pox. Fish, especially young ones when heavily infested, show skin lesions, emaciation, and anaemia, and, where the gills are affected, signs of asphyxia with a consequent heavy mortality.

These parasites can be controlled by the use of 1 : 4000 formalin, 1 : 10,000,000 benzene hexachloride (Gammexane), or 1 : 50,000,000–100,000,000 DDT. (Note, the last two may kill off the natural crustacean foods present.)

Leeches

Piscicola goemetra is the main fish leech encountered. It attaches to the fish and sucks blood and, when gorged, leaves the fish. Severe infestations cause an anaemia. Leeches transmit fish trypanosomes.

Miscellaneous Conditions

There are several conditions of which only two will be mentioned here.

Asphyxia

Different species of fish have different requirements for dissolved oxygen, e.g., trout need about 8 p.p.m. and carp 5 p.p.m. When the levels fall much below these figures they suffer from asphyxia. The amount of dissolved oxygen decreases with increasing temperature, excess of organic matter, over-population, etc. Asphyxiated fish die with the gill covers and mouth wide open.

Hepatoma

One specific form of neoplasia is caused by a fungal toxin, aflatoxin, produced by *Aspergillus flavus*. This toxin is well known as a liver toxin in many species of animals and trout are very susceptible. Until the discovery of this toxin, the appearance of hepatoma had all the characteristics of an epizootic and was thought at first to be an infectious disease. The histological changes are similar to those in other animals, e.g., turkeys, and feeding tests with the pure aflatoxin reproduced the condition in trout.

BIBLIOGRAPHY

AMLACHER, E. (1961), *Taschenbuch der Fischkrankheiten.* Jena: Fischer.

BREED, R. S., MURRAY, E. G. D. and SMITH, N. R. (1957), *Bergey's Manual of Determinative Bacteriology*, 7th ed. Baltimore: Williams & Wilkins.

BYCHOWSKY, B. E. (1957), *Monogenetic Trematodes.* American Institute of Biological Sciences, 1962.

DAVIS, H. S. (1945), *Care and Diseases of Trout.* Washington, D.C.: U.S. Department of Interior Research, Report No. 12 (1962).

— — (1961), *Culture and Diseases of Game Fish.* Berkeley: University of California Press.

GHITTINO, P. (1970), *Piscicoltura e Ittiopatologia*, Vols. 1 and 2. Sesto: Edizione Rivista di Zootecnia.

LEITRITZ, E. (1960), *Trout and Salmon Culture.* Sacramento: California Department of Fish and Game Fish, Bulletin 107.

REICHENBACH-KLINKE, H., and ELKAN, E. (1965), *The Principal Diseases of the Lower Vertebrates.* New York: Academic.

SCHÄPERCLAUS, W. (1954), *Fischkrankheiten.* Berlin: Akademie.

VAN DUIJN, C., jun. (1967), *Diseases of Fishes*, 2nd ed. Springfield, Ill.: Thomas.

HUSBANDRY PRACTICES AND ANIMAL PERFORMANCE WITH SPECIAL REFERENCE TO PIG-KEEPING

S. R. Wragg, M.A.

The proposition that there exists a corpus of proved principles and practices in respect of each branch of animal husbandry could imply that these same principles and practices, and the degree of their adoption or non-adoption by individual farmers, must provide the main components of any formula intended to explain, in quantitative terms, the causes of the variations in performance which are well known to exist between technical production units, considered either as individual animals or as whole herds or flocks. It follows from this that it should be theoretically possible to define an output function for a specific animal production unit in terms of the nature, quantities, and qualities of the inputs used, the environmental situation, and the practices and procedures attending the production process itself, the latter usually being included under the omnibus term 'management'. All these things are in fact subsumed in the concept of giving technical and management advice to livestock farmers, directed towards raising the efficiency of their animals either by reducing costs or by raising output.

It would not be unreasonable to assume also that the competent adviser will carry in his mind a clear idea and a firm estimate of the nature and size of the 'pay-off' which he associates with each particular practice to which he gives his approval and commendation. Of course, there are many aspects of each animal production process about which an adviser may be in a position to recommend a preferred practice; so in aggregate, the 'pay-off' associated with doing everything in the right and best of all possible ways is theoretically enormous. In practice, however, the consequences which flow from the advice-purveying activity not infrequently fall far short of expectations. One reason for this is a strong tendency for estimates of the outcome of particular practices and procedures to be conditioned by the size of the somewhat ideal and unique treatment effects obtained in the course of controlled experiments. To say the least, these are likely to be highly optimistic when placed in the context of average expectations in commercial production units.

As far as commercial livestock enterprises are concerned, no one in this country, to the writer's knowledge, has yet succeeded in establishing the presence of a substantial degree of correlation between technical or financial success on the one hand and the apparent quality of the corresponding husbandry practices, environment, and stock on the other hand. On the contrary, the magnitude of such estimated relationships can often turn out to be disconcertingly low. But these general statements in no way conflict with the fact that there are, of course, many successful farmers who follow recommended and approved husbandry practices very closely indeed, and who have also invested quite heavily in the provision of a high standard of environment and livestock. But if, in a multivariate model, using the recorded experiences of a reasonably representative cross-section of commercial livestock producers, it is impossible to identify the existence of a significant and substantial association between the level of inputs, the adoption of approved practices, and sound environments on the one hand and the accompanying level of technical or economic performance on the other hand, on what basis, other than the experimental evidence, can one rationally make technical recommendations, which are of interest and value to the recipient only if he can be reasonably certain that they will be accompanied by commensurate gains in technical and economic efficiency. The purpose of this article is to elaborate and examine these notions in greater detail with special reference to pig-keeping.

Annual surveys of production methods, costs, and returns in pig-keeping have been carried out on an almost continuous basis in this country over the past 40 years. Anyone at all conversant with the results will be well aware of the very wide range in performance encompassed by these studies. The coefficient of variability in profit per unit of output for a typical sample of herds is usually in the order of about 70 per cent. This means that if the sample average profit is £3 per pig, approximately one-sixth of all the herds in the sample will be making less than £1 per pig, while at the opposite end of the distribution another sixth will be making profits of more than £5 per pig. But it would be quite wrong to suppose that the same herds occupy approximately the same positions in the distribution from one year to the next, or indeed anything like it. For there is, in fact, a very high degree of instability in the year-to-year performance of individual herds. And quite obviously this is not unconnected with the low levels of correlation evident between performance and management practices, etc., referred to above.

Given the annual figures of profit per unit of output for each member of an identical sample of herds for each of a number of years, they can be set out in the form of a rectangular array in which the rows represent herds and the columns represent years. If the total variation over the whole array of profits is calculated, then by the use of analysis of variance this total can be divided into components which measure the variation attributable to different sources: in this case to differences between herds (between rows), differences between years (between columns), and an unexplained residual variance (within rows and columns). On *a priori* grounds one would expect that the first two of these sources would together account for most of the total variation present in the array. But as the results of the two accompanying analyses of variance tables show quite clearly, this is not the case.

Tables I and *II* are based on 5 years' annual results for an identical sample of 62 herds* which has been divided into two equal subsamples containing the 31 least profitable and the 31 most profitable herds, profit being measured per £100 of output and averaged over the 5-year period. In *Table I*, which relates to the least profitable subsample, the total variance in profits per £100 output is only reduced from £51·7 to £49·2 by accounting for the variation present between herds and between years. This illustrates the quite remarkable degree of instability and inconsistency in the performance of individual herds. *Table II* relates to the 31 most profitable herds, and although

* The data used to calculate the results in *Tables I* and *II* were extracted from a report entitled *The Results in Pig Management Scheme*, published by the Agricultural Economics Unit, Cambridge University, in 1970.

it shows that variability was significantly less than in the subsample of poorer herds it will be noted that most of the variation present again occurs within rows and columns, which means that it is unexplained residual variance. In standard deviation form it amounts to £5·1 per £100 output, equal to a coefficiency of variation of 27 per cent in relation to a subsample mean profit of £18·9 per £100 output.

Table I.—ANALYSIS OF VARIANCE IN PROFITS PER £100 OUTPUT FOR 31 LEAST PROFITABLE HERDS OVER 5 YEARS

SOURCE OF VARIATION	DEGREES OF FREEDOM	SUM OF SQUARES	ESTIMATED VARIANCE
Between rows (herds)	30	1413	47·1
Between columns (years)	4	643	160·8
Within rows and columns (residual)	120	5903	49·2
Total	154	7959	51·7

Mean profit per herd over 5 years=£9·1 per £100 output.

Table II.—ANALYSIS OF VARIANCE IN PROFITS PER £100 OUTPUT FOR 31 MOST PROFITABLE HERDS OVER 5 YEARS

SOURCE OF VARIATION	DEGREES OF FREEDOM	SUM OF SQUARES	ESTIMATED VARIANCE
Between rows (herds)	30	1834	61·1
Between columns (years)	4	1159	289·7
Within rows and columns (residual)	120	3152	16·3
Total	154	6145	39·9

Mean profit per herd over 5 years=£18·9 per £100 output.

The relationship between husbandry practices and economic performance in pig production has recently been examined in considerable detail in a small purposive sample of commercial herds, thanks to a grant received from the Meat and Livestock Commission for this purpose by Bristol University.* Fourteen herds were selected for study, and over a period of approximately 3 years they and their management were subjected to continuous and detailed scrutiny to the fullest extent possible without allowing the process of making regular observations to become a nuisance or an embarrassment to the herd owner; and also without allowing the presence of the observer to change the management or influence decisions during the diagnostic period. The sample, selected on the basis of known past performance records, contained 7 financially unsuccessful units (Category 1) in which the stock, environment, health,

* This has been treated as an interdisciplinary project for which the Department of Animal Husbandry, School of Veterinary Science, and the Agricultural Economics Research Unit, Department of Economics, were jointly responsible. The Research Fellow working on the project was Dr. M. G. Trapnell.

nutrition, and day-to-day management appeared to be at least satisfactory; and 7 financially successful units (Category 2) in which the factors referred to above appeared to range from less than satisfactory to most unsatisfactory. The average size of breeding herd was between 50 and 60 sows of the white breeds and their crosses, entirely or almost entirely self-contained. The main end-product was bacon pigs. In the 2 years prior to the start of the project the average rates of profit were £11·3 per £100 output for Category 1 herds and £22·6 per £100 output for Category 2 herds. The average profit during this same period, according to similar but much larger surveys, was about £16 per £100 output.

Selection of the sample was quite a lengthy procedure, not made any easier by the outbreak of foot-and-mouth disease in 1967–8. The period of diagnostic observation and recording lasted for approximately a whole year, and because of the large amount of information collected, evaluation and interpretation also took longer than had been expected, all of which delayed the next stage which consisted of reporting back to participating herd owners and commending to them such remedial advice as seemed appropriate under the circumstances. The final stage, still to be completed at the time of writing this paper, is concerned with the extent to which the advice has been accepted and made fully operational, and its eventual effectiveness in increasing productivity and profits. However, some conclusions have emerged from the results of the study so far. They are mostly in keeping with the initial thinking and hypothesis.

All herds, regardless of their average performance over time, displayed the same degree of instability in performance from year to year as that already noted as being present in other samples of recorded herds. It is not at all easy to diagnose the cause of these fluctuations, partly because they are difficult to detect immediately and partly because one is dealing with a situation which is subject to almost continual change, sometimes in one direction and sometimes in another. But it was possible, on the basis of some of the more static elements in the situation, to draw certain conclusions. It became evident during the course of the study that in order to obtain an accurate description and evaluation of the policy, goals, operational procedures, and environmental circumstances associated with an individual herd it will usually be necessary to devote far more time and resources to this task than are likely to be available in the course of conventional advisory activities. For, by no means immediately but well into the second half of the diagnostic period, the whole of which lasted for at least 12 months, it became apparent that conditions and practices in Category 2 herds were better, and those in Category 1 herds were less good, than the original assessment. The reappraisal is a matter of fundamental significance if it is assumed that a correct diagnosis and a complete understanding of all the circumstances affecting a unit are essential prerequisites to the formulation of appropriate and effective remedial action.

Nine important measures of technical or economic efficiency were selected, in connexion with which a total of 42 management and environmental criteria were identified as being likely to have a significant bearing on performance. Some of these were more conveniently divided into subclasses. In the context of individual herd situations, criteria can be either positive or negative; and, according to the nature of the particular criterion in question, this will determine whether it is likely to contribute to a good or to a poor performance. An example of this procedure is given in *Table III.* It relates to the average liveweight of piglets at weaning and the relevant management and environmental criteria.

Table III.—EFFICIENCY FACTOR: AVERAGE LIVEWEIGHT OF PIGLETS WEANED

CRITERIA	FAVOURABLE	CAT. 1	CAT. 2	UNFAVOURABLE	CAT. 1	CAT. 2
Age at weaning	⩾56 days	4	4	<56 days	3	3
System	Outdoors	1	—	Indoors	5	7
	Early weaning	1	—			
Disease	Absent	5	4	Present	2	3
Environment	Good	4	—	Poor	3	7
Nutrition						
Milk yields	Average/good	6	5	Poor	1	2
Palatability	Good	5	4	Poor	2	3
Meal	Fresh	6	7	Stale	1	—
Water	Clean	5	7	Dirty	2	—
Creep feeding	Before 3 weeks	3	5	3 weeks or later	4	2
Food as fed	Pellets	3	3	Meal	4	4
Total		43	39		27	31

Although the extremely terse nature of the descriptions used in *Table III* may tend to suggest that there was a strong element of spontaneity in the evaluation process, this part of the investigation was, in fact, based on very meticulous observation and recording, such as the use of thermographs and hydrographs for measuring environmental conditions, laboratory analysis of feedingstuffs, post-mortems, and other pathological work.

The distribution of herds in relation to favourable/unfavourable criteria situations was analysed with respect to each of the nine selected efficiency factors. A very condensed summary of the results is given in *Table IV.* The first point worth noting in this table is the fact that these nine efficiency factors alone involved, on average, as many as 61 criteria situations per herd, of which 34 were considered to be favourable and 27 unfavourable. Although Category 1 herds (financially less successful) had rather fewer criteria situations favouring a good performance and rather more favouring a poor performance than had Category 2 herds (financially more successful), the differences were not sufficiently important to constitute a really significant advantage or disadvantage. In effect, therefore, the analysis lends support to the hypothesis that differences in performance between herds arise quite independently of any differences there may be in the husbandry and environment.

In terms of husbandry, managerial and environmental deficiencies, it is also quite clear that the more profitable herds are as much in need of advice on these matters as are the less profitable herds. But if, as seems to be the case, high and low levels of profitability are not associated with correspondingly high and low standards of management practices and environments, how relevant is the advice likely to be, and how confident can the adviser be that its adoption will take the herd owner a significant step nearer to his goal of a better performance and higher profits?

In spite of the underlying train of thought contained in the previous paragraph, a total of 247 separate, although often related, pieces of advice

Table IV.—THE DISTRIBUTION OF FAVOURABLE AND UNFAVOURABLE CRITERIA RELATED TO EFFICIENCY FACTORS

EFFICIENCY FACTOR	NO. OF CRITERIA USED INCLUDING SUBCLASSES	FEATURES FAVOURING GOOD PERFORMANCE — *No. of Herds*			FEATURES FAVOURING POOR PERFORMANCE — *No. of Herds*		
		Cat. 1	Cat. 2	Total	Cat. 1	Cat. 2	Total
Average litters per sow and gilt per annum	9	12	27	39	30	14	44
Average live pigs born per litter	6	16	21	37	19	14	33
Pre-weaning mortality-rate	6	16	13	29	5	8	13
Average live-weight of piglets at weaning	11	43	39	82	27	31	58
Meal consumed per sow per gilt including creep feed	6	28	26	54	14	16	30
Cost per unit of sow and creep feed	10	31	39	70	32	24	56
Feed conversion of growing and fattening pigs	12	40	34	74	36	40	76
Cost per unit of growers fattening meal	6	17	21	38	18	14	32
Receipt per score of pigs sold	7	20	32	52	26	15	41
Total	73	223	252	475	207	176	383

were given to participants in the study after the diagnostic stage had been completed; an average of 16 items per Category 1 herd and 17 items per Category 2 herd. The overall rates of adoption, at the time the advice was presented, were estimated to be 44 per cent in Category 1 herds and 70 per cent in Category 2 herds, from which it would appear that pig-keepers initially operating at a low profit may be less willing to adopt recommendations designed to raise profits than those with herds showing a fairly good profit.*

Some very tentative analyses have been made relating to the progress of these herds since the owners either accepted or rejected the advice which was offered following the period of observation and diagnosis. These are summarized briefly in *Table V*.

Considering the results in *Table V* the most that can be said about them is that they add up to something which appears to be just a little better than

* Twelve months later the adoption rates were 49 per cent for Category 1 herds and 71 per cent for Category 2 herds but many accepted recommendations still remained unimplemented.

what would in all probability have happened without any intervention at all. But in view of what was said earlier about the presence of a major element of random variability in the performance of pig herds, a considerably longer period of evaluation is really necessary in order to authenticate the presence of any permanent changes in performance.

Table V.—CHANGES IN TECHNICAL PERFORMANCE IN CATEGORY 1 AND 2 HERDS: POST-ADVICE SITUATION COMPARED WITH PRE-ADVICE SITUATION*

DIRECTION OF CHANGE	BREEDING HERDS			FATTENING HERDS		
	Category 1	Category 2	All Herds	Category 1	Category 2	All Herds
	No.	No.	No.	No.	No.	No.
Improving	—	2	2	1	2	3
Deteriorating	1	1	2	—	1	1
No change	3	3	6	5	4	9
Discontinued breeding	2	1	3	—	—	—
Ceased production	1	—	1	1	—	1
Total	7	7	14	7	7	14

* Only the following simple criteria were used in construction of this table: (*a*) number of young pigs weaned per sow and gilt per annum; (*b*) lb. of meal fed per lb. live-weight gain. The classification of herds into the first three change categories was judged subjectively on the basis of the observed changes, their magnitude, and apparent consistency.

The subject of advice, approved practices, and their adoption by farmers has also been investigated in the course of another recent study carried out at Bristol by Mitchell (1970). This was concerned with an examination of farmers' factual beliefs and values in relation to the acceptance or non-acceptance of approved practices in pig-keeping. It was based on a survey, by personal interviews, of a stratified random sample of pig-keepers in Somerset and Wiltshire. The results indicate that the degree of acceptance by herd owners of established and generally approved practices was often well below expectations. Moreover, owners of large herds were not seen to be invariably more willing to adopt a particular practice than were owners of much smaller herds. *Table VI* contains an extract from the data relating to the adoption level of five of the approved practices included in the study.

This same survey also dealt with the beliefs and values which both adopters and non-adopters attached to approved practices. Almost all herd owners acknowledged their general validity and potential benefits. But non-adopters also claimed to recognize situational barriers which prevent them, in the context of their particular situations, from adopting the practices, or deriving any worth-while benefits if they did so. Adopters did not rate the approved practices much more highly than did non-adopters. The essential difference between them was that the former did not recognize any situational barriers to adoption, or if they had done so initially they had taken whatever action was necessary to remove them.

These findings are in very close agreement with various attitudes towards approved practices observed among herd owners in the course of the study of husbandry practices and performance in pig production. The majority of the recommendations made to participants in this latter study were basically a repetition of advice already given by other advisers on one or more previous occasions. In this connexion it is interesting to note that among the reasons given to explain their earlier rejection of the same recommendations, the most

Table VI.—ESTIMATED PERCENTAGE OF HERD OWNERS IN SOMERSET AND WILTSHIRE USING CERTAIN APPROVED PRACTICES*

APPROVED PRACTICE	HERD SIZE: SOWS AND GILTS			
	5–19	20–49	50 and over	All Herds
	(per cent)	(per cent)	(per cent)	(per cent)
1. Cleaning, disinfecting, and resting houses between batches of pigs	62	46	33	57
2. Removal of the sow from piglets at weaning	59	72	56	62
3. Provision of farrowing aids	82	96	80	85
4. Provision of insulation for houses	37	60	80	45
5. Early weaning	24	40	56	29

* Based on raised sample estimates.

frequent were those falling into the category of situational barriers. In some instances it was discovered that recommendations had been accepted in principle as a course for future action but little or nothing had been done to implement the decision. Poor communications between the pigman and herd owner was a frequent underlying reason why policy decisions were not implemented. If the pigman's attitude towards the proposed change fell within a range described as neutral to hostile, the owner's decision to introduce the change could be partially or wholly circumvented unless his oversight was both rigorous and well informed. But quite often this was not the case.

The results obtained from various studies, using both sample surveys and national data, designed to monitor progress in livestock farming, lend strong support to the view that, in most branches of livestock production, standards of performance on the generality of commercial farms are well below the standards which research workers and advisers in animal husbandry believe are readily attainable by the majority of commercial producers, given the present state of knowledge in this field. An example of this, again relating to pig farming, is illustrated by the graph in *Fig.* 22, which shows the trend in the estimated average number of weaned piglets produced per sow and gilt per annum in the national herd for the period 1949–69.*

The picture is one of steady progress during the 1950's—a compound annual rate of increase in productivity per sow and gilt of 2·6 per cent per annum. But in the following decade the rate of progress first declines and then follows a period in which absolute productivity declines, the trend value in

* The estimates are based not on sample data but on national census data and information on slaughterings. The height of the curve is very slightly underestimated because the figures do not include weaned piglets which died on the farm prior to sale as fat pigs.

1969 being 0·6 piglet below its maximum value in 1962. It was interesting to find that when a linear trend was fitted to the period 1949 to 1962 and then extrapolated to 1969, the extrapolated trend value was 18·3 piglets weaned per sow, which is, in fact, about the standard of productivity that animal scientists and husbandry advisers usually have in mind as a norm for applying to the generality of commercial producers. Had the extrapolated trend value

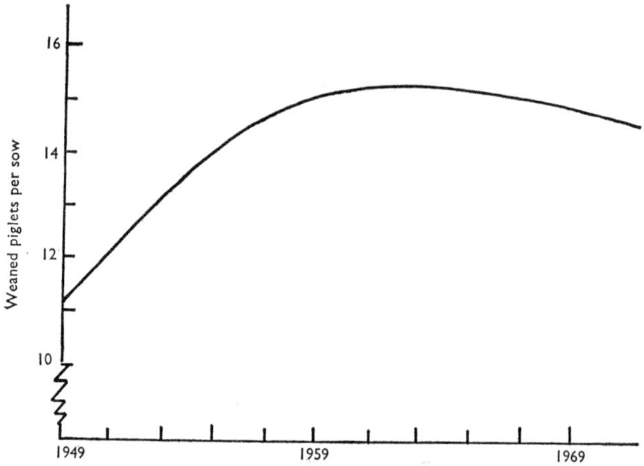

Fig. 22.—National trend in the average number of weaned piglets produced per sow and gilt per annum, 1949–69.

been borne out in practice there would have been an additional 3 million weaned pigs per annum in 1969 from the same total sow population.

A further important point of interest in connexion with the trend values described in *Fig.* 22 is the coexistence of a declining rate of growth in productivity per sow, to a point where the rate of growth is certainly not better than zero, with substantial changes in the size structure of pig farming occurring during the same period. In 1960, 61 per cent of all sows and gilts in the United Kingdom were in breeding herds of less than 20 sows and gilts, while only 16 per cent of the national total were to be found in breeding herds of 50 or more. But by 1969 these proportions had changed to 42 per cent and 30 per cent respectively. Whatever may be the economic advantage of large-scale units in pig farming, higher productivity in the breeding herd does not appear to be one of them.

The conclusion to be drawn from this review is that there is an urgent need to discover the reasons for the existence of this obvious gap between precept and practice and between scientific norms and the most probable outcome under the generality of commercial farm conditions. This conclusion most likely applies not only to pigs but also to dairy cows, beef cattle, and sheep (Wragg, 1970).

REFERENCES

MITCHELL, G. F. C. (1970), *Farmers' Factual Beliefs and Values related to the Acceptance of Approved Practices in Pig-keeping.* Agricultural Economics Research Unit. Bristol University.

WRAGG, S. R. (1970), *J. agric. Econ.*, **21**, 85.

PLATE VIII

LIPIDOSES AND LEUCODYSTROPHIES

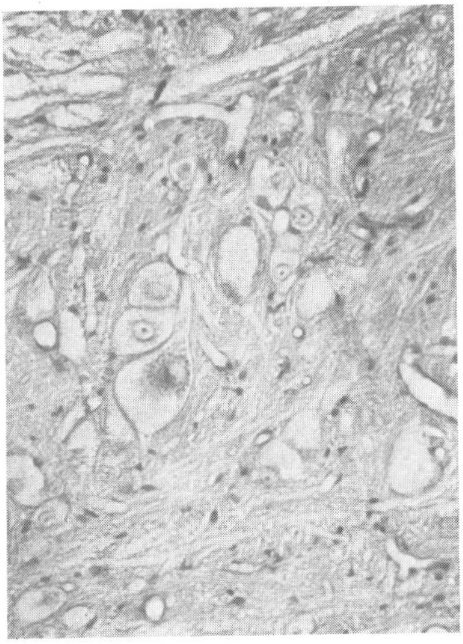

Fig. A.

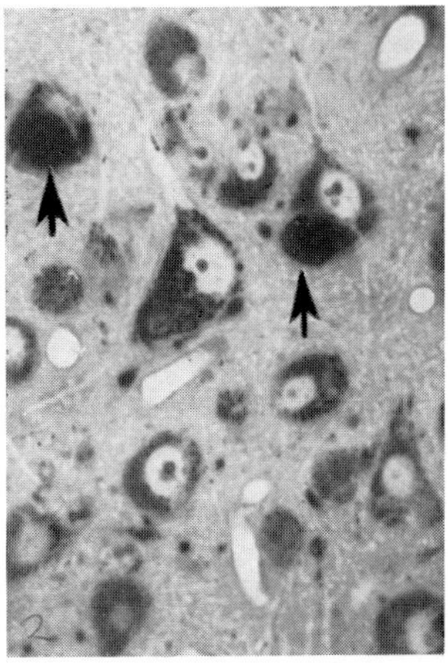

Fig. B.

Fig. A.—GM_1 gangliosidosis. Vacuolated nerve cells in the reticular formation. The lipid has been lost during dehydration. Paraffin section, PAS—haematoxylin. (×400.)

Fig. B.—GM_1 gangliosidosis. Neurons in the cerebral cortex full of stained inclusions; the large inclusions (arrowed) are in glial cells. Toluidine blue, Araldite section. (×900.)

PLATE IX

LIPIDOSES AND LEUCODYSTROPHIES—*continued*

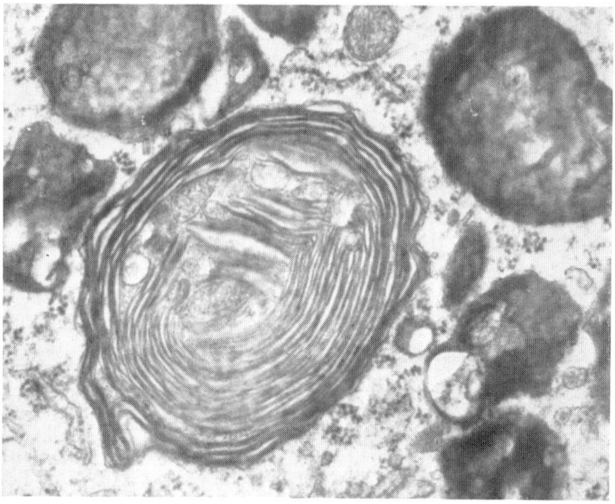

Fig. C.—GM_1 gangliosidosis. Electron micrograph of neuronal membranous cytoplasmic bodies. (×33,000.)

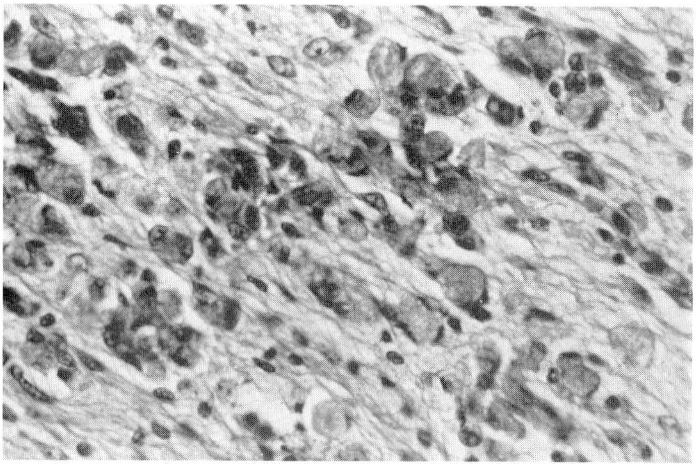

Fig. D.—Collections of globoid cells in cerebral white matter from dog affected with Krabbe-type leucodystrophy. H. and E. (×275.)

CEREBRAL LIPIDOSES AND LEUCODYSTROPHIES IN ANIMALS

W. F. Blakemore, M.A., Ph.D., B.V.Sc., M.R.C.V.S., and A. C. Palmer, M.A., Ph.D., F.R.C.V.S.

Infectious diseases of the nervous system of animals command attention for economic and zoonotic reasons, but as veterinary neurology develops it becomes plain that there is a variety of other conditions affecting the nervous system, some of which are brought about by defective metabolism. Amongst these are the disorders of lipid metabolism, the lipidoses and leucodystrophies, conditions characterized by progressive degeneration of neural tissue and accumulation of adventitious material within lysosomes. In cerebral lipidoses, often referred to as 'amaurotic familial idiocies', degeneration and storage primarily involve neurons, while in the leucodystrophies involvement of white matter is more prominent.

The stored material accumulates because a deficiency of a particular acid hydrolase halts its breakdown. Thus in GM_1 gangliosidosis, GM_1 ganglioside accumulates in neurons as the result of a deficiency of β-galactosidase. As lysosomal enzymes display a linkage, rather than a substrate specificity, several different substances may become stored as the result of a single enzyme deficiency. The site of storage, as well as the substance stored, reflects the metabolic and functional activity of affected tissues. Therefore deficiencies in myelin lipid catabolism are seen as the leucodystrophies (sulphatides and cerebrosides being mainly found in myelin), while lipids associated with general cell structure (the gangliosides and sphingomyelin) accumulate in the lipidoses. Likewise the involvement of the reticulo-endothelial system in many lipidoses reflects the extent to which these cells participate in lipid catabolism (Hers and Van Hoof, 1969).

Our purpose in this article is to draw attention to these diseases in animals, some of which have been reported in this country, hoping that this may lead to their early recognition and elimination. As comparable conditions affect man, the animal counterpart may offer opportunities for research into fundamental aspects of these diseases.

In man the unsatisfactory classification of lipidoses is based on clinical manifestations, morphological changes, and the chemistry of the 'stored substance'. However, a start has been made in characterizing these conditions on the basis of the specific enzyme abnormalities present. This is leading to a more comprehensible classification; a comparable development has not yet been achieved in comparative studies. Some of the major human lipidoses and leucodystrophies are listed in *Table I.* Most conditions have one or more variant, thus non-cerebral Gaucher's disease and Niemann-Pick's disease have been described. In addition, each may manifest itself at different ages; therefore, infantile, juvenile, and adult types may be recognized.

Lipidoses

Only a limited number of lipidoses have been reported in the veterinary literature.

Table I.—Major Human Lipidoses and Leucodystrophies

	Predominant Substance stored in the Brain	Enzyme Deficiency in Man	Visceral Involvement	Disease in Animals
Niemann-Pick's	Sphingomyelin	Sphingomyelinase	Severe	Cat
Gaucher's disease	Glucocerebroside	Glucocerebrosidase	Severe; reticulo-endothelial system	Sheep (visceral only)
GM_1 gangliosidosis	GM_1 ganglioside	β-Galactosidase	May be severe; polysaccharide storage	Cat
GM_2 gangliosidosis	GM_2 ganglioside	Hexosaminidase A	Little involvement	Dog, cat ?, pig
Gargoylism	Glycolipids		Severe; polysaccharide storage	None
Ceroid lipofuscinosis	Ceroid or lipofuscin		Not severe	Dog, cattle
Globoid or Krabbe's leucodystrophy	Cerebroside	β-Galactocerebrosidase	None	Dog
Metachromatic leucodystrophy	Sulphatide	Arylsulphatase A	None	Mink

GM_1 Gangliosidosis

The condition known as 'GM_1 gangliosidosis' (Suzuki, Suzuki, and Kamosita, 1969) or 'generalized gangliosidosis' in man (O'Brien, 1969) has been seen in a cross-bred cat by one of us (Blakemore, 1972). The cat was seen when 3 months old. It was smaller than its litter mates and showed signs of dullness and inactivity, and motor deficiency (ataxia and tremor). On post-mortem examination the only abnormality was an enlarged and pale liver. Histologically, neurons throughout the central nervous system contained glycolipid inclusions (*Plate VIII*). Liver hepatocytes contained glycolipid inclusions and were vacuolated due to storage of an extremely labile unidentified substance—probably a polysaccharide. Electron microscopy showed neurons and glia to contain membranous cytoplasmic bodies (*Plate IX, Fig. C*) typical of ganglioside storage conditions (Terry and Weiss, 1963; Aleu, Terry and Zellweger, 1965; Gonatas and Gonatas, 1965). An excess of GM_1 ganglioside was demonstrated in the brain and liver by thin-layer chromatography. Excess ceramide tetrahexoside was also demonstrated in cerebral tissue.

GM_2 Gangliosidosis

A disease resembling Tay-Sachs disease in man, in which there is cerebral accumulation of GM_2 ganglioside, has been reported in the German short-haired Pointer by several workers (Karbe and Schiefer, 1967; McGrath, Kelly, and Steinberg, 1968; Bernheimer and Karbe, 1970; Gambetti, Kelly, and Steinberg, 1970). The condition is usually first noticed at about 6 months of age when signs of mental deterioration and auditory and visual deficiencies are seen. With time motor signs develop, and as the disease progresses seizures may be seen. Death occurs 6–12 months after the onset of signs. Thin-layer chromatography of cerebral tissue (Bernheimer and Karbe, 1970; Gambetti and others, 1970) show an increase of GM_1 ganglioside.

Other Gangliosidoses

Two further examples of gangliosidoses have been reported, but in each the exact type of ganglioside was not characterized. Read and Bridges (1968) reported a ganglioside-storage condition in Yorkshire swine, and Kuruhara and Mochizuki (1969) reported a similar condition in a line of Siamese cats. Neither of these groups of workers demonstrated visceral storage. Both diseases were seen in young animals and could be further examples of GM_2 gangliosidosis.

Sphingomyelin Storage (Niemann-Pick's disease)

Chrisp and others (1970) documented a case of sphingomyelin storage in a Siamese cat. The animal presented at 6 months of age with a history of retarded growth and decreased appetite. It showed no nervous signs at 3 months of age, but on examination there was a coarse tremor of the head and trunk, hypermetria, and ataxia. Nervous signs progressed over the next 3 months and the animal was killed; no fits were reported. No gross pathological changes were seen, but on histological examination vacuolated nerve cells were present in the central and autonomic nervous systems. Reticulo-endothelial cells throughout the body were also swollen and vacuolated as were the hepatocytes. Thin-layer chromatography indicated an increase in sphingomyelin and gas chromatography showed an increase in 16:0 and 24:1 fatty acids. These findings are similar to those found in a case of human Niemann-Pick's disease analysed by these workers.

Neuronal Ceroid Lipofuscinosis

In man the neuronal ceroid lipofuscinoses form a group of conditions linked by the common finding of neuronal storage of ceroid or lipofuscin. A similar condition in the dog has been extensively studied in the English Setter by Koppang (1966, 1970) and by Bernheimer and Karbe (1970). Affected dogs show no specific signs up to 12 months of age; from 12 to 15 months there is reduced vision and dullness and by 15–18 months vision and hearing are often severely affected. The animals become stiff, ataxic, and develop muscular spasms which become generalized. The animals are debilitated due to feeding difficulties and often die by 2 years of age. Although signs of defective vision are apparent, the pupilloconstriction reflex is present until the terminal stages. Little can be seen at necropsy, but histological examination reveals storage of ceroid and/or lipofuscin in both central and autonomic neurons. The ultrastructural appearance of the stored material is similar to that seen in the condition in man (Duffy, Kornfeld, and Suzuki, 1968; Gonatas, Gambetti, and Baird, 1968). Biochemical studies of Bernheimer and Karbe (1970) revealed no specific abnormality in the lipid content of the brain.

A case of ceroid lipofuscinosis has been reported in the Beefmaster breed of cattle by Read and Bridges (1969). The time course of the disease and the onset of neurological signs at 12 months of age, together with a progression over 6 months, are similar to those seen in the dog. The histological findings are also similar.

Gaucher's Disease

No case of cerebral Gaucher's disease has been reported in the veterinary literature, but Laws and Saal (1968) have reported a case of visceral Gaucher's disease in the sheep. The liver was the only organ examined. It was of normal size but contained light-grey areas, up to 5 mm. in size, evenly distributed throughout the organ, and on histological examination these areas contained typical Gaucher cells.

Gargoylism

Gargoylism in man comprises a complex of conditions in which there is a disorder of polysaccharide metabolism. This manifests itself in skeletal malformations and visceral storage of mucopolysaccharide. In some cases there is cerebral storage of ganglioside. No cases have been reported in the veterinary literature.

Undefined Lipidoses

Three other dogs with lipidosis have been described (Ribelin and Kintner, 1956; Fankhauser, 1965), but the reports contain insufficient data to make comparisons with the known lipidoses. It is of interest that they all involve Cocker Spaniels or dogs with Cocker Spaniel blood.

Pseudolipidoses

The condition reported in the literature as 'pseudolipidosis', because of its histological resemblance to the lipidoses (Whittem and Walker, 1957), has recently been shown to be the result of an absolute deficiency of α-mannosidase (Jolly, 1971). This disease occurs in Aberdeen Angus cattle and is inherited as a recessive. Jolly and his co-worker have demonstrated a lower level of α-mannosidase in heterozygotes. As there is no abnormality of lipid metabolism it should no longer be classed with the lipidoses, and the term 'pseudolipidosis' should be dropped.

Diagnosis of Lipidoses

These are all rare, progressive encephalopathies of young animals. The age of onset of the disease is dependent on the type or its variant. Clinical signs usually progress for 6–12 months, the rate of deterioration being related to the age of onset; a more fulminating disease may be seen in younger animals. In young animals, retarded growth is a consistent feature. At all ages, affected animals show signs of progressive mental, motor, and sensory deficiency. If there is a visceral involvement (e.g., GM_1 gangliosidosis, Gaucher's disease) this may be manifested by non-neurological signs (e.g., hepatomegaly, lymphadenopathy, or skeletal changes). It should be stressed that considerable variation exists within each specific lipidosis, particularly with regard to the age of onset and the speed of progression of the clinical signs.

Diagnosis of the lipidoses depends on demonstrating the presence of the specific stored material, the products of defective metabolism, or, when this is known, an enzyme deficiency. Thus in man urine analysis is used to detect excess urinary sulphated mucopolysaccharide in gargoylism and excess sulphatide in metachromatic leucodystrophy. In lipidoses blood smears may be examined for vacuolated cells and lymph-node or bone-marrow biopsies are useful in the diagnosis of lipidoses which involve the reticulo-endothelial system, such as Niemann-Pick's and Gaucher's disease. When the autonomic nervous system is involved, as is seen in some but not all cases of lipidoses, a rectal biopsy may be examined for neuronal storage in the cells of Meissner's plexus. Examination of cerebral biopsies by chemical and histological methods probably offers the most reliable method for differentiating the lipidoses. At death all cases of cerebral lipidoses should be examined histopathologically and fresh tissue taken, and stored at −20° C. for chemical and enzyme assays. The detection of the specific enzyme abnormality underlying these conditions is of the utmost importance, because until these are known a satisfactory classification cannot be made.

Leucodystrophies

Of the four types of human leucodystrophy only two have been reported in animals. Globoid cell leucodystrophy (Krabbe's disease) in the dog was first described by Fankhauser, Luginbühl, and Hartley (1963); metachromatic leucodystrophy in mink was extensively documented by Andersen and Palludan (1968).

The original report on leucodystrophy in the dog concerned a West Highland bitch and a dog of uncertain breeding. Since that time there have been a number of papers from the United States indicating that the disease affects essentially the West Highland and Cairn Terrier breeds (Fletcher, Kurtz, and Low, 1966; Hirth and Nielsen, 1967; Austin, Armstrong, and Margolis, 1968; Jortner and Jonas, 1968; McGrath and others, 1969; Fletcher, 1970; Kurtz and Fletcher, 1970; Suzuki and others, 1970). Although these are British breeds of dog the first 2 cases in this country were not reported until 1972 by Howell and Palmer.

Clinical signs of leucodystrophy in the dog are usually noticed by 3–6 months of age although incoordination may be present as early as 6 weeks, perhaps described by the owner as stiffness. Both sexes are affected and in the animals reported from North America several of the groups were related and there was obviously a familial component. Hindlegs become progressively weak; there may be blindness, nystagmus, and tremor. Usually the animals die within 3 months of onset of the disease. Electro-encephalographic recordings were reported by Fletcher (1970), who considers that the abnormalities (generalized cerebral hemisphere asymmetry, asymmetrical spindling and spiking, excessive high voltage–low frequency activity, decrement of E.E.G. arousal to sound stimuli) are of diagnostic value in the early stage of the disease because they indicate cerebral involvement at a time when the clinical signs suggest cerebellar and spinal cord involvement only.

Pathologically, changes are present in the central and peripheral nervous systems. In the brain accumulations of globoid cells occur, particularly associated with blood-vessels, in the white matter or the cerebrum, cerebellum, brain-stem, and spinal cord (*Plate IX*, *Fig. D*). The cells are found densely gathered in the more dorsal parts of the cerebrum and cerebellum, whereas in the brain-stem and spinal cord collections occur at the peripheral margin. In appearance the globoid cells bear resemblance to lipid phagocytes, but may contain two to five nuclei and their contents do not stain positively for lipid but give a positive periodic acid-Schiff reaction. Myelin depletion occurs in areas with large populations of globoid cells. A neuropathy was reported by Kurtz and Fletcher (1970) to affect a number of peripheral nerves and some cranial nerves (II, V) and there was evidence of muscle atrophy. Chromatolysis of motor nuclei could not be found in either the brain or spinal cord by Howell and Palmer (1972).

Biochemical analysis has shown that the globoid cells probably contain cerebroside-bound protein. Affected white matter from human cases has a low lipid content and a cerebroside : sulphatide ratio higher than that of normal brain. A similar elevation has been shown to occur in the dog by McGrath and others (1969) and Howell and Palmer (1972) and also by Suzuki and others (1969, 1970) who reported a β-galactocerebrosidase deficiency in affected dogs as well as a slightly low value in an apparently healthy litter mate (perhaps a heterozygote carrier). β-Galactocerebrosidase deficiency also occurs in the human disease and Suzuki and colleagues point out that the canine disorder is an authentic enzyme model and not a facsimile of the human condition. The lowered β-galactocerebrosidase activity in the dogs occurred not only in the brain but also in the liver and kidney.

Although Howell and Palmer were unable to show a familial connexion in their 2 cases, Suzuki and colleagues presented evidence that the disease is inherited as an autosomal recessive. There can be little doubt that leucodystrophy in the Cairn and West Highland Terriers is more prevalent in this country than the 2 reported cases would indicate. Progressive paralysis of the hindlegs in puppies of these breeds should be sufficient to arouse suspicions of the disease: confirmation can be obtained by cerebral biopsy.

Eradication

Most of the lipidoses and leucodystrophies are inherited by means of recessive genes and the detection of heterozygotes is therefore important. When the specific enzyme derangement has been established, it is possible to detect heterozygotes because they usually show similar but less severe abnormalities. Once the heterozygotes are identified, selective breeding should eradicate the condition.

REFERENCES

Aleu, I. P., Terry, R. D., and Zellweger, H. (1965), *J. Neuropath. exp. Neurol.*, **24**, 304.

Andersen, H. A., and Palludan, B. (1968), *Acta Neuropath.*, **11**, 347.

Austin, J., Armstrong, D., and Margolis, G. (1968), *Trans. Am. neurol. Ass.*, **93**, 181.

Bernheimer, H., and Karbe, E. (1970), *Acta Neuropath.*, **16**, 304.

Blakemore, W. F. (1972), *J. comp. Path. Ther.*, in the press.

Chrisp, C. E., Ringler, D. H., Abrams, G. D., Radin, N. S., and Boenkert, A. (1970), *J. Am. vet. med. Ass.*, **156**, 616.

Duffy, P. E., Kornfeld, M., and Suzuki, K. (1968), *J. Neuropath. exp. Neurol.*, **27**, 351.

Fankhauser, R. (1965), *Schweiz. Arch. Tierheilk.*, **107**, 73.

— — Luginbühl, H., and Hartley, W. J. (1963), *Ibid.*, **105**, 198.

Fletcher, T. F. (1970), *J. Am. vet. med. Ass.*, **157**, 190.

— — Kurtz, H. J., and Low, D. G. (1966), *Ibid.*, **149**, 165.

Gambetti, L. A., Kelly, A. M., and Steinberg, S. A. (1970), *J. Neuropath. exp. Neurol.*, **29**, 137.

Gonatas, N. K., Gambetti, P., and Baird, H. (1968), *Ibid.*, **27**, 371.

— — and Gonatas, J. (1965), *Ibid.*, **24**, 318.

Hers, H. G., and Van Hoof, F. (1969), in *Lysosomes in Biology and Pathology* (ed. Dingle, S. T., and Fell, H. B.), Vol. 2, p. 19. *Frontiers of Biology*, Vol. 14B. Amsterdam: North Holland.

Hirth, R. S., and Nielsen, S. W. (1967), *J. small Anim. Pract.*, **8**, 569.

Howell, J. McC., and Palmer, A. C. (1972), *Ibid.*, in the press.

Jolly, R. D. (1971), personal communication.

Jortner, B. S., and Jonas, A. M. (1968), *Acta Neuropath.*, **10**, 171.

Karbe, E., and Schiefer, B. (1967), *Path. vet.*, **4**, 223.

Koppang, N. (1966), *Ergebn. allg. Path. path. Anat.*, **47**, 1.

— — (1970), *J. small Anim. Pract.*, **10**, 639.

Kurtz, H. J., and Fletcher, T. F. (1970), *Acta Neuropath.*, **16**, 226.

Kuruhara, Y., and Mochizuki, H. (1969), *Adv. neurol. Sci., Tokyo*, **13**, 268.

LAWS, L., and SAAL, J. R. (1968), *Aust. vet. J.*, **44**, 416.
MCGRATH, J. T., KELLY, A. M., and STEINBERG, S. A. (1968), *J. Neuropath. exp. Neurol.*, **27**, 1414.
— — SCHUTTA, H., YASEEN, A., and STEINBERG, S. A. (1969), *Ibid.*, **28**, 171.
O'BRIEN, J. (1969), *J. Pediat.*, **75**, 167.
READ, W. K., and BRIDGES, C. H. (1968), *Path. vet.*, **5**, 67.
— — — — (1969), *Ibid.*, **6**, 235.
RIBELIN, W. E., and KINTNER, L. D. (1956), *Cornell Vet.*, **46**, 532.
SUZUKI, Y., AUSTIN, J., ARMSTRONG, D., SUZUKI, K., SCHLENKER, J., and FLETCHER, T. (1970), *Expl Neurol.*, **29**, 65.
— — SUZUKI, K., and KAMOSITA, S. (1969), *J. Neuropath. exp. Neurol.*, **28**, 25.
TERRY, R. D., and WEISS, M. (1963), *Ibid.*, **22**, 18.
WHITTEM, J. H., and WALKER, D. (1957), *J. Path. Bact.*, **74**, 281.

REVIEW OF THE CURRENT LITERATURE

DISEASES RELATED TO VIRUSES

G. R. Scott, B.Sc., M.S., Ph.D., M.R.C.V.S.

DISEASES RELATED TO VIRUSES

DIFFERENTIATION OF VIRAL DISEASES OF HORSES

G. R. Scott, B.Sc., M.S., Ph.D., M.R.C.V.S.

In a paper read at a meeting of the British Equine Veterinary Association in 1970 I listed 58 viruses known to infect horses and I predicted that every year more would be added to the list (Scott, 1971). Today, less than 12 months later, amendments and additions have raised the total to nearly 80; a precise count is impossible because viral taxonomy is in a state of flux and, moreover, the viral aetiology of some of the infections has yet to be confirmed.

Some 30–40 of the viruses cause disease in horses. Most of the other viruses are incriminated serologically and many of these are arthropod-borne viruses. Others probably cause disease, for example para-influenza-1 and para-influenza-2. Currently a plethora of herpesviruses isolated from healthy horses and equine tissues is causing taxonomic embarrassment; some are classic herpesviruses, others are cytomegaloviruses, and the rest form a heterogeneous group sharing properties with both the classic herpesviruses and cytomegaloviruses (Erasmus, 1970).

A few viruses known from antibody surveys to infect horses have provoked disease when injected parenterally into horses; for example Calovo virus (Bardos, 1967), Murray Valley encephalitis virus (Miles, 1952), St. Louis encephalitis virus (Ferguson, 1954), and Wesselbron virus (Weiss, Haig, and Alexander, 1956). In addition, Mucambo virus, an arthropod-borne virus related to Venezuelan encephalitis virus but which has not, to date, been incriminated as infecting horses naturally, induced fever, leucopenia, and antibodies when injected into a horse (Shope and others, 1964). On the other hand, Tahyna virus, which commonly infects horses in Czecho-Slovakia, does not induce disease when injected into susceptible foals (Bardos, Cupkova, and Jakubik, 1965).

Differentiation of viral diseases of horses is not easy; often, it is impossible. Nevertheless, there are several epidemiological, clinical, and pathological features that help to narrow the range of possibilities (*Fig.* 23).

Transmission and Geographical Distribution

Viruses are transmitted either by contact or by vectors (*Table I*). The distribution of the contagions is world-wide whereas that of the vector-borne infections is restricted to areas where suitable vectors exist. A key factor in the distribution and spread of the viral contagions is the high volume of the intercontinental traffic in horses. A new serotype of influenza A, for example, emerged in Florida in 1963 and caused havoc among horses in the United States of America (Waddell, Teigland, and Sigel, 1963). It was designated Influenza A/Equi 2/Miami 1/63. The virus spread to horses in South America in 1963 (Vallone, Somma, and Tosi, 1964) and to France in 1964 (Brion and others, 1966). Thereafter it spread rapidly in the spring of 1965 throughout Europe disrupting the racing industry (Beveridge, Mahaffey, and Rose, 1965).

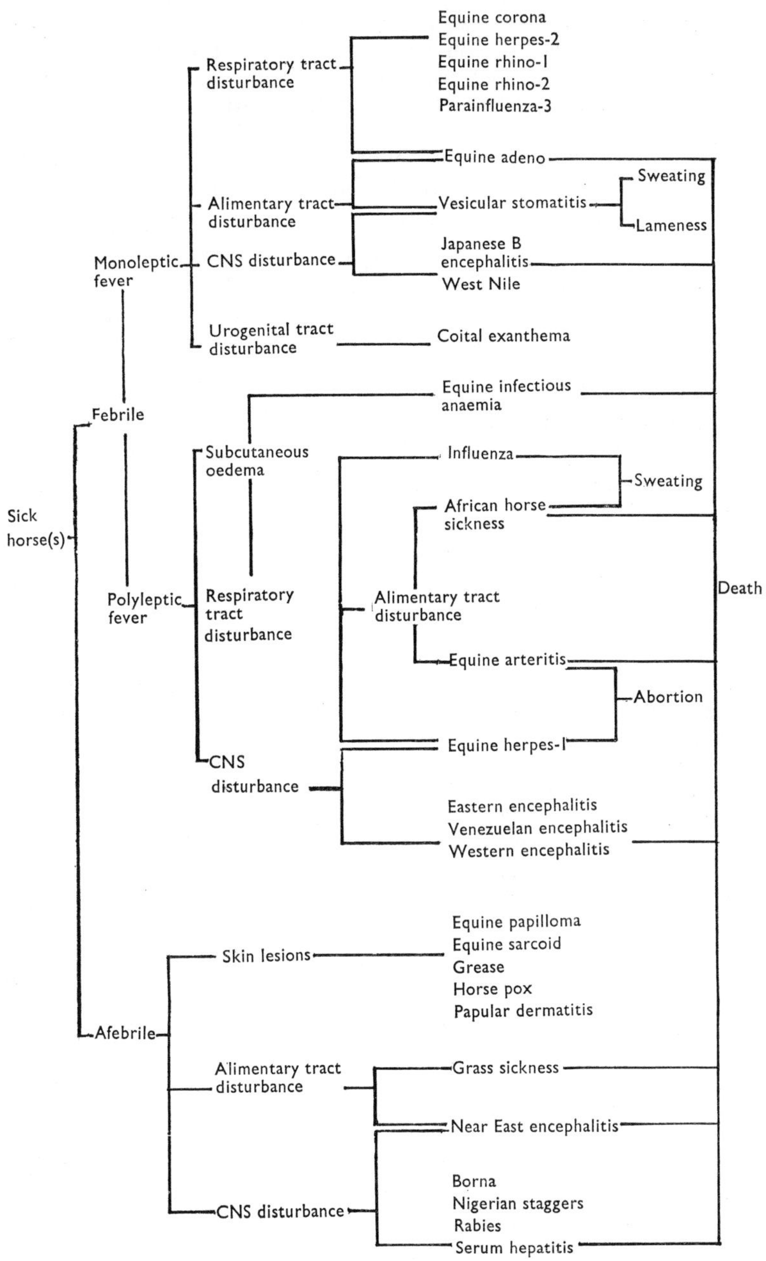

Fig. 23.—Flow diagram differentiating the viral diseases of horses.

The geographical boundaries of the vector-transmitted viruses are not static; for example, Venezuelan encephalitis, a mosquito-borne virus, is spreading northwards from its locus in northern South America through Central America and into the southern states of North America (Work, 1964). Similarly, West Nile, another mosquito-borne virus, has spread out of Africa and has established itself in the horse population of the Camargue, the delta of the Rhône in the south of France (Joubert and others, 1970).

Table I.—MODE OF TRANSMISSION OF VIRUSES THAT INDUCE DISEASES IN HORSES

Contagious	*Vector-borne*	*Unknown*
Coital exanthema	African horse sickness	Aborted foal
Equine adeno	Eastern encephalitis	Borna
Equine arteritis	Japanese B encephalitis	Grass sickness
Equine corona	Near East encephalitis	Serum hepatitis
Equine herpes-1	Nigerian staggers	Vesicular stomatitis, New Jersey
Equine herpes-2	Rabies	Virus diarrhoea
Equine infectious anaemia	Venezuelan encephalitis	
Equine papilloma	Vesicular stomatitis, Indiana	
Equine rhino-1	West Nile	
Equine rhino-2	Western encephalitis	
Equine sarcoid		
Grease		
Horse pox		
Influenza-A		
Influenza-B		
Influenza-C		
Papular dermatitis		
Para-influenza-3		

Periodically the occurrence of abnormal meteorological conditions favouring the spread and survival of vectors enables an arthropod-borne virus to spill out of its enzootic focus. African horse sickness virus, for example, spread into Aden in 1906, Yemen in 1930, North Africa and the Middle East and the Indian subcontinent in 1959, North Africa in 1965, and thence into Spain in 1966 (Stellmann and others, 1967; Chalmers, 1968). The epizootics temporarily devastated the horse populations of the invaded countries but new enzootic foci were not established.

Morbidity Rate

Outbreaks of viral contagions occur at any season of the year, are linked to animal movements, and are characterized by high morbidity rates. There are three apparent exceptions; coital exanthema, equine arteritis, and equine herpes-1 or rhinopneumonitis. The regular seasonal occurrence of these three infections is a managemental artefact which stems from the need of the racing industry to age horses as from an arbitrary date.

Diseases caused by arthropod-borne viruses tend to be seasonal and sporadic, being governed by vector behaviour. Thus increased humidity stimulates insect activity such that the 'horse sickness year' in South Africa begins in February and in the Sudan in May. When the 'rains' are late the advent of horse sickness is delayed (Henning, 1956). Some arthropods have a seasonal pattern of host preference; for example, in the U.S.A. *Culex tarsalis* feeds primarily on birds in the spring, but in the summer it feeds increasingly upon mammals and the incidence of Western encephalitis in horses rises accordingly (Hess and Hayes, 1967).

Most of the infections induced by most arthropod-borne viruses in horses are inapparent. Often the horse is a true natural host which has evolved an equilibrium with the virus to the mutual advantage of both. An example is St. Louis encephalitis virus which causes disease in man but circulates harmlessly in mosquitoes, birds, and horses (Razenhofer and others, 1957). The sporadic character of the arthropod-borne diseases stems from the accidental nature of the infections; the horse is not the natural host and the resulting infection is often a 'dead-end' so far as survival of the virus as a species is concerned. At least one arthropod-borne virus, Venezuelan encephalitis virus, can also spread by contact between sick and healthy horses and so confound the sporadic incidence of the infection (Kissling and others, 1956).

The age of the host influences the morbidity rate. The viral abortions and coital exanthema obviously affect mature horses. Most of the viral contagions, however, attack immature horses because their world-wide prevalence is such that immature horses are the only animals at risk; the adults are immune from earlier infection or vaccination and the suckling foals are protected passively. The age incidence of equine papillomatosis, on the other hand, appears to be governed by innate resistance; the disease only affects horses up to 3 years of age (Cook and Olson, 1951). Equine sarcoid virus, however, affects horses aged from 6 months (Ragland, Keown, and Gorham, 1966) to 20 years (Olson, 1963).

The virulence of the strain of virus influences the morbidity rate. The equi-1 strain of influenza-A, for example, provokes a much milder disease than the equi-2 strain (Waddell and others, 1963). Similarly marked variations exist among wild strains of African horse sickness virus in their virulence for horses (Howell, 1963).

Incubation Period

Incubation periods of equine viral diseases may be short, moderate, or long; most are less than 10 days but those of the American and Japanese encephalitides range from 1 to 3 weeks, that of Borna disease is at least 4 weeks, and those of equine papillomatosis, equine sarcoid, equine serum hepatitis, and rabies are measured in months. The most variable is that of equine infectious anaemia; it is usually 12–15 days but it can vary from 4 days to 3 months or longer (Stein, 1963). The incubation periods of a few of the diseases are unknown, namely, aborted foal virus, grass sickness, Near East encephalitis, and Nigerian staggers. Two viruses, equine arteritis virus and equine herpes-1 or rhinopneumonitis virus, induce respiratory signs in non-pregnant animals and abortions in pregnant mares. The incubation periods of both respiratory syndromes last only a few days, but there is a significant difference of differential diagnostic import in the periods between infection and abortion; abortion induced by arteritis virus occurs 12–30 days after infection (Doll and others, 1957) whereas that caused by rhinopneumonitis virus occurs 1–4 months after infection (Dimock and Edwards, 1936).

Duration of Illness

Most illnesses induced by viruses in horses are transient, recovery or death occurring 2–3 weeks after the onset of illness. An exception is equine serum hepatitis which is usually manifested as a peracute illness that terminates within 48 hours (Marsh, 1937). A few viral infections have peracute, acute, and chronic courses; the pulmonary form of African horse sickness, for example, is a peracute manifestation which often terminates fatally within 12 hours whereas the cardiac form is an acute illness lasting approximately 2 weeks (Howell, 1963). Similarly, grass sickness may be peracute with death within hours of the onset, acute with death after 1 week, or chronic with ill-health persisting for weeks (Boddie, 1966). Hyperacute cases of Near East encephalitis die within 48 hours, acute cases last for 6 or 7 days, and chronic cases survive for several months (Daubney and Mahlau, 1967). In equine infectious anaemia the course of the acute syndrome ranges from 5 to 20 days, whereas the course of the chronic syndrome lasts for weeks (Gainer and others, 1965). Virus diarrhoea also may be acute or chronic (Rooney, 1969).

Two virus diseases of horses have protracted courses; lesions of equine papillomatosis persist for up to 18 months and those of equine sarcoid last for up to 8 months (Olson, 1963).

The virus of at least one infection, equine infectious anaemia, often, but not always, persists for the life of the animal (Gainer and others, 1965) and acute fatal relapses have been observed (Lemetayer, 1949). There is also some evidence that equine herpesviruses persist in horses as latent infections (Burrows, 1970). Rhinovirus is harboured in pharyngeal tissues for at least 1 month after infection and can be recovered from the faeces (Plummer and Kerry, 1962).

Fever

All but 11 of the virus diseases of horses are febrile (*Table II*). Monoleptic fevers tend to be low grade and transient. Polyleptic fevers, on the other

Table II.—EQUINE VIRUS FEVERS

Afebrile	*Monoleptic Fever*	*Polyleptic Fever*
Borna	Coital exanthema	African horse sickness
Equine papilloma	Equine adeno	Eastern encephalitis
Equine sarcoid	Equine corona	Equine arteritis
Grass sickness	Equine herpes-2	Equine herpes-1
Grease	Equine rhino	Equine infectious anaemia
Horse pox	Japanese B encephalitis	Influenza
Near East encephalitis	Para-influenza-3	Venezuelan encephalitis
Nigerian staggers	Vesicular stomatitis	Western encephalitis
Papular dermatitis	West Nile	
Rabies		
Serum hepatitis		

hand, often exhibit peaks of 106° F. The first wave of a polyleptic fever is frequently prodromal; in infections with Eastern encephalitis virus, for example, overt clinical signs are delayed until the second febrile wave begins (Byrne and others, 1964).

Sweating

Sweating, often patchy, occurs in horses infected with African horse sickness, grass sickness, influenza-B, and vesicular stomatitis. It is profuse in cases of serum hepatitis.

Skin Lesions

Five viruses cause skin lesions in horses and they are readily differentiated. Grease is a pox affecting the lower limbs and it is first manifested as vesicles which rapidly turn into confluent crust-covered pustules. The pocks of horse pox, on the other hand, are limited to the muzzle, lips, gums, and cheek mucosa. Papular dermatitis is probably also a pox, but vesicles and pustules are not manifest and instead multiple, firm papules up to 0·5 cm. in diameter develop in the skin on any body site. The papules become encrusted within 7 days and persist for 10–40 days (McIntyre, 1949). Equine papilloma virus forms small horny warts on the skin around the lips and muzzle of young horses. Equine sarcoids are locally aggressive fibroblastic tumours of the skin. They are often multiple and can spread to secondary sites.

Mucosal Lesions

Five viruses induce mucosal lesions in addition to the congestion attendant upon fever. Vesicular stomatitis, as the name implies, is characterized by the development of vesicles on the lips, gums and tongue. The vesicles often coalesce and rupture quickly leaving red ulcers that always stimulate a profuse flow of saliva. On occasions, the only pocks present in cases of horse pox are on the gums and buccal mucosa. Petechiae stud mucosal surfaces in African horse sickness and equine infectious anaemia.

Equine coital exanthema has been known as a venereal plague for at least 150 years. In European horses the exanthema is characterized more by papules than by vesicles, whereas in Australian horses the lesions progress from vesicles to ulcers. Differing serotypes of equine herpesviruses explain the difference; the German isolate has a relationship with equine herpes-1 (Petzoldt, 1970) but the Australian virus has not (Pascoe, Spradbrow, and Bagust, 1969).

Subcutaneous Oedema

Subcutaneous odema is a prominent feature of the cardiac form of African horse sickness. It first involves the temporal fossae and then the intermandibular space. When, on occasion, the oedema extends to the throat, brisket, and forelegs, the head and neck appear strikingly smooth and round.

Dependent oedema occurs in horses infected with equine infectious anaemia and influenza-A viruses and, less often, with equine herpes-1 virus. It is also a feature of equine arteritis. Palpebral oedema, however, is the significant lesion in equine arteritis.

Lameness

One virus, vesicular stomatitis virus, lames horses. Vesicles developing on the coronary band coalesce and rupture forming deep, bleeding ulcers. Separation of the hoof wall may follow.

Respiratory Illness

The commonest clinical syndrome in virus-infected horses is respiratory illness, the commonest lesion rhinitis in association with conjunctivitis (*Table III*). The infections are difficult to differentiate hence the confusing terminology based on clinical or epidemiological features; catarrhal fever, contagious pleuropneumona, epizootic cough, infectious bronchitis, influenza, pink-eye, rhinopneumonitis, stable fever, shipping fever, summer snots, typhoid fever, etc. The nasal discharge is usually serous, clear, and transitory but it may become mucopurulent because of secondary bacterial invaders. It may be copious as in equine rhinovirus infections or frothy as in African horse sickness. Rhinitis is not a feature of acute grass sickness but, at intervals, green gastric fluid is regurgitated through the nostrils. Lacrimation is most dramatic in equine arteritis.

Table III.—Virus-induced Respiratory Illness

Rhinitis	*Coughing*	*Pneumonia*
African horse sickness	African horse sickness	African horse sickness
Borna	Equine corona	Equine adeno
Equine adeno	Equine herpes-2	Equine arteritis
Equine arteritis	Influenza-A	Influenza-A
Equine corona	Para-influenza-3	
Equine herpes-1		
Equine herpes-2		
Equine rhino-1		
Equine rhino-2		
Influenza-A		
Influenza-B		
Influenza-C		
Para-influenza-3		

A frequent dry, harsh cough is the most common symptom of equine influenza. Coughing also commonly occurs in African horse sickness, coronavirus, herpes-2, and para-influenza-3 infections. It occurs occasionally in herpes-1 infection.

Severe pharyngitis is a common lesion in horses infected with rhinoviruses.

Pneumonia is a feature of equine adenovirus and equine arteritis virus infections and can occur in influenza-A infection particularly when the equi-2 strain is involved. Pulmonary oedema is a characteristic of African horse sickness and influenza-A infection.

Encephalitis

The second commonest clinical syndrome in virus-infected horses is disturbance of the central nervous system. All but two of the viruses, equine herpes-1 and equine serum hepatitis, are exotic to Great Britain. Nevertheless, even in Great Britain, the possibility of rabies must always be entertained when equine encephalitis is encountered. Elsewhere rabies in horses is probably more prevalent than present reports indicate; rabies virus, for example, was isolated from 14 out of 79 cases diagnosed as equine encephalitis in Egypt and yet there had been no reports of equine rabies in the previous 25 years (Badiali and others, 1967).

Equine serum hepatitis is manifested suddenly by hyperexcitability, impaired vision, muscular tremors, and profuse sweating. Usually there is no prostration and horses die on their feet.

Serious nervous symptoms probably complicate equine herpes-1 infections more commonly than records indicate (Saxegaard, 1966). Affected animals suffer from posterior paralysis and usually have to be destroyed.

Gastro-enteritis

Colic is a prodromal symptom of Near East encephalitis and a common feature of African horse sickness and equine arteritis, but it does not occur in grass sickness despite severe intestinal impaction which results in regurgitation of the stomach contents. Diarrhoea is provoked by equine adeno, equine arteritis, and Venezuelan encephalitis viruses, and by virus diarrhoea virus. It occurs infrequently as a symptom of herpes-1 infection.

Death

Case mortality-rates are notoriously influenced by the virulences of the strains of virus involved and by the innate resistances of the hosts. In general,

9 viruses induce fulminating fatal infections, 3 kill about half the animals clinically affected, and 2 kill occasionally (*Table IV*).

Table IV.—CASE MORTALITY-RATES OF EQUINE VIRAL DISEASES

>75 *Per Cent*	10–75 *Per Cent*	<10 *Per Cent*
African horse sickness	Equine infectious anaemia	Equine arteritis
Borna	West Nile	Japanese B encephalitis
Eastern encephalitis	Western encephalitis	
Grass sickness		
Near East encephalitis		
Nigerian staggers		
Rabies		
Serum hepatitis		
Venezuelan encephalitis		

Equine adenovirus infections kill foals, but not enough is known about the prevalence of adenovirus infections to make a valid estimate of the case mortality-rate (Todd, 1969).

Abortion

Two viruses, equine arteritis and equine herpes-1, induce abortion in pregnant mares. The incidence of abortion is 50–70 per cent in arteritis infections and ranges from a few per cent to 100 per cent when herpes-1 virus is implicated. Arteritis abortion is linked to systemic illness and occurs late in the course of the fever or in the early phase of convalescence. In herpes-1 infections, on the other hand, mares abort 1–4 months after exposure.

Confirmation of a Provisional Diagnosis

Confirmation of a provisional diagnosis usually requires specialized laboratory facilities and serological reagents possessed by few investigation centres, research institutes, or universities. Clinicians, therefore, must often rely on their own skills. The greatest challenge is presented by respiratory illness, but, in the absence of confirmatory tests, it would be wise to avoid specific labels.

REFERENCES

BADIALI, L., FERRIS, D. H., ABOU-YOUSSEF, M., RADWAN, A., and HAMDY, F. (1967), *Vet. ital.*, **18**, 166.

BARDOS, V. (1967), *Catalogue of Arthropod-borne Viruses of the World* (ed. TAYLOR, R. M.), p. 385. Washington: U.S. Public Health Service,.

— — CUPKOVA, E., and JAKUBIK, J. (1965), *Acta virol.*, **9**, 555.

BEVERIDGE, W. I. B., MAHAFFEY, L. W., and ROSE, M. A. (1965), *Vet. Rec.*, **77**, 57.

BODDIE, G. F. (1966), *International Encyclopedia of Veterinary Medicine* (ed. DALLING, T., and others), p. 1183. Edinburgh: Green.

BRION, A., FONTAINE, M., FONTAINE, M. P., and MORAILLON, R. (1966), *Rec. Med. vet.*, **12**, 269.

BURROWS, R. (1970), *Equine Infectious Diseases* (ed. BRYANS, J. T., and GERBER, H.), Vol. II, p. 1. Basel: Karger.

BYRNE, R. J., FRENCH, G. R., YANCEY, F. S., GOCHENOUR, W. S., RUSSELL, P. K., RAMSBURG, H. H., BRAND, O. A., SCHEIDER, F. G., and BUESCHER, E. L. (1964), *Am. J. vet. Res.*, **25**, 24.

CHALMERS, A. W. (1968), *Equine vet. J.*, **1**, 83.

COOK, R. H., and OLSON, C. (1951), *Am. J. Path.*, **27**, 1087.

DAUBNEY, R., and MAHLAU, E. A. (1967), *Res. vet. Sci.*, **8**, 375.

DIMOCK, W. W., and EDWARDS, P. R. (1936), *Cornell Vet.*, **26**, 231.

DOLL, E. R., BRYANS, J. T., MCCOLLUM, W. H., and CROWE, M. E. W. (1957), *Cornell Vet.*, **47**, 4.
ERASMUS, B. J. (1970), *Equine Infectious Diseases* (ed. BRYANS, J. T., and GERBER, H.), Vol. II, p. 46. Basel: Karger.
FERGUSON, F. F. (1954), *Biological Factors in the Transmission of American Arthropod-borne Virus Encephalitides.* Washington: U.S. Public Health Service Monograph No. 23.
GAINER, J. H., AMSTER, R. L., HALL, KUHNS, L. J., and NELSON, S. L. (1965), *Proc. U.S. live Stk sanit. Ass.*, p. 254.
HENNING, M. W. (1956), *Animal Diseases in South Africa*, 3rd ed., p. 785. Pretoria: Central News Agency.
HESS, A. D., and HAYES, R. O. (1967), *Am. J. med. Sci.*, **253**, 333.
HOWELL, P. G. (1963), *Emerging Diseases of Animals*, p. 71. Rome: F.A.O.
JOUBERT, L., OUDAR, J., HANNOUN, C., BEYTOUT, D., CORNIOU, B., GUILLON, J. C., and PANTHIER, R. (1970), *Ann. Inst. Pasteur*, **118**, 239.
KISSLING, R. E., CHAMBERLAIN, R. W., NELSON, D. B., and STAMM, D. D. (1956), *Am. J. Hyg.*, **63**, 274.
LEMETAYER, E. (1949), *Int. Vet. Congr.*, **2**, 322.
MCINTYRE, R. W. (1949), *Am. J. vet. Res.*, **10**, 229.
MANAHAN, F. F. (1970), *Aust. vet. J.*, **46**, 231.
MARSH, H. (1937), *J. Am. vet. med. Ass.*, **91**, 88.
MILES, J. A. R. (1952), *Aust. J. exp. Biol.*, **30**, 341.
OLSON, C. (1963), in *Equine Medicine and Surgery*, 1st ed. (ed. BONE, J. F., and others), p. 119. Wheaton, Illinois: American Veterinary Publishers.
PASCOE, R. R., SPRADBROW, P. B., and BAGUST, T. J. (1969), *Aust. vet. J.*, **45**, 166.
PETZOLDT, K. (1970), *Berl. Münch. tierärztl., Wschr.*, **83**, 93.
PLUMMER, G., and KERRY, J. B. (1962), *Vet. Rec.*, **74**, 967.
RAGLAND, W. L., KEOWN, G. H., and GORHAM, J. R. (1966), *Nature, Lond.*, **210**, 1399.
RAZENHOFER, E. R., ALEXANDER, E. R., BEADLE, L. D., BERNSTEIN, A., and PICKARD, R. C. (1957), *Am. J. Hyg.*, **65**, 147.
ROONEY, J. R. (1969), quoted by MANAHAN, F. F. (1970).
SAXEGAARD, F. (1966), *Nord. VetMed.*, **18**, 504.
SCOTT, G. R. (1971), *Equine vet. J.*, **3**, 1.
SHOPE, R. E., CAUSEY, O. R., DE ANDRADE, A. H. P., and THEILER, M. (1964), *Am. J. trop. Med.*, **13**, 723.
STEIN, C. D. (1963), in *Equine Medicine and Surgery*, 1st ed. (ed. BONE, J. F., and others), p. 147. Wheaton, Illinois: American Veterinary Publishers.
STELLMANN, C., MIRCHAMSY, H., GILBERT, H., and SANTUCCI, J. (1967), *Bull. Off. int. Épizoot.*, **67**, 887.
TODD, J. D. (1969), *J. Am. vet. med. Ass.*, **155**, 387.
VALLONE, E. F., SOMMA, R. E., and TOSI, H. C. (1964), *Publnes. trimest. Centro invest. Vet. 'Miguel C. Robino'*, **2**, 12. Abstr. *Vet. Bull.* (1966), **36**, 20.
WADDELL, G. H., TEIGLAND, M. B., and SIGEL, M. M. (1963), *J. Am. vet. med. Ass.*, **143**, 587.
WEISS, K. E., HAIG, D. A., and ALEXANDER, R. A. (1956), *Onderstepoort J. vet. Res.*, **27**, 183.
WORK, T. H. (1964), *Science, N.Y.*, **145**, 270.

DISEASES RELATED TO PROTOZOA

S. B. KENDALL, B.Sc., Ph.D., M.R.C.V.S., A.R.C.S., F.I. Biol.
L. P. JOYNER, B.Sc., Ph.D., F.I.Biol.

DISEASES RELATED TO PROTOZOA

PROTOZOAL INFECTIONS OF POULTRY

S. B. Kendall, B.Sc., Ph.D., M.R.C.V.S., A.R.C.S., F.I.Biol.

Coccidiosis

A good many papers have been published on chemotherapy and these are reviewed elsewhere (p. 212). In other fields of research the main attention seems to have been concentrated on trying to induce species of *Eimeria* to develop in tissue culture and in chick embryos. Doran (1970) has been successful in following the complete development, as normally seen in the chick, of *Eimeria tenella* in cell culture. Excysted sporozoites were inoculated into chick kidney and into chick-embryo kidney monolayer cultures. Development through two schizogonous stages occurred in cell suspensions where there were few cell aggregates but if there were abundant cell aggregates, development could proceed through gametocytes to oocysts. There was better development in the chick-kidney culture than in the culture of embryo tissue. Oocysts obtained from culture were sporulated and later proved infective to chickens.

Work of this type may be designed to offer the opportunity of more precise observations on the different developmental stages of the parasite and the factors which influence their appearance. There is the possibility also of devising new models for the standardized screening of drugs. The use of chick embryos makes the model more likely to approximate to the situation in the bird itself, and Long (1970) has suggested that counting the macroscopic focal lesions associated with schizogony in the chorioallantois gives a measure of the severity of infection and can be used as an index of the response to therapeutic agents.

A possible relationship between avian leucosis and coccidiosis has been the subject of investigation at intervals during the past 30 years, and there has been a little evidence that birds suffering from the former may prove less resistant to the latter. Jeffers, Challey, and McGibbon (1969) have investigated the response to infection with *E. tenella* among lines of fowls selected for differential resistance to leucosis, but were unable to demonstrate a correlation.

Histomonas

The interesting advances in our understanding of the development and transmission of *Histomonas* reported in the 1970 review (VETERINARY ANNUAL, 179) have been extended by the work of Ruff, McDougald, and Hansen (1970) who have finally isolated *H. meleagridis* from the embryonated egg of *Heterakis gallinarum. Histomonas* was recovered from *Heterakis* by culturing the artificially hatched eggs in a modified De Volts alkaline serum medium. The protozoon was seen microscopically in the culture and intracaecal inoculation of turkeys produced histomoniasis. Lund and Chute (1970) have looked into the relative importance of young and mature turkeys and chickens in contaminating soil with *Histomonas*-bearing *Heterakis* eggs. Young chickens were many times more important than were mature fowls, and young turkeys excreted so few *Heterakis* eggs that they could be regarded as of no importance. Mature turkeys were nearly as important as young chickens in contaminating soil with *Heterakis* capable of transmitting *Histomonas*, although the disease that followed seemed less severe. These results can be considered with the knowledge that *Heterakis* appears not to thrive in caeca that are acutely affected by *Histomonas* but that they are better able to establish in a bird which is resistant to *Histomonas*. An adult turkey is likely to be resistant to *Histomonas*; young chickens are more susceptible than are old ones to *Histomonas*. There is obviously a complicated relationship which affects the epidemiological picture.

The virulence of strains of *Histomonas* may vary according to treatment after isolation and it is well known that culture *in vitro* may reduce and indeed quite rapidly eliminate the infectivity of a field strain. Dwyer and Honigberg (1970) have shown that a highly virulent strain may be attenuated by cultivation at 41·5° C. for 9 weeks until it is no longer fatal for susceptible birds, but that the original virulence may be restored by passage through susceptible birds. Freeze preservation does not seem to affect virulence and, as shown also by Chute and Chute (1969), is satisfactory for about a year or more.

Trichomonas

Trichomoniasis is of particular interest where domestic and racing pigeons are of economic importance and also in a range of wild Columbiformidae which are susceptible particularly, so it seems, under captive conditions. It is usually accepted that infection, although not necessarily clinical disease, is widespread. Transmission occurs mainly in the nest and morbidity is most evident in young birds. Kocan and Knisley (1970) used challenge infections in domestic pigeons and American mourning doves, apparently free from infection, to determine the percentage of resistant birds in the population. More than 80 per cent of both species were resistant, presumably an indication of earlier infection.

Some years ago 2-amino-5-nitrothiazole was reported as a satisfactory therapeutic agent and more recently dimetridazole and metronidazole have been recommended. Devos, Viaene, and Devriese (1969) have reported on the use of several drugs in pigeons. Ronidazole added to the drinking water for 5 days at 0·6 g./litre was effective as was metronidazole at 1 g./litre. Carbarsone (1 g./litre) was less effective.

REFERENCES

CHUTE, M. B., and CHUTE, A. M. (1969), *Poultry Sci.*, **48**, 2189.

DEVOS, A., VIAENE, N., and DEVRIESE, L. (1969), *Vlaams diergeneesk. Tijdschr.*, **38**, 297.

DORAN, D. J. (1970), *Proc. helminth Soc. Wash.*, **37**, 84.

DWYER, D. M., and HONIGBERG, B. M. (1970), *J. Parasit.*, **56**, 694.

JEFFERS, T. K., CHALLEY, J. R., and MCGIBBON, W. H. (1969), *Poultry Sci.*, **48**, 1604.

KOCAN, R. M., and KNISLEY, J. O. (1970), *J. Wildl. Dis.*, **6**, 13.

LONG, P. L. (1970), *Z. ParasitKde*, **33**, 329.

LUND, E. E., and CHUTE, A. M. (1970), *Avian Dis.*, **14**, 342.

RUFF, M. D., MCDOUGALD, L. R., and HANSEN, M. F. (1970), *J. Protozool.*, **17**, 10.

DISEASES RELATED TO PROTOZOAL INFECTIONS

L. P. Joyner, B.Sc., Ph.D., F.I.Biol.

Babesiasis

Cattle

After a single experimental tick-transmitted infection with *Babesia argentina*, young cattle maintained in a tick-free environment showed recurrences of parasitaemia for 1½ to 2 years. With *B. bigemina*, shorter periods and fewer recurrences were observed in a study by Mahoney (1969) of some of the factors concerned in transmission. Young cattle were able to infect ticks with *B. argentina* for up to a year after removal from an infected environment, but with *B. bigemina* infectivity was retained for only 4–7 weeks. In infected environments the incidence of *B. argentina* parasitaemia rose from zero at birth to a maximum at 1–2 years of age and then declined. A similar pattern occurred with *B. bigemina* but maximum values were reached at 6–12 months of age. An analysis of age-incidence data suggested that one infection of each animal occurred every 200–500 days depending upon the degree of infestation to which the herd was exposed. For *B. bigemina* the frequency of transmission was estimated at one infection every 110–330 days. These values suggest that in endemically stable environments the incidence of babesial infection in ticks is low.

Johnston and Tammemagi (1969) infected 20 susceptible shorthorn heifers with *B. argentina* and kept them either free from ticks or continuously exposed to *Boophilus microplus* capable of transmitting the infection. The animals were tested periodically for the presence of babesial infection (indirect F.A. tests proved very sensitive). All animals retained the infection for 13 months after initial infection irrespective of the presence of ticks and were immune to challenge. Those challenged with a heterologous strain developed a parasitaemia while those challenged with the homologous strain did not.

In trials of an improved vaccine against *B. argentina* using controlled numbers of parasites (20 millions per dose) Meehan (1969) observed 3488 cattle removed from tick-free areas of N.S.W. and tick-infested properties in Queensland. Although there were heavy losses among local unvaccinated animals only 0·05 per cent of vaccinated animals succumbed to babesiasis. There were severe reactions to vaccination in 1·3 per cent of the cattle and 0·8 per cent of them died.

Callow and McGregor (1969) investigated the possibility of reducing the risks of vaccination by the use of quinuronium. Two grammes of the drug were injected subcutaneously from 4 weeks before to 1 week after inoculation with *B. argentina* vaccine and the cattle developed a lower parasitaemia than untreated animals. An adequate immunity was present in the treated animals 15 weeks after vaccination. Treatment given at the time of inoculation or at the onset of parasitaemia did not eliminate the parasitaemia. No drug resistance was observed in *B. argentina* after passage in 7 treated animals. Kidney damage was observed in 4 animals which died 2–10 weeks after treatment.

Pipano (1969) noted that the reaction to immunization against *B. berbera* by the inoculation of infected blood varied from mild to moderate in animals from one particular herd while animals from another all reacted severely and had to be treated. By treating with amicarbalide isethionate (10 mg. per kg.) on the ninth and tenth days after the inoculation of infected blood, severe reactions could be controlled (Pipano, Raz, and Klinger, 1970).

The protection given by a bivalent vaccine containing *B. bigemina* and *B. bovis* may last for less than 1 year in the case of the former species to more than 2 years for the latter. The premunity is boosted by tick reinfestation which may decrease with systematic dipping. Treatment of *B. bigemina* may sterilize the infection and render the animals fully susceptible (Neitz, 1969).

An analysis of the serum from calves infected with *B. argentina* revealed two substances from serum from uninfected calves. One was immunologically identical with bovine fibrinogen and its presence was probably due to intravascular coagulation and subsequent fibrinolysis. The other appeared to be a pigmented macromolecular complex containing a number of proteins found in the tissues of normal cattle. Mahoney and Goodger (1969) also found this substance in the serum of a calf with chemically induced haemolytic anaemia. It therefore is not of parasitic origin. It is possible that this material may stimulate antibodies in the host which play a part in the removal of damaged erythrocytes from the circulation.

Ludford (1969) studied the staining of piroplasms with fluorescein-conjugated globulins from serum from animals recovered from infections with *B. argentina*, *B. bigemina*, *B. canis*, or *B. rodhaini*. Certain features of the parasitized cells were indicated by the antibody staining which were not seen by the conventional Giemsa staining. Specific fluorescence of the margins of erythrocytes parasitized by *B. argentina* and *B. canis* and of granules in erythrocytes parasitized by *B. bigemina* and to a lesser extent in those parasitized by *B. argentina* and *B. canis* was observed. It has been suggested that reactions between antibodies and the parasitized cells are part of the host's reaction to parasitization.

Adapting a capillary agglutination test originally devised for anaplasma-antibodies, Löhr and Ross (1969a) used antigens derived by sonication from *B. bigemina* separated from lysed red blood-cells. The results given by 223 serum samples agreed with those given by parasitological examination. There were no cross reactions with other micro-organisms nor with serum from cattle infected with *B. divergens*. The test was used to follow the antibody responses in 4 cattle experimentally infected with *B. bigemina*. Antibodies were first detected soon after the parasites appeared in the blood and reached a peak (titres of 1 : 160–1 : 320) 5–12 days later. Positive reactions were still clearly recognizable after 18–26 months.

Using the records of 7500 cases in a veterinary practice in South Devon from 1955 to 1967, Donnelly and Mackellar (1970) showed that the case-incidence followed a bimodal seasonal curve reflecting the periods of activity of the vector *Ixodes ricinus*. A relationship was established between the incidence and the temperature and rainfall recorded a fortnight previously. A similar relationship was demonstrated from the records of a practice in the Llyn Peninsula in N. Wales.

Clinical infections with *B. divergens* in adult female cattle were shown by Jerichow and Jungmann (1969) to be accompanied by raised blood-potassium and iron levels and lowered blood-calcium levels. Blood-magnesium concentrations were not significantly changed. The changes in calcium level could be controlled by Berenil treatment.

Horses

The concept of the strong host specificity of species of *Babesia* has tended to become eroded by recent experimental data (Barnett and Brocklesby, 1968). Unsuccessful attempts by Frerichs, Johnson, and Holbrook (1969) to transmit *B. equi* to a large series of splenectomized animals indicated that host specificity must still be accepted as a general characteristic of the group.

In the course of the preparation of antigens for use in complement fixation tests for *B. equi* or *B. caballi*, Frerichs, Holbrook, and Johnson (1969) encountered a number of problems. With *B. caballi* the greatest difficulty arose from the low yield of antigen due to the low levels of parasitaemia. The use of splenectomized horses or donkeys and the administration of corticosteroids greatly reduced the problem. *B. equi* lost its serological specificity after passage in horses, so suitable antigens of this species were best obtained by using fresh isolates from the field or low-temperature stabilates.

Anthony and Holbrook (1969) have continued their studies of the transmission of *B. caballi* by the horse tick *Dermacentor nitens.* Transmission was effected by six generations of the tick. The piroplasm is probably transmitted late in the larval feeding period or soon after the larva–nymph moult. The tick probably acquires the infection during the engorgement of the female. Cyclic transmission therefore occurs by reinfection of ticks and their immediate progeny from horses which they originally infected. Engorged females from infected horses were smaller and laid fewer eggs and had a higher mortality-rate than uninfected ticks.

Laboratory Rodents

Serum antigens prepared from rats acutely infected with *Babesia rodhaini* and from dogs similarly infected with *B. canis* were studied by Sibinovic and others (1969). One antigen (designated B), which was associated with beta-globulin, was the principal immunogenic component and was partly involved in the production of anaemia in acutely infected animals. After intravenous injection it is quickly bound to the erythrocytes which are then rapidly removed from the circulation causing temporary anaemia. Antiserum to antigen B selectively agglutinated and eventually disintegrated erythrocytes containing more mature parasites but the parasites released remained intact. The infectivity of the parasites was destroyed after infected cells had been incubated with antiserum for longer than 30 minutes at 37° C. The antibody was directed against the infected erythrocytes rather than against the parasites themselves.

In a comparison of *B. rodhaini*-infected rat erythrocytes with red blood-cells from normal rats Rickard (1969) observed appreciably increased rates of oxygen uptake and glycolysis in the parasitized cells. Lactate was always the major end-product of glucose metabolism but the ratio of oxygen uptake to glucose utilization was the same as that in normal erythrocytes and less than that reported with *Plasmodium* spp. This suggests a greater dependence of *B. rodhaini* on anaerobic metabolism.

COCCIDIOSIS

Cattle

Niilo (1969) infected 4 new-born calves orally five times with 100 oocysts of *Eimeria zuernii*. Each calf was isolated with its dam until weaned at 13 weeks of age. The calves were then challenged with 300,000 sporulated oocysts at the age of 5, 7, and 9 months. Their response was compared with that of similar uninfected calves which developed clinical coccidiosis after the first challenge and resisted the second and third. The neonatally exposed calves were susceptible to infection at the first and subsequent challenges although the clinical signs were milder after the second and third infections. It was suggested that calves which become infected in early life may retain their susceptibility for long periods, shedding large numbers of oocysts providing a source of infection for other animals.

In a later experiment Niilo (1970) compared the response to infection with *E. bovis* and *E. zuernii* of calves housed in a heated building or left unsheltered with uninoculated animals. Clinical coccidiosis developed in most calves but whereas the sheltered, 'in contact', animals remained unaffected, mild coccidiosis developed in the unsheltered controls. It is suggested that exposure may increase susceptibility but not the severity of the disease.

The endogenous development of *E. auburnensis* was studied by Chobotar and Hammond (1969). Trophozoites and immature second generation schizonts were found in calves killed 10 and 12 days after infection. Mature second generation schizonts were found after 12–15 days and gametocytes were first seen on the fourteenth day after infection. Fully formed oocysts appeared after 18–19 days. The mean prepatent period of 6 calves was 17·5 days and the patent period averaged 3·3 days.

Cell line cultures of bovine kidney, human intestine, embryonic bovine trachea, and embryonic bovine spleen were used in attempts to establish *in vitro* cultures of *E. auburnensis*. Clark and Hammond (1969) observed that cell penetration by sporozoites occurred rapidly but development did not proceed appreciably beyond the first generation merozoite stage. Degeneration in both culture cells and parasites began after 9–17 days.

Horses

Eimeria leuckarti oocysts were detected by Dunlop (1970) in the faeces of horses from three different locations in Washington State. None of the infected animals showed clinical symptoms.

Barker and Remmler (1970) administered doses of approximately 50,000 sporulated oocysts of *E. leuckarti* to two yearling Shetland ponies. Relatively small numbers of oocysts were produced sporadically by the two animals. Oocysts from one of them were collected, sporulated, and given in doses of 200,000 and 100,000 to two more ponies which began excreting oocysts on days 34 and 35 respectively. In one of the animals the patent period was 12 days with oocyst numbers reaching a maximum of 4600 per g. of faeces on day 39. No clinical signs were observed.

Rabbits

Very young animals are generally considered to be difficult to infect with coccidia. This is partly due to incompletely established digestive enzyme systems resulting in incomplete sporulation. Dürr and Pellérdy (1969a) were able to confirm this in unweaned rabbits experimentally infected with *Eimeria stiedae* and intestinal species. The rabbits were susceptible from birth to both oral and parenteral infection when large numbers of oocysts were given. Experimental infections could be established more readily with excysted than with intact oocysts. Resistance was strongest at birth and subsequently tended to decline. Pellérdy (1969b) found in Hungary that only 4–6 of the known species of *Eimeria* in the rabbit occurred on any given farm. There is no cross-immunity between species. Although coccidiosis in rabbits may be controlled by strict attention to hygiene it is not always possible to achieve optimum conditions. Acute intestinal coccidiosis was accompanied by diarrhoea, poor food utilization, meteorism, and impaction. These changes may facilitate secondary infections and absorption of toxic metabolic products.

Davies and Joyner (1962) first showed that coccidial infections could be induced in chicks by parenteral inoculation of oocysts or excysted sporozoites of *E. tenella.* Pellérdy (1969a) has carried out similar experiments with *E. stiedae* in rabbits. Oocysts or sporozoites injected intravenously, intraperitoneally, or intramuscularly induced hepatic lesions, but the infections were always milder than those which followed oral inoculation. The intraperitoneal route was the most successful. Merozoites obtained on the fourteenth day after infection also induced coccidiosis when injected intravenously.

Pigs

The size and morphological characteristics of oocysts are often considered to be absolutely constant. In fact, size and conformation may depend upon the weight of infection, immunity of the host, and the phase of the patent period. Rommel (1970) observed this with two pure strains of *Eimeria scabra* and *E. polita.* When the infective dose was small, in the absence of immunity and in older hosts the oocysts became larger during the course of the patent period. Both species produced some smooth and colourless oocysts. From a detailed morphological study Rommel considered *E. cerdonis* (Vetterling, 1965) to be a synonym of *E. polita.*

General Studies

Oxygen is an essential requirement for sporulation. Dürr and Pellérdy (1969b) estimated the oxygen requirement for the complete sporulation of *Eimeria stiedae* to be between 30·2 and 39·5 μl. per 100,000 oocysts.

Generally oocysts will not survive prolonged exposure to near-body temperatures or above. Oocysts of the sheep species *Eimeria ninaekohlyakimovae, E. parva, E. arloingi,* and *E. faurei* were studied by Rakhmatullina and Svanbaev (1969). They concluded that oocysts were able to survive incubation at 40–50° C. for 4 hours, 60° C. for 2½ hours, and 70° C. for 30 minutes, although only 12–36 per cent completed sporulation after heat treatment. For the disinfection of premises 80° C. for 30 minutes or 100° C. for 20 minutes were considered necessary.

From their studies on the oocysts of *E. bovis*, Hibbert, Hammond, and Simmons (1969) found that satisfactory excystation could be obtained with pretreatment for 24 hours at 39° C. in 50 per cent air-CO_2 mixture and treatment for 4 hours in *tris*-maleate-buffered medium at *p*H 7·5–8·5 containing 0·25 per cent trypsin and 1 per cent of one of the bile acids (or 10 per cent bile).

Theileriasis

Cattle

A species of *Theileria* commonly occurs in cattle in Japan, frequently in mixed infections with *Babesia* sp. It is transmitted by *Haemaphysalis neumanii* and a comparison with strains from Africa and Australia suggests that it resembles *T. sergenti* rather than *T. mutans*. The presence of the *Theileria* infection has been shown to inhibit the babesial infection (Ishihara, 1968).

Pipano and Cahana (1969) applied the indirect fluorescent antibody test using a slide antigen prepared from emulsified livers from experimentally infected animals. The results indicated that serum with a titre of 1 : 50 or more can be considered as positive and that a titre of 1 : 26 may be considered doubtful.

It has been suggested that some bovine species of *Theileria* may be strains of a single species. This is supported by the observations of Brocklesby (1969), who isolated a parasite which behaved initially like *Theileria mutans*. After five passages in cattle transmitted by *Rhipicephalus appendiculatus*, the infections proved indistinguishable from those due to *T. parva*.

Pirie, Jarrett, and Crighton (1970) were able to immunize a high proportion of cattle against East Coast Fever by the innoculation of preparations of macroschizonts extracted from lymphoid tissue. Only 1 of the 57 inoculated animals died after vaccination. They were challenged 5–6 weeks later by application of ticks (*R. appendiculatus*) infected with *T. parva*. Survival following single vaccination with 10^8 macroschizonts was 20 per cent and with 10^9 macroschizonts 57 per cent survived. Two animals given 10^{10} schizonts were fully protected. Of 10 animals given two doses of 10^9 macroschizonts, 80 per cent survived the tick challenge.

An indirect fluorescent antibody test for the detection of antibodies against *Theileria parva* was described by Löhr and Ross (1969b). Piroplasm and schizont preparations were compared as antigens. The former proved to be more satisfactory. Cross-reactions only occurred with serum from other theilerial infections. With *T. parva* antigen there was no difference in serum titres of cattle recovered from either *T. parva* or *T. lawrencei* infections, while those from *T. mutans* cases were lower. By using the two antigens, antibodies to the one species could be titrated in the presence of those to the other.

Antibodies appeared 8–14 days after initial infection rising to peaks at about the thirtieth day followed by a gradual decline in titre which was still detectable for at least 12 months. After natural reinfection with *T. lawrencei* responses were less but similar in pattern. In 15 cattle fatally infected with *T. parva* there was little or no detectable antibody.

A satisfactory vaccine prepared from tissue cultures of *T. annulata* has been in use for several years. It produces no clinical response and intra-erythrocytic forms do not develop. Pipano and others (1969) showed that an immunological response to vaccination may be detected by the indirect fluorescent antibody test: 39 to 48 days after vaccination titres up to 1 : 150 were recorded.

Schindler and Mehlitz (1969) used the complement-fixation test and the indirect fluorescent antibody tests to study the immunological relationships between *T. mutans* and *T. parva*. Cattle infected with *T. mutans* developed serum antibodies but were susceptible to infection with *T. parva* and the antibodies to *T. mutans* were reduced. In the indirect fluorescent antibody test there were cross-reactions between *T. parva* and *T. mutans*, although the serum titres were highest with the homologous antigen.

Toxoplasmosis

Cats

Following the discovery of a cystic stage of *Toxoplasma gondii* in cats (*see* VETERINARY ANNUAL, 1970, 192) a number of confirmatory reports have been published. Overdulve (1970a, b) has reported his experiments with experimental infections in cats which largely agree with the observations of others. Following the feeding of toxoplasma-infected mice to cats, the *Isopora*-like oocysts appeared in the faeces on the fourth day, the numbers increasing to a maximum on day 6, and falling to very few by day 11. Oocysts recovered during days 3–10 were very infective for mice producing positive serum titres (Sabin-Feldman dye test). The cats themselves gave positive serum titres from day 11 onwards.

Pigs

A survey of the brains and diaphragm muscles of pigs in a slaughter house in Bratislava (Czecho-Slovakia) indicated a high incidence of infection. *Toxoplasma* was isolated from 11 out of 15 pools of 5 pigs each and in another series of tests, 13 out of 30 individual pigs were positive. The organisms were isolated from animals with complement-fixation test titres of 1 : 4 or higher. Eight out of 85 cattle from the same source were found to be positive (Čatár, Bergendi, and Holková, 1969). Weisstanner (1969) also found a high incidence in diaphragm muscle of pigs: 13 out of 105 slaughtered pigs were found by mouse inoculation to be infected. There was no evidence of infection in the throat lymph-nodes.

Fuhr (1970) found that antibodies were present in the juice from heart and diaphragm muscles and from the iliac lymph-nodes. The titres of the juice from the muscles of mice and from the heart, diaphragm, and iliac lymph-nodes of pigs were 1 to 2 dilutions below the corresponding serum titre. The titre of skeletal muscle juice from pigs was 2 to 4 dilutions below the serum titre. In samples from 302 slaughtered pigs fresh muscle-juice titre was 1 to 2 dilutions below the serum titre and was reduced by storage and freezing. Iliac lymph-nodes gave the most reliable results.

Using a modification of the haemagglutination test, Nobuto and others (1969) studied the levels of toxoplasma antibodies in sows and their progeny. Little fluctuation of titre occurred in positive sows. Antibody was found in piglets 7 days after ingesting colostrum, but it disappeared by 90 days of age. On contaminated farms new positive reactors were recorded among the piglets and the rise in titre with age was demonstrated. One-third of these animals showed clinical symptoms between 150 and 180 days of age.

In order to study the pathology of the infection Moller and others (1970) infected 8 pigs and 6 pregnant sows with cysts of a porcine strain or trophozoites of the R.H. strain of *T. gondii*. The lesions did not appear to be influenced by the infecting strain but they were more extensive in the younger than in the older animals. Lesions in acute fatal infections of retained or stillborn piglets, in liveborn congenitally infected piglets, and in 1 pig and 1 sow were characterized by exudative and degenerative changes with focal necrosis. *Toxoplasma* was demonstrable morphologically in all animals that died after clinical disease and non-viable *Toxoplasma* was demonstrable in 17 of 24 retained or stillborn piglets with pathological changes. The lesions in chronic infections showed reactive changes with the formation of granulomas, though the organisms were difficult to demonstrate. In certain circumstances it is suggested that *Toxoplasma* may provoke a tissue reaction of 'specific' granulomatous nature.

Sheep

In attempts to detect *Toxoplasma* in the milk of infective ewes Schurian (1969) tested daily samples of blood and milk for 8 weeks with negative results. Lambs from 7 of the latently infected ewes showed no evidence of the infection. When 1 ewe was reinfected intraperitoneally 4 weeks before parturition, organisms were recovered from the placenta and organs of the lamb.

Domestic Animals—General

Piper, Cole, and Shadduck (1970) have reported on their study of ocular lesions in *Toxoplasma* infections in dogs, cats, pigs, sheep, and cattle. Lesions were found most frequently in the iris, ciliary body, and retina. Focal necrosis especially of the retina was frequently observed. Ovine and bovine ocular lesions differed from those of other species by the predominance of epitheloid cells in sheep and plasmacytes in cattle. Masses of organisms, severe necrosis, and suppurative myositis occurred in the extra-ocular muscles of dogs, cats, and sheep. The lesions generally were similar to those reported for several species of domestic and laboratory animals but differed from those seen in man.

The epidemiology of toxoplasmosis was studied by Wallace (1969) on three remote atolls in the Western Pacific. According to dye-test antibodies, human infection was prevalent on Ifalik, less common on Woleai, and almost absent from Eauripik. On the first two there was also serological evidence of infection in rats, the only wild mammal present, and in domestic animals including cats, dogs, and pigs. On Eauripik rats and cats had not become established and the dogs and pigs were serologically negative except for 1 dog that had been imported from Woleai. Cats or rats appeared to be the most likely reservoir. The consumption of raw meat did not appear to be an important source of human infection.

The Sabin-Feldman dye test has been the most widely used test in serological surveys. Several alternatives are now available and Hübner and Uhlikova (1969) claimed that the micro-gel diffusion test using serum or whole blood with centrifuged peritoneal exudate from infected mice as antigen was as accurate as the dye-test. They also claimed that this test was also simpler, quicker, and easier to read. Only small volumes of reagents were required and the stained slides could be kept as a permanent record.

Continuing a study of uterine toxoplasma infection and its importance in pregnancy, Werner and Egger (1969) studied 232 female mice latently infected with an avirulent strain, which had little affinity for the reproductive organs: 52 per cent became pregnant as did 51–53 per cent of uninfected females. Of the 120 infected pregnant females 6 had uterine infection without demonstrable foetal infection and 35 had both uterine and foetal infections. With few exceptions no developmental disturbances were noted and no pregnancy disorders were noted.

Rašín (1970) studied 12 strains of *Toxoplasma* isolated from hares (*Lepus europaeus*). Four strains proved to be of low pathogenicity for mice and were suitable for the hyperimmunization of rabbits. Six were highly pathogenic and 2 were classified as of intermediate pathogenicity.

Although *T. gondii* was shown to survive in nymphal *Ornithodorus moubata* for up to 10 days and in adults for 2 days, ticks which had fed on infected guinea-pigs failed to transmit the infection. Jagow and Hoffmann (1970) concluded that this soft tick played little or no part in the epidemiology of the infection.

Vivier and Petitprez (1969) have studied the membrane structure of *Toxoplasma*. They recognized three membranes of which only the outer is considered to be the plasma membrane. During reproduction by fission or more commonly by endodiogeny the membranes of the daughter individuals are formed from those of the parent. The 3-membrane complex of the endozoites is completed at their liberation and the plasma membrane of the daughter cells is derived from that of the parent.

The sporozoites obtained by excystation of the *Isospora*-like cysts obtained from infected cat faeces were studied by Sheffield and Melton (1970). They were shown to be infective for monkey kidney cell cultures and their ultrastructure was similar to that previously described for the proliferative stages of *Toxoplasma*.

TRYPANOSOMIASIS

Cattle

By studying 2444 cattle passing through 10 crushes in the Teso District of Uganda, Mwambu (1969) attempted to assess the prevalence of trypanosome infections. Wet blood films were examined and the indirect fluorescent antibody test was applied using thick blood films and blood samples on filter paper. In addition mice, goats, and sheep were inoculated with suspected positive samples.

Of 1192 cattle examined by the wet film method 1·1 per cent were found to be infected with trypanosomes (9 with *Trypanosoma theileri* and 42 with *T. vivax*). The indirect fluorescent antibody test was positive for 57·5 per cent of cattle but only 12 out of the 1406 positive samples gave maximum fluorescence. Isolates in the sheep and goats were identified as *T. vivax* which proved to be only mildly pathogenic in test cattle. It appears that mildly pathogenic strains of this species are fairly widespread in cattle in this area.

Krampitz (1970) studied the course of infection with *T. congolense* alone or with *T. brucei* and *T. vivax* in East African Zebu cattle using trypanosomes derived from tsetse flies. Mixed infections were not invariably more severe than pure *T. congolense* and whether the infection became acute or chronic did not depend on age or weight. An acute infection lasted for about 4 months. There was a steady fall in haematocrit values and body-weight, unrelated to the degree of parasitaemia. Spontaneous recovery did not depend on the physical condition of the animal nor on haematocrit values or body-weight. Disseminated micro-haemorrhages, pigment deposits in tissues, perivascular round-cell infiltration (particularly in the kidney), and myocardial lesions were found in the tissues of animals dying from acute or subacute infections.

Woo, Soltys, and Gillick (1970) have reported the finding of trypanosomes in the blood of cattle in southern Ontario. The incidence varied from about 8 to 85 per cent. Two species were identified; one was *T. theileri* and the other resembled the smaller *T. uniforme*. Both species could be transmitted to chick embryos.

Sheep

Sheep infected with a rodent-adapted strain of *Trypanosoma vivax* showed relapsing infections for about 3 months after which no further detectable parasitaemia occurred. Clarkson and Awan (1969) separated the trypanosome populations from each parasitaemia by mouse inoculation and showed that they were antigenically distinct by agglutination or immune lysin tests against serum samples from the infected sheep. In sheep inoculated with blood from one of the original sheep, lytic antibodies developed to several trypanosome populations, suggesting that each population was a mixture of several antigenic types.

Soluble and bound antigens were studied in rats infected with 3 of the trypanosome populations. The soluble antigens produced specific precipitin lines against homologous antisera and the bound antigens contained common antigens in addition to the specific ones. The rodent-adapted strain evidently is still capable of antigenic variation in the natural host.

Game Animals

Keymer (1969) has published the results of his survey of trypanosome infections in wild ungulates in the Luangwa Valley of Zambia. Of 43 animals examined in 1962, 10 were found to be infected with trypanosomes (*Trypanosoma congolense*, *T. vivax*, *T. brucei*, *T. rhodesiense*, and *T. megatrypanum*). The results were essentially the same as those obtained by Bruce, working in the same area in 1912, although they incorrectly identified *T. caprae* from a waterbuck. From this observations of the parasite which he isolated from the same species, Keymer considered this to be a subspecies of *T. vivax* which he has named *T. vivax ellipsiprymni* subs. nov.

Dogs

Pathological changes in dogs experimentally infected with *Trypanosoma evansi* were studied by Srivastava, Mathotra, and Iyer (1969): intense congestion and enlargement of the spleen, congestion of lung, liver, and kidney with accumulations of fluid in the pericardial, pleural, and peritoneal cavities. In the spleen enlargement was due to hyperaemia and obstructive pressure on the venules and sinuses with mesenchymal hyperplasia, mobilization of macrophages and intense phagocytic activity, and haemosiderosis. In the liver there were retrogressive changes in hepatic cells around the central veins, hypertrophy and hyperplasia of endothelial lining cells and Kupffer cells, and their transformation into free macrophages were observed. Extensive tubular degeneration was evident in the kidneys; in the lungs oedema with the presence of macrophages in the alveoli were noted.

Pigs

English pigs were shown by Marsden and others (1970) to be susceptible to infection with a virulent Peruvian strain of *Trypanosoma cruzi*. Three out of 4 pigs became infected when 18,000–250,000 organisms were inoculated subcutaneously or conjunctivally. Xenodiagnosis and cultural tests were negative but the presence of the organisms was demonstrated by the inoculation of blood into mice. The infection was clinically inapparent and few histological changes were noted.

In Brazil, *T. cruzi* has been found in the peripheral blood of 47 species of mammals. Dogs and cats are considered to be the main reservoirs followed by rats and opossums (Corrêa, 1968). In Mexico opossum, armadillos, dogs, and cats have been identified as vertebrate hosts (Tay and others, 1969).

General Laboratory Studies

The effect of different hosts upon the infectivity of *Trypanosoma congolense* and its viability in cultures was studied by Yesufu (1970). Six strains of *T. congolense* were infective for rats, mice, rabbits, sheep, goats, and dogs but only 3 were infective for guinea-pigs and 2 for domestic pigs. The trypanosomes caused heavy infections in rats and mice but those in other species were less virulent. When the 6 strains were cultured from rats and rabbits, 5 developed, only 2 grew from sheep, and 1 from goats. All 3 strains from guinea-pigs grew, as did isolates from domestic pigs.

Trypanosomes (*T. brucei* and *T. congolense*) artificially maintained in mice multiply exclusively by longitudinal fission. Soltys and Woo (1969) found that in rabbits, guinea-pigs, and sheep they have, in addition to multiplication by binary fission, a developmental cycle which includes leishmanial, leptomonad, crithidial, and multinucleate forms. Since some of these forms were seen dividing, these authors have suggested that they may be part of a developmental cycle in the vertebrate host.

Soltys, Woo, and Gillick (1969) attempted to separate the tissue forms from the blood stages by filtration and found that infective forms of *T. brucei* from the liver and spleen of mice will pass through filters of pore-size of 0·8–1·0 μ diameter. On sub-inoculation into mice infective forms appeared in filtrates of liver or spleen after 72 hours, while blood-stream forms were present after 24 hours. When blood-stream forms were inoculated, tissue forms appeared in the liver and spleen in about 24 hours.

The antigenic types present in trypanosome populations derived from a single *T. brucei* stabilate may be studied by cloning the variant populations arising from the first relapses of parasitaemia and preparing monospecific antisera to them. McNeillage, Herbert, and Lumsden (1969) used this method and were able to recognize six different antigenic types. Variant populations sometimes consisted of mixtures of more than one type. The first antigenic variants arising from a single stabilate were not always of the same antigenic type.

It has been suggested that the variable specific 'exoantigens' associated with successive relapse populations are related to structures of the surface envelope. To investigate this, immune globulins to two specific variants were conjugated with ferritin. Electron microscopy of sections of trypanosomes treated with homologous conjugated globulin revealed ferritin granules adhering to the surface coat of the organisms, their flagella, and free plasmanemes, but rarely on the surface membrane of trypanosomes which had lost the surface coat. There was no reaction with heterologous globulin (Vickerman and Luckins, 1969). Wright, Lumsden, and Hales (1970) have described long filaments arising from both the posterior end and the tip of the flagellum of blood-stream forms of *T. brucei* which may become attached to various substrates by these filaments. They appeared to have a structure resembling filopodia and it has been suggested that these structures may have a role in the release of antigenic material and in the mediation of attachment.

The blood-stream forms of a number of strains of *T. rhodesiense*, *T. brucei*, *T. vivax*, and *T. congolense* were studied in chick embryos by Goedbloed and Kinyanjui (1970). Following supra-chorioallantoic inoculation all strains of *T. brucei* subgroup multiplied readily, but *T. vivax* and *T. congolense* did not. The degree of parasitaemia produced by *T. brucei* subgroup trypanosomes varied with the different strains and with the inoculation period. Five attempts at serial passage with a clone of *T. rhodesiense* failed, although the initial passage multiplied well. Egg-cultured trypanosomes retained their infectivity for mice, rats, and rabbits in which they showed normal characteristics. Parasitaemic chicks which hatched from infected embryos occasionally showed relapses and because the embryos exhibited no antibody response the authors suggested that fluctuations in parasitaemia and polymorphism in *T. brucei* may occur independently of the antibody response of the host.

From the results of tests on serum samples from 467 cattle in two different regions of East Uganda, Wilson (1969) concluded that the agglutination test was of limited value. The indirect fluorescent antibody test was useful in determining the stage of the disease process and in detecting cases of chronic infection.

REFERENCES

ANTHONY, D. W., and HOLBROOK, A. A. (1969), *Proc. 2nd Int. Congr. Acarology*, Sutton Bonington, 1967, p. 621.
BARKER, I. K., and REMMLER, O. (1970), *Vet. Rec.*, **86**, 448.
BARNETT, S. F., and BROCKLESBY, D. W. (1968), *Symp. zool. Soc. Lond.*, No. 24, 159.
BROCKLESBY, D. W. (1969), *Expl Parasit.*, **25**, 258.
CALLOW, L. L., and MCGREGOR, W. (1969), *Aust. vet. J.*, **45**, 408.
ČATÁR, G., BERGENDI, L., and HOLKOVÁ, R. (1969), *J. Parasit.*, **55**, 952.
CHOBOTAR, B., and HAMMOND, D. M. (1969), *Ibid.*, **55**, 1218.
CLARK, W. N., and HAMMOND, D. M. (1969), *J. Protozool.*, **16**, 646.
CLARKSON, M. J., and AWAN, M. A. Q. (1969), *Ann. trop. Med. Parasit.*, **63**, 515.
CORRÊA, R. R. (1968), *Revta bras. Malar. Doenç. trop.*, **20**, 39. (Abstr. *Vet. Bull., Weybridge*, **40**, 367.)
DAVIES, S. F. M., and JOYNER, L. P. (1962), *Nature, Lond.*, **194**, 996.
DONNELLY, J., and MACKELLAR, J. C. (1970), *Agric. Met.*, **7**, 5.
DUNLOP, J. S. (1970), *J. Am. vet. med. Ass.*, **156**, 623.
DÜRR, U., and PELLÉRDY, L. (1969a), *Acta vet. hung.*, **19**, 453.
— — — — (1969), *Ibid.*, **19**, 307.
FRERICHS, W. M., HOLBROOK, A. A., and JOHNSON, A. J. (1969), *Am. J. vet. Res.*, **30**, 1337.
— — JOHNSON, A. J., and HOLBROOK, A. A. (1969), *Ibid.*, **30**, 1333.
FUHR, R. (1970), Inaugural Dissertation, Faculty of Veterinary Science, Freie Universität, Berlin.
GOEDBLOED, E., and KINYANJUI, H. (1970), *Expl Parasit.*, **27**, 464.
HIBBERT, L. E., HAMMOND, D. M., and SIMMONS, J. R. (1969), *J. Protozool.*, **16**, 441.
HÜBNER, J., and UHLIKOVA, M. (1969), *J. Hyg. Epidem. Microbiol. Immun.*, **13**, 514.
ISHIHARA, T. (1968), *Jap. agric. Res.*, *Q.* **3**, 23.
JAGOW, M., and HOFFMANN, G. (1970), *Z. ParasitKde*, **33**, 246.
JERICHOW, H., and JUNGMANN, R. (1969), *Mh. VetMed.*, **24**, 732.
JOHNSTON, L. A. Y., and TAMMEMAGI, L. (1969), *Aust. vet. J.*, **45**, 445.
KEYMER, I. F. (1969), *Ann. trop. Med. Parasit.*, **63**, 195.
KRAMPITZ, H. E. (1970), *Z. Tropenmed. Parasit.*, **21**, 3.
LÖHR, K. F., and ROSS, J. P. J. (1969a), *Ibid.*, **20**, 287.
— — — — (1969b), *Res. vet. Sci.*, **10**, 453.
LUDFORD, C. G. (1969), *Expl Parasit.*, **24**, 327.
MCNEILLAGE, G. J. C., HERBERT, W. J., and LUMSDEN, W. H. R. (1969), *Ibid.*, **25**, 1.
MAHONEY, D. F. (1969), *Ann. trop. Med. Parasit.*, **63**, 1.
— — and GOODGER, B. V. (1969), *Expl Parasit.*, **24**, 375.
MARSDEN, P. D., BLAICKIE, E. J., ROSENBERG, M. E., RIDLEY, D. S., and HAGSTROM, J. W. C. (1970), *Trans. R. Soc. trop. Med. Hyg.*, **64**, 156.
MEEHAN, J. F. (1969), *Qd agric. J.*, **95**, 768.
MOLLER, T., FENNESTAD, K. L., ERIKSEN, L., WORK, K., and SIIM, J. C. (1970), *Acta path. microbiol. scand.*, **78A**, 241.
MWAMBU, P. M. (1969), *Bull. épizoot. Dis. Afr.*, **17**, 395.
NEITZ, W. O. (1969), *J. S. Afr. vet. med. Ass.*, **40**, 419.

NIILO, L. (1969), *Can. J. comp. Med.*, **33**, 287.
— — (1970), *Ibid.*, **34**, 20.
NOBUTO, K., HANAKI, T., KOIZUMI, T., and YONEMOCHI, K. (1969), *Natn. Inst. Anim. Hlth Q., Tokyo*, **9**, 136.
OVERDULVE, J. P. (1970a), *Tijdschr. Diergeneesk.*, **95**, 149.
— — (1970b), *Proc. K. ned. Akad. Wet.*, Ser. C, **73**, 129.
PELLÉRDY, L. (1969a), *Acta vet. hung.*, **19**, 171.
— — (1969b), *Parasit. hung.*, **2**, 175.
PIPANO, E. (1969), *Refuah vet.*, **26**, 113.
— — and CAHANA, M. (1969), *J. Parasit.*, **55**, 765.
— — FELLER, B., SHABAT, Y., and DAVID, E. (1969), *Refuah vet.*, **26**, 145.
— — RAZ, A., and KLINGER, I. (1970), *Ibid.*, **27**, 1.
PIPER, R. C., COLE, C. R., and SHADDUCK, J. A. (1970), *Am. J. Ophthal.*, **69**, 662.
PIRIE, H. M., JARRETT, W. F. H., and CRIGHTON, G. W. (1970), *Expl Parasit.*, **27**, 343.
RAKHMATULLINA, N. K., and SVANBAEV, S. K. (1969), *Izv. Akad. Nauk. kazakh. SSR, Ser. biol.*, 1969 (5), 47. (Abstr. *Vet. Bull., Weybridge*, **40**, 368.)
RAŠÍN, K. (1970), *Vet. Med.,, Praha*, **15**, 127.
RICKARD, M. D. (1969), *Expl Parasit.*, **25**, 16.
ROMMEL, M. (1970), *Z. ParasitKde.*, **34**, 141.
SCHINDLER, R., and MEHLITZ, D. (1969), *Z. Tropenmed. Parasit.*, **20**, 459.
SCHURIAN, E. (1969), Inaugural Dissertation, Faculty of Veterinary Science, Freie Universität, Berlin.
SHEFFIELD, H. G., and MELTON, M. L. (1970), *Science, N.Y.*, **167**, 892.
SIBINOVIC, K. H., MILAR, R., RISTIC, M., and COX, H. W. (1969), *Ann. trop. Med., Parasit.*, **63**, 327.
SOLTYS, M. A., and WOO, P. (1969), *Trans. R. Soc. trop. Med. Hyg.*, **63**, 490.
— — — — and GILLICK, A. C. (1969), *Ibid.*, **63**, 495.
SRIVASTAVA, R. V. N., MALHOTRA, M. N., and IYER, P. K. R. (1969), *Indian J. Anim. Sci.*, **39**, 307.
TAY, J., ONTIVEROS, D., ORTEGA, M., and TORRES, J. (1969), *Boln Of. sanit. pan-am.*, **47**, 310. (Abstr. *Vet. Bull., Weybridge*, **40**, 367.)
VETTERLING, J. M. (1965), *J. Parasit.*, **51**, 897.
VICKERMAN, K., and LUCKINS, A. G. (1969), *Nature, Lond.*, **224**, 1125.
VIVIER, E., and PETITPREZ, A. (1969), *J. Cell. Biol.*, **43**, 329.
WALLACE, G. D. (1969), *Am. J. Epidem.*, **90**, 103.
WEISSTANNER, T. (1969), *Path. Microbiol.*, **33**, 44.
WERNER, H., and EGGER, I. (1969), *Zentbl. Bakt. ParasitKde*, I (Orig.) **212**, 155.
WILSON, A. J. (1969), *Trop. Anim. Hlth Prod.*, **1**, 89.
WOO, P., SOLTYS, M. A., and GILLICK, A. C. (1970), *Can. J. comp. Med.*, **34**, 142.
WRIGHT, K. A., LUMSDEN, W. H. R., and HALES, H. (1970), *J. cell. Sci.*, **6**, 285.
YESUFU, H. M. (1970), *J. comp. Path.*, **80**, 1.

PARASITOLOGY

J. DONNELLY, B.Sc.

T. E. GIBSON, D.V.Sc., F.R.C.V.S., F.I. Biol.

S. B. KENDALL, B.Sc., Ph.D., M.R.C.V.S., A.R.C.S., F.I. Biol.

PARASITOLOGY

ARTHROPOD PARASITOLOGY

J. Donnelly, B.Sc.

Ticks

Sometimes we need reminding that ticks are of economic importance primarily in terms of the diseases they carry. Williams and Gonzalez (1968) have investigated the situation in Trinidad with respect to tick-borne diseases of imported cattle and found babesiasis and anaplasmosis to be important. Ticks of the genus *Boophilus* which are vectors of these two diseases are known to occur in Trinidad. Uilenberg (1967) has reported 5 cases of equine babesiasis in Madagascar in 1965 and 1966, caused by *B. equi*. No recognized vector of this organism is known to occur in Madagascar.

In a study of African Swine Fever (ASF) virus in Tanganyika, Plowright and his coworkers (Plowright, Parker, and Peirce, 1969) surveyed warthog burrow populations of the tick *Ornithodoros moubata* and measured infection rates in them. Inoculation of suspensions of infected ticks from the warthog burrows produced typical and fatal ASF in domestic pigs which spread by contact to other pigs housed with the primary recipients.

Transmission of *Theilera annulata* in calves has been induced by injection of triturated, unfed but infected *Hyalomma dromadarii* (Mazlum, 1969). The disease pattern so induced more resembled that following natural infection than did disease produced by syringe passage. Russian investigations (Meshcheryakova, 1967) showed that transmission of *T. sergenti* was effected by larvae of *Rhipicephalus bursa* resulting from adults fed on infected hosts. No transmission resulted from adults fed as nymphs or from nymphs fed as larvae on infected hosts. The same organism was transmitted by *Ixodes ricinus* but only by nymphs which had fed on infected hosts as larvae. There was no transovarial transmission as with *R. bursa*. The incubation period of *T. sergenti* as transmitted by *R. bursa* and *I. ricinus* was comparable to that when transmitted by *Haemaphysalis neumanni*.

Other Russian work described by Krylov and Krylova (1967) involved transmission of *Babesia* (*Nuttalia*) *tadzhikistanica* among gerbils (*Meriones libycus erythrourus*) by the tick *H. anatolicum*. At extremely low levels of parasitaemia in the mammalian host, such as occur during the prepatent phase of infection, larvae and nymphs were not infected when fed on such hosts. Nymphs resulting from larvae which were fed on the host when the parasitaemia was at levels between 30 and 2142 parasites per 100,000 erythrocytes proved to be infected. Branagan, at Muguga in Kenya, has shown (Branagan, 1969) that the maintenance of *T. parva* depends on the severity of the fever reaction, the pattern of behaviour of the emerging nymph, and the level of infection acquired by the tick, and that all of these factors show considerable variation. Precision in transmission studies was greatly limited by these effects.

Feeding by *Boophilus microplus* was enhanced when their bovine hosts were sedated with antihistaminic promazine hydrochloride, according to Tatchell and Bennett (1969). The yield of ticks from 8 out of 12 animals was significantly increased as a result of treatment by this drug. Presumably the protective reaction to remove the ticks was in some way inhibited. Musatov (1967a) has studied protective mechanisms impeding successful feeding of ticks in the long wool of sheep. He found that *R. bursa* and *H. marginatum* tended to attach themselves in an area containing the least lanolin. He also concluded that attack stimulated a protective reaction to remove the ticks and found that attached ticks were inhibited from normal feeding by some host-produced factor. The same worker (Mustaov, 1967b) showed that when *R. bursa*, *H. marginatum*, *H. asiaticum*, and *R. sanguineus* were fed on rabbits, which had been sensitized by prior experience of tick feeding or by injection of preparations of tick salivary glands, poor development of the ticks resulted.

German workers (Köhler and others, 1967) demonstrated an immunological reaction, in the rabbit, which was a response to repeated infestations of *H. anatolicum* and *R. sanguineus*. Ticks, when fed on such rabbits, ingested less blood and had lowered fertility. Specific serum antibodies were demonstrable by gel-diffusion, electrophoresis, and fluorescence techniques in these rabbits, and also in rabbits which had been injected with salivary gland preparation from ticks.

Trapping experiments, carried out in America by Sonenshine and Stout (1968), showed that the tick burdens of the white-footed deer-mouse *Peromyscus leucopus* were related to the distance travelled by the host between release and recapture. Male mice were more heavily infested than female mice.

Mating in the soft tick, *O. tholozani*, was shown to be a stimulus to oogenesis (Galun and Warburg, 1967). The accessory gland secretion of the male was shown to contain catecholamine, and drugs of this group including dopa (dihydroxyphenylalanine) were shown to initiate oogenesis in the female tick. Parasympathomimetic drugs are shown to stimulate salivation in ticks. The Muguga workers, Purnell, Branagan, and Radley (1969), tested the effect of such drugs on *R. appendiculatus*. Pilocarpine nitrate and arecoline hydrobromide at 10 per cent in 6 per cent saline gave the best results when such substances were used in studies on the measurement of the level of *T. parva* infection of salivary gland acini. The infective particles were successfully harvested by stimulation of salivation.

Malysheva (1967) has demonstrated the usefulness of certain plants as indicators of activity periods of the tick *T. persulcatus*. The idea is very appealing. There is nothing quite like plants for telling us what time of year it is, and by extension of the idea they should be able to tell us what kind of year it is or may be about to be, if only we could read the signs. Seasonal tick rises and their variation from year to year are presumably under the same climatological influences as is vegetation pattern.

Several workers have reported on the use of CO_2 as a method of attracting ticks for population assessments. Nosek and Kosuch (1969) suggest the placement of lumps of dry ice on the herbage, Korenberg (1969) got attraction of ticks over a $1\frac{1}{2}$ m. radius by using dry ice in bags, and Garcia (1969), using a CO_2 gas generator near an elk carcass, collected unfed and fed ticks whereas only the few engorged ones have been detected on the animal. The last author suggested that a response to CO_2 is part of the normal host-finding reaction in *Dermacentor albipictus*. A successful method of radioactive labelling of

D. andersoni and *D. variabilis* (Sonenshine and Clark, 1968) used glucose or glycine labelled with radioactive carbon which was injected into the ticks.

The occurrence of the exotic tick *R. sanguineus* continues to be reported in northern European cities. According to Winding, Willenberg, and Haarløv (1970) there were 29 sightings of this tick in Denmark during a period of a few months. It was also found (Best, Butt, and Rohrbach, 1969) in London on two dogs and as unengorged adults in the flat in which they lived.

Diapause studies on *I. ricinus* (Belozerov, 1967a) showed that the rate of feeding of nymphs, after being kept prior to feeding under short-day conditions (12 hr. photoperiod) was only about 30 per cent of the feeding rate of those kept under long-day conditions (20 hr. photoperiod). Older nymphs of 9 months or more showed no difference in feeding rate resulting from difference in pre-engorgement photoperiod. Increase in diapause occurred as a result of short-day conditions after engorgenemt. Other studies by the same worker (Belozerov, 1967b) showed that the water content of females tended to increase at the beginning of feeding with a subsequent decrease as feeding went on. Two mechanisms of water regulation were involved. The fluid balance during the early stage is regulated by cuticular transpiration; in the final stages the cuticle is less permeable and water balance and concentration of the blood meal is under the control of the matured salivary glands.

The activity of *D. marginatus* was studied also by Belozerov (1967c). Old ticks (7½ months) held at 10° C. and corresponding to spring ticks were compared with newly emerged ticks in their ability to remain active when subjected to different combinations of temperature (18° or 25° C.) and photoperiod (10 hr. or 20 hr.). Both age-groups became inactivated more readily at 25° C. and 20 hr. photoperiod and this effect was more severe in the newly emerged group. Activity was generally more sustained in both groups under the shorter photoperiod conditions, and similarly under the lower temperature conditions. These findings provide some explanation of the phenomenon of inactivity of tick populations during high summer.

Unfed adults of *R. simus sinus* were kept by Branagan and Bailey (1968) for 32 months under laboratory conditions. Although the tick can transmit both *T. parva* and *Anaplasma marginale*, these authors did not consider it to be important as an alternative vector of East Coast Fever. They suggested that it might, however, play a part in the dissemination of rickettsial infections such as tick typhus.

Multiple mating of *D. andersoni* females has been reported by Gregson (1969). In his experiments, males were irradiated with ^{60}Co at a level that partially sterilized them without interfering with their ability to mate. Females, which were mated with them, laid eggs of which only 1 per cent were fertile. If normally fertile males were offered after their mating with a partially sterile male then these females laid normally fertile eggs masses. This multiple mating could nullify the effect of a first mating with a sterile male during a release programme aimed at control by the sterile males method. Rechar and Oppenheim (1969) have demonstrated that males of *H. excavatum* are capable of fertilizing more than one female each.

A useful account of methods for the laboratory rearing of a range of tick species has been published by Hadani and a group of Israeli workers (Hadani and others, 1969). Rehacek and Brzostowski (1969) were able to cultivate cells of *R. sanguineus* in a culture medium based on an analysis of tick haemolymph. It contained the usual components of such media—sugars, amino-acids, cations, etc.—along with 1 per cent of haemolymph from the moth *Antheraea peryni* and 1 per cent bovine serum.

Two Indian workers (Divakaran and Barat, 1970) have studied the tenacity of attachment of ticks by measuring the force required to dislodge them. Brevirostrate adult ticks require a force equal to 62 *g* to remove them from the host's body and 50 *g* to remove them from the ear; longirostrate adults needed forces of 100 *g* and 75 *g* respectively to remove them.

A new canine disease syndrome noted in Royal Air Force dogs in Singapore has been reported on (Wilkins, Bowden, and Wilkinson, 1967). The syndrome is haemorrhagic, transmissible, and affects imported dogs worse. Serum neutralization tests seem to implicate a virus isolated from the tick *Boophilus microplus* which resembles the Wad Medani virus of Egyptian sheep.

Mites

Insecticidal control of *Dermanyssus avium* has been shown by Schneider and Haas (1969), in Germany, to improve egg output and reduce losses in intensively reared poultry. Before control of the mite, egg production was 5–10 per cent below normal and losses were 3–5 per cent per month.

The distribution of the itch mite *Psorergates ovis* on merino sheep has been studied by Sinclair and Gibson (1970). The mite is to be found in greatest numbers on the upper parts of the sheep and is more frequent in the spring than in the autumn. The immature forms generally lie under the stratum corneum on the upper surface of the stratum granulosum, often near the opening of a wool follicle.

Faecal flotation is recommended by Derwelis (1967) for the diagnosis of demodicosis in dogs. Of 71 dogs examined for *Demodex canis*, 18 showed mites in both skin scrapings and faeces. In all but one case the mites were more frequent and more easily demonstrable in the faeces. Baker (1970), on the other hand, recommends skin scrapings for diagnosis. Because of the degree to which this mite penetrates the skin acaricidal control is difficult. Eradication would require the removal of pups by Caesarean section and artificial rearing of them away from the dam.

Mites of the genus *Demodex* have been found in the eyelids of various mammalian species. Baker and Fisher (1969) conducted a survey in southern U.S.A. and found this mite in the eyelids of 8 out of 70 cattle examined, 44 out of 75 horses, and 2 out of 18 goats. None was found in 40 sheep and 66 deer examined.

Grono (1969) showed a correlation between infestation of ear mite, *Otodectes cynotis*, and ear type among dogs in Brisbane. Semi-erect ears were the type usually infected. There was a correlation between mite infestation and otitis externa, but mites were not found where the otitis had become suppurative.

An epidemic of spirochaetosis in fowls in the Soviet Union occurred in the absence of the usual vector *Argas persicus* (Reshetnikov, 1967). However, large numbers of *D. gallinae* were present and these, when confined under the wings of hens, appeared to transmit spirochaetosis.

Gräfner and Nietzow (1969) surveyed 143 herds of pigs in East Germany for ectoparasites and found 39 per cent with *Sarcoptes suis*; 83 per cent of the smaller fattening herds had severe mange whereas in larger breeding or fattening herds there was only 39 per cent with light or moderate infestations. *Demodex suis* was found in two herds.

Fleas and Lice

Dogs and cats were rendered less sensitive to flea bites by treating them with weekly injections of 2 ml. of a haptenic fraction of flea saliva in 1 per cent solution of sodium alginate (Michaeli and Goldfarb, 1968). Three or four injections gave 5–6 weeks' protection to 47 out of 61 animals treated.

The mechanism by which the hen flea finds its host has been investigated by Humphries (1968). Negative geotactic responses lead the flea to the tips of the vegetation, where it orientates itself towards the light. Passage of the host's shadow reduces the light intensity which stimulates a jumping response. Those fleas that miss the host fall to the ground where they repeat the whole process. Host finding activity increases during the first few days after emergence and thereafter declines probably as a result of water loss.

Goat lice, *Damalinia crassipes* and *D. limbata*, have been reared *in vitro* by Hopkins and Chamberlain (1969) using scrapings from goat skin as food. *D. crassipes* was reared at 72 per cent R.H. and 35° C. and took about 37 days to develop; 94 per cent of eggs hatched and 66 per cent developed to adults. For *D. limbata* at 76 per cent R.H. and 35° C. a generation took 32 days with 87 per cent of the eggs hatching and 67 per cent reaching adulthood.

Lice infestations were severe in 120 of the herds in East Germany surveyed by Gräfner and Neitzow (1969) (*see* p. 167); 67 per cent were infested with *Haematopinus suis*. *Pulex irritans* was seen in one herd.

Hereford cattle, kept on low rations and regularly infested with *B. microplus*, supported higher levels of infestation by *Damalinia bovis*. The effect of the low plane of nutrition was considered by Utech and his fellow workers (Utech, Wharton, and Wooderson, 1969) to have an effect on self-grooming and time of shedding of the coat.

Tsetse

An account of the tsetse problem for the general reader has been published by Nash (1969). The book covers the historical and social aspects of trypanosomiasis as well as the biology and ecology of the fly and research on the problem. The same author and his fellow workers at Bristol continue to report on their work on laboratory rearing of tsetse. Incubator rearing in the dark (Jordan, Nash, and Boyle, 1968) of tsetse fed on lop-eared rabbits is suggested as a method suitable for production of tsetse for such studies as trypanosome transmission. This is not so satisfactory for larger-scale rearing as the method they have described in another paper (Nash, Jordan, and Boyle, 1968). This large-scale rearing technique involves feeding on goats and rearing in cages in an insectary. Curtis and Jordan (1970) have reported on comparative productivity of *Glossina austeni* when maintained on goats and on lop-eared rabbits. Output per week from colonies could be 20–30 per cent of the breeding population. For a given output, feeding on goats would require a colony some 18–20 per cent larger than would feeding on rabbits.

Other workers have reported on similar studies of laboratory rearing. Laboratory studies by Phelps and Burrows (1969) gave results permitting the prediction of the duration of the puparial stage to within 5 per cent of actual values in specific sites, provided that adequate climatological information is available. The developmental state of host guinea-pigs was shown by Odhiambo (1969) to have an effect on the feeding activity of *G. pallidipes*.

Pregnant females and mature males were the most favoured hosts; infants and suckling mothers the least. Attempts to find a suitable membrane for artificial feeding of the tsetse have been reported by Langley and Maly (1969). Greatest success was achieved using a membrane constructed by pouring a 2–5 per cent solution of agar in boiling water over a terylene net to give a membrane about 2 mm. thick. Better results were obtained when the membrane was covering plastic foam or cotton-wool soaked in blood than when the membrane was over a pool of blood.

Baldry's (1970) observations, that in south-eastern Nigeria the resting sites of *G. tachinoides* were around the villages and especially the animal enclosures, led him to the view that control, if not eradication, could be achieved by concentrating control measures on these 'peri-domestic' sites. Cattle rearing is prohibited on about 14 per cent of the potential grazing land of Rhodesia because of tsetse. Lovemore (1969) has suggested that, rather than turning these areas over to game farming, some attempt should be made at eradication by extending the control measures now operating at the boundaries of these lands. However, selective elimination of game would have to be carried out, and successful elimination of the fly would raise the question of future land use.

Ford and Clifford (1968) have considered the effect of the spread of *G. morsitans morsitans* on the build-up of Ankole cattle populations after their serious depletion by the Rinderpest catastrophes of 1890–1 and 1919–30. Tsetse had an effect on limiting the rate of herd build-up, but this effect was limited to restriction of suitable grazing. *T. parva* had a much greater and more direct controlling effect on the rate of increase of numbers of cattle.

Male and female *G. morsitans* were caught on a moving vehicle in two areas, in one of which sleeping sickness was endemic and one where it was unknown (Geigy, Kauffmann, and Diehl, 1968). Trypanosome infections were found in 11·2 per cent of the males in the first area and in 9·5 per cent of males in the second. All but one were of the *Trypanosoma vivax* or *T. congolense* type.

Infection rates of *T. brucei* in *G. austeni* after 1–2 days' feeding on infected guinea-pigs were examined by Ward (1968). Those fed when 1 day old had 25 per cent of their number showing infection of the midgut and 3 per cent with infection of the salivary glands when dissected from 1 to 2 months later. Of those fed when 2 days old only 1 out of 173 had midgut infections and none had infected salivary glands. The susceptibility of this species of tsetse to trypanosome infection is clearly influenced by the age at which the infective meal is taken. Three tsetse species, *G. morsitans*, *G. pallidipes*, and *G. fuscipes*, were infected with *T. congolense* and then fed on a pool of defibrinated blood at intervals. The blood remaining after feeding was titrated in mice to find the amount of infective material extruded into it by the fly during feeding (Harley and Wilson, 1968). All individuals of *G. morsitans* and *G. pallidipes* extruded infective trypanosomes throughout their life though not necessarily at every meal. The two *G. fuscipes* individuals which were studied extruded infective trypanosomes on a single occasion only followed by a series of feeds which produced no infective material.

Nodules were observed to develop at sites of infection on cattle bitten by *G. morsitans* infected with *T. congolense* (Roberts, Gray, and Gray, 1969). The skin reactions were seen at the sites of fly-bites 7–11 days after the cattle were bitten and some 4–12 days before trypanosomes were to be seen in the blood. Many normal blood forms similar to those seen in the tsetse were also found.

Curtis (1969) attempted to produce, in *G. austeni*, chromosomal translocations which might be used ultimately for control of the species. Males were irradiated at a ^{60}Co source when they were 9 days old, and their progeny bred from. The pattern of inheritance and high frequency of induced lethal mutations suggested that translocations were probably involved.

Mitotic metaphase chromosomes from the circumoesophageal tissue of early puparial stages of *G. palpalis* showed two long pairs and one short pair of chromosomes (Riordan, 1968). This suggested a closer affinity of *G. palpalis* with *G. tachinoides* which also has three pairs, than with *G. morsitans* (5 pairs) or *G. pallidipes* (4 pairs).

Partially sterilized males of *G. morsitans orientalis*, produced by treatment with tepa, were capable of transmitting *T. congolense* according to Dame and McKenzie (1968).

Warble-fly

During the months of October to March, Hiepe and his fellow workers in Germany (Hiepe and others, 1969) examined 1303 head of cattle for the presence of *Hypoderma bovis* in the back. Most of the warbles (79 per cent) found on 622 cattle were in the lumbar region. Eleven 1st instar larvae were found between the 5th and 6th lumbar vertebrae. Larval tunnels were found as far back as the 4th sacral vertebra. Further work reported by Beesley (1969) on his study of *H. bovis* and *H. lineatum* showed that larvae migration was more due to their lytic activity than to mechanical action of the mouth parts. Boulard (1969) found that collagenase which is produced by 1st instar *Hypoderma* larvae is reabsorbed along with the host tissues on which it has acted. This collagenase can be found in the blind midgut of larvae, especially the 1st instars. This collagenase extract was collected and purified by ultrafiltration and addition of aluminium gel (Boulard, 1970) to give a concentration of 5 larval equivalents per ml. Cattle were injected with 7–20 ml. of this extract in December or January. Spring warble burdens in these animals was 6–19 per head as compared with 11–72 per head of control animals.

A case of human infestation by *H. lineatum* has been reported by Krivko (1969) from Kazakhstan. Larvae were found under the scalp and in the back of a female patient who had no contact with cattle.

Blow-fly and Bots

Males of the sheep blow-fly *Lucilia cuprina* were found to be sexually stimulated by the presence of females of their own species (Bartell, Shorey, and Barton-Browne, 1969). Odours from the female provided partial stimulus, but tactile contact produced a greater effect. The strongest stimulus was provided by sexually mature females and the strongest response was from sexually active males.

It is believed that *Oestrus ovis* passes the winter as a quiescent larva within the nasal sinuses of the sheep. A study by an American team (Rogers and others, 1968) showed that ambient air temperatures as low as 10° F. do not affect the temperature in the nasal sinuses of sheep, at depths of 2 in. or more, sufficiently to produce quiescence in larvae of *O. ovis*, Other American work reported by Meleney and Apodaca (1969) observed the regeneration of *O. ovis* populations following treatment of the sheep in two successive years by intramuscular injections of dimethoate. It was found that population levels were some 55 per cent of their original pre-treatment value (of 50 per head) 7 years or 14 fly-generations later.

Keds and Biting Flies

The biting mechanism of the ked *Melophagus ovinus* has been observed by Nelson and Petrussia (1969), using the transillumination technique on mouse ears. Feeding was from blood-vessels near the apocrine glands and follicle bases. The haustellum could be seen to penetrate the stratum corneum and sub-epidermal tissue, assisted by the movements of the prestomal teeth. On contact with a small vessel, penetration occurred and the prestomal teeth were everted to anchor the labella to the vessel wall. Sucking of blood began at once and continued for 5–10 minutes. Jets of saliva were seen to enter the vessel several times during feeding.

Roberts (1968) found that the small eye-frequenting flies of the genus *Hippelates* contained bovine blood ingested from wounds made by tabanids. It is known that anaplasmosis can be transmitted to cattle by flooding the ocular membranes with infected blood. Roberts suggests that *Hippelates* can become infected from open punctures on infected cattle and then infect other cattle via the eye. In a later paper (Roberts and others, 1969) this hypothesis was tested by caging cattle in such a way as to exclude access by tabanids and *Hippelates*. Of control animals exposed to all Diptera 32 per cent contracted anaplasmosis and of those protected from *Hippelates* and *tabanids* none contracted the disease.

American work (Sanders and Dobson, 1969) has shown the preference for bovine dung as a breeding site for *Haematobia irritatus*, the horn fly. Thin cow pats or very thick ones tended to be avoided as oviposition sites. Preference was shown for larger pats of 2 lb. or more.

REFERENCES

Baker, D. W., and Fisher, W. F. (1969), *J. econ. Ent.*, **62**, 942.
Baker, K. P. (1970), *Vet. Rec.*, **86**, 90.
Baldry, D. A. T. (1970), *Bull. ent. Res.*, **59**, 585.
Bartell, R. J., Shorey, H. H., and Barton-Browne, L. (1969), *Anim. Behav.*, **17**, 576.
Beesley, W. N. (1969), *Ann. trop. Med. Parasit.*, **63**, 157.
Belozerov, V. N. (1967a), *Parazitologiya, Leningr.*, **1**, 279.
— — (1967b), *Zool. Zh.*, **46**, 1182.
— — (1967c), *Parazitologiya, Leningr.*, **1**, 13.
Best, J. M. J., Butt, K. M., and Rohrbach, J. A. (1969), *Vet. Rec.*, **85**, 633.
Boulard, C. (1969), *Annls Soc. ent. Fr.*, **5**, 371.
— — (1970), *C. r. hebd. Séanc. Acad. Sci., Paris*, **270B**, 728.
Branagan, D. (1969), *Trop. Anim. Hlth Prod.*, **1**, 119.
— — and Bailey, K. P. (1968), *E. Afr. med., J.*, **45**, 203.
Curtis, C. F. (1969), *Genet. Res.*, **13**, 289.
— — and Jordan, A. M. (1970), *Bull. ent. Res.*, **59**, 651.
Dame, D. A., and McKenzie, P. K. I. (1968), *Ann. trop. Med. Parasit.*, **62**, 372.
Derwelis, S. K. (1967), *Illinois Vet.*, **10**, 10.
Divakaran, S., and Barat, S. K. (1970), *Indian vet. J.*, **47**, 309.
Ford, J., and Clifford, H. R. (1968), *J. appl. Ecol.*, **5**, 301.
Galun, R., and Warburg, M. (1967), *Věst. Čsl. Spol. Zool.*, **31**, 329.
Garcia, R. (1969), *J. med. Ent.*, **6**, 286.
Geigy, R., Kauffmann, M., and Diehl, P. (1968), *Acta trop.*, **25**, 72.
Gräfner, G., and Nietzow, E. W. (1969), *Mh. VetMed.*, **24**, 773.
Gregson, J. D. (1969), *J. Parasit.*, **55**, 260.
Grono, L. R. (1969), *Vet. Rec.*, **85**, 6.
Hadani, A., Cwilich, R., Rechav, Y., and Dinur, Y. (1969), *Refuah Vet.*, **26**, 87.
Harley, J. M. B., and Wilson, A. J. (1968), *Ann. trop. Med. Parasit.*, **62**, 178.

HIEPE, T., RIBBECK, R., GATHOW, I., GRAMANN, F., and HORST, J. (1969), *Mh. VetMed.*, **24**, 289.
HOPKINS, D. E., and CHAMBERLAIN, W. F. (1969), *Ann. ent. Soc. Am.*, **62**, 826.
HUMPHRIES, D. A. (1968), *Parasitology*, **58**, 403.
JORDAN, A. M., NASH, T. A. M., and BOYLE, J. A. (1968), *Ann. trop. Med. Parasit.*, **62**, 331.
KÖHLER, G., HOFFMAN, G., HÖRCHNER, F., and WEILAND, G. (1967), *Berl. Münch. Tierärztl. Wschr.*, **80**, 396.
KORENBERG, E. I. (1969), *Medskaya Parazit.*, **38**, 427.
KRIVKO, A. M. (1969), *Ent. Obozr.*, **48**, 144.
KRYLOV, M. V., and KRYLOVA, A. P. (1967), *Parazitologiya, Leningr.*, **1**, 329.
LANGLEY, P. A., and MALY, H. (1969), *Nature, Lond.*, **221**, 855.
LOVEMORE, D. F. (1969), *Rhod. Sci. News*, **3**, 342.
MALYSHEVA, T. V. (1967), *Medskaya Parazit.*, **36**, 469.
MAZLUM, Z. (1969), *Parasitology*, **59**, 597.
MELENEY, W. P., and APODACA, S. A. (1969), *J. Am. vet. med. Ass.*, **155**, 136.
MESHCHERYAKOVA, V. D. (1967), *Veterinariya*, No. 1, 59.
MICHAELI, D., and GOLDFARB, S. (1968), *Aust. vet. J.*, **44**, 161.
MUSATOV, V. A. (1967a), *Veterinariya*, No. 4, 52.
— — (1967b), *Parazitologiya, Leningr.*, **1**, 288.
NASH, T. A. M. (1969), *Africa's Bane: The Tsetse Fly.* London: Collins.
— — JORDAN, A. M., and BOYLE, J. A. (1968), *Ann. trop. Med. Parasit.*, **62**, 336.
NELSON, W. A., and PETRUSSIA, D. M. (1969), *Expl Parasit.*, **26**, 308.
NOSEK, J., and KOSUCH, O. (1969), *Zentbl. Bakt. ParasitKde*, **211**, 400.
ODHIAMBO, T. R. (1969), *Bull. ent. Res.*, **59**, 519.
PHELPS, R. J., and BURROWS, P. M. (1969), *J. Appl. Ecol.*, **6**, 323.
PLOWRIGHT, W., PARKER, J., and PEIRCE, M. A. (1969), *Nature, Lond.*, **221**, 1071.
PURNELL, R. E., BRANAGAN, D., and RADLEY, E. (1969), *Parasitology*, **59**, 709.
RECHAR, Y., and OPPENHEIM, J. (1969), *Refuah Vet.*, **26**, 71.
REHACEK, J., and BRZOSTOWSKI, H. W. (1969), *J. Insect Physiol.*, **15**, 1431.
RESHETNIKOV, P. T. (1967), *Veterinariya*, No. 3, 48.
RIORDAN, K. (1968), *Parasitology*, **58**, 835.
ROBERTS, C. J., GRAY, M. A., and GRAY, A. R. (1969), *Trans. R. Soc. trop. Med. Hyg.*, **63**, 620.
ROBERTS, R. H. (1968), *Mosquito News*, **28**, 236.
— — POUND, W. A., MCCRORY, H. F., SCALES, J. W., and COLLINS, I. (1969), *Ann. ent. Soc. Am.*, **62**, 863.
ROGERS, C. E., KNAPP, F. W., COOK, D., and CROWE, M. V. (1968), *J. Parasit.*, **54**, 164.
SANDERS, D. P., and DOBSON, R. C. (1969), *J. econ. Ent.*, **62**, 1362.
SCHNEIDER, J., and HAAS, K. (1969), *Arch. Geflügelk.*, **33**, 279.
SINCLAIR, A. N., and GIBSON, A. J. F. (1970), *Aust. vet. J.*, **46**, 311.
SONENSHINE, D. E., and CLARK, G. M. (1968), *J. med. Ent.*, **5**, 229.
— — and STOUT, J. (1968), *Ibid.*, **5**, 49.
TATCHELL, R. J., and BENNETT, G. F. (1969), *Expl Parasit.*, **26**, 369.
UILENBERG, G. (1967), *Rev. Élev. Méd. vét. Pays trop.*, **20**, 497.
UTECH, K. B. W., WHARTON, R. H., and WOODERSON, L. A. (1969), *Aust. vet. J.*, **45**, 414.
WARD, R. A. (1968), *Trans. R. Soc. trop. Méd. Hyg.*, **62**, 672.
WILKINS, J. H., BOWDEN, R. S. T., and WILKINSON, G. T. (1967), *Vet. Rec.*, **81**, 57.
WILLIAMS, H. E., and GONZALEZ, F. O. (1968), *Trop. Agric. Trin.*, **45**, 23.
WINDING, D., WILLENBERG, P., and HAARLØV, V. N. (1970), *Nord. VetMed.*, **22**, 48.

HELMINTHOLOGY

T. E. Gibson, D.V.Sc., F.R.C.V.S., F.I.Biol.

Parasitic Diseases of Cattle

Gastro-intestinal Parasites

Pathogenesis

Ostertagia ostertagi.—Murray, Jennings, and Armour (1970) studied the changes in gastric structure and function in relation to worm burden in calves infected with a single dose of 300,000 *O. ostertagi.* When the parasites began to emerge from the gastric mucosa, the functional cells in the gastric glands had been replaced by undifferentiated cells. Morphological changes indicative of reduced activity were observed in the differentiated cells which remained. The biochemical and clinical consequences of these changes were elevation of the *p*H of the abomasal fluid, raised plasma pepsinogen levels, anorexia, diarrhoea, and weight-loss. When the worm burden was thrown off, there was a gradual return to normal structure and function. Allen and others (1970) studied the effects of daily infections of 200–1600 third-stage larvae of *O. ostertagi* given for 6 months. Only the highest level of infection produced clinical disease. The only haematological effect observed was a slight fall in packed-cell volume. No significant changes were seen in plasma-electrolyte level. Plasma-pepsinogen levels showed large variations within groups but the levels increased with increased numbers of larvae administered. A seven-fold increase was seen in the group receiving the most larvae and this persisted for three months after, when there was a decrease in spite of the continued administration of larvae. Thus in continuing infections the rate of damage must decrease or the rate of repair increase. From the third month onward increased activity of plasma pepsinogen was related to the number of larvae maturing with the abomasum. The increase in plasma-pepsinogen and glycoprotein values bore no constant relationship to the number of infective larvae being ingested at a particular time. The increased pepsinogen activity was correlated with the raised serum-glycoprotein concentration and both were related to tissue damage associated with the adult worm as indicated by increased abomasal *p*H.

Oesophagostomum radiatum.—Using ^{51}Cr-labelled erythrocytes Bremner (1970) estimated the blood-loss into the intestine in *O. radiatum* infections. Bleeding began 19–20 days after infection of the calves with the parasite when the stage of the fourth larval ecdysis had been reached. Maximum blood-loss occurred in the seventh week of infection when a mean worm burden of 2500 was present. After the seventh week haemorrhage decreased slowly, but was still present 12 weeks after infection. Faecal blood-loss was markedly reduced following anthelmintic medication but persisted up to 6 days after treatment. Intestinal haemorrhage appears to be the chief cause of anaemia in oesophagostomiasis.

Trichostrongylus axei.—Ross, Purcell, and Todd (1970a) studied the effects of infections with *T. axei* in cannulated calves. An increase in abomasal *p*H was observed together with increase in sodium-ion concentration and decrease in potassium- and chloride-ion concentrations. Similar changes were seen in duodenal, ileal, and caecal fluid constituents. A significant rise in the bacterial flora of the duodenal fluid followed these changes. In acute cases these changes result in severe diarrhoea, anorexia, dehydration, and rapidly developing hypo-albuminaemia followed by death about 8 weeks following infection. Further studies by Ross, Todd, and Purcell (1970) suggest that imbalance of albumin and electrolytes is a critical factor, which results from protein and electrolyte loss from the gastro-intestinal tract during the diarrhoea phase. In acute, subacute, and chronic fatal infections water imbalance may be important.

Neoascaris vitulorum.—Prenatally infected calves were studied by Enyenihi (1969), who found that high worm burdens were correlated with poor weight-gain, loss of appetite, and anaemia. The animals showed a progressive reduction in weight-gain during the second and third months of life. Excessive faecal fat was observed in heavily infected calves between the fifth and eleventh weeks of life and indicates an interference with the nutrition of the host by the worm infection. The author estimates that *N. vitulorum* infection results in the loss of many millions of pounds of meat and urges the importance of control measures.

Ecology of Larvae on Pasture

Goldberg (1970) studied the development and survival of the eggs and larvae of various species of gastro-intestinal nematodes of cattle at Beltsville during 1968. Larvae were recovered within a week of the deposition of the eggs of *O. ostertagi*, *Cooperia punctata*, and *O. radiatum*. Maximum numbers were recovered 1–2 weeks after deposition and 9½ weeks later all larvae had died out. *O. ostertagi* developed in larger quantities than the other two species. Little lateral migration occurred, the majority of the larvae being found within 13 cm. of the faecal pats. The dry conditions in the area were responsible for the rapid death of the larvae and for the restricted lateral migration. Rose (1970) studied the fluctuations of larvae on the pasture herbage under field conditions. Residual herbage larval infection is responsible for the initial infection of calves turned out in the spring. Eggs passed out in the faeces as a result develop at varying speeds and result in a marked increase in pasture larval population in early July. The timing of this increase varies from year to year according to the temperature and the distribution of rainfall. This variability does not, however, necessitate changes in the timing of control measures which are normally applied in mid-July.

Epidemology and Control

Michel, Lancaster, and Hong (1970) studied the fluctuations in the numbers of larvae in cattle pastures in the north-east and in the south-west of England. Pasture larval population falls to a low level at the end of April and calves turned out in early May cause a rise in pasture larval count in mid-July. In the south-west calves turned out before this time may produce heavy pasture larval infections by early June. This is best avoided by turning out calves initially on to clean pastures where they remain until the end of April or by ensuring that the area they graze up to the middle of May is not grazed after the third week in June. Michel and Lancaster (1970) described field experiments carried out over 3 successive years on the control of parasitic gastro-enteritis in calves. Calves kept in the same pasture during the season were compared with others moved to clean pasture in July, with a third group moved to clean pasture in July and treated with an efficient anthelmintic, and with a fourth group treated weekly with anthelmintic but kept on the same ground throughout. The first group became severely affected with parasitic gastro-enteritis and suffered a mid-season check in weight-gain. The other three groups gained weight in linear fashion throughout, but the best results were most consistently obtained with the group both dosed and moved in mid-July. Van Adrachem (1970) treated 7-month-old calves with thiabendazole before they were housed for the winter. Treated calves gained more weight during the winter and the subsequent summer grazing period than untreated calves. Trials carried out during the winter showed that treated calves consumed less food per unit of weight-gain. Winks (1970) treated beef calves in central Queensland with trichlorphon either after rainfall exceeding 50 mm. or monthly. He found no significant difference between the weight-gains of these groups and untreated controls and concluded the use of anthelmintic was uneconomic.

Immunity

In a study of acquired resistance to *Trichostrongylus axei* Ross (1970e) showed that calves acquired resistance under conditions of continuing infection but that animals treated with anthelmintic so that the parasites they acquired never reached maturity developed a lower level of resistance. Smith (1970) compared the resistance to infection of *O. ostertagi*, *Cooperia oncophora*, and *Nematodirus helvetianus* in 15-month-old cattle and 3-month-old calves. The former had greater resistance as manifested by the establishment of smaller worm burdens, the stunting of worms, and a lower worm-egg output.

Parasitic Bronchitis

Gupta and Gibbs (1970) studied the epidemiology of parasitic bronchitis of cattle on six farms in Ontario and Quebec. It was found that infection was perpetuated both by larvae which survived the winter and by carrier animals. The latter were considered to be the more important source of infection. In order to control infection it is recommended that calves should be grazed on clean pastures not grazed by cattle the previous year, or should be reared indoors for the first year of their lives. Adult stock should be grazed separately from young stock.

Cornwell and Jones (1970a) showed that triethylene melamine (TEM) could be used for the attenuation of *Dictyocaulus viviparus* larvae, the optimum concentration being 0·7 per cent to which the larvae were exposed for 1 hour. Using these attenuated larvae as a vaccine, it was shown that a high degree of immunity was produced. In further experiments, Cornwell and Jones (1970b) compared the vaccine with the irradiated larval vaccine which has been used for some years and found that both gave good protection. Two doses of 1000 of the attenuated larvae are given either at a two- or 4-week interval. Cornwell and Jones (1970c) also used the TEM-attenuated larvae as a vaccine successfully under field conditions. A similar level of immunity was stimulated to that produced when using irradiated larval vaccines.

Miscellaneous

Trichuris discolor

Smith and Stevenson (1970) describe an outbreak of trichuriasis in calves, in which the important symptoms were diarrhoea, accompanied by tenesmus, foamy faeces containing mucus and anorexia. The diagnosis was made at autopsy of a 10-month-old animal which died. Treatment with methyridine controlled the outbreak.

Schistosomiasis

Hussein, Saeed, and Nelson (1970) showed that exposure of calves to cercariae of *Schistosoma mansoni* protected them when they were subsequently exposed to *S. matheii* infection. This suggests that exposure of cattle to *S. mansoni* may reduce the severity of bovine schistosomiasis in endemic areas.

Parasitic Diseases of Sheep

Gastro-intestinal Parasites

Pathogenesis

Trichostrongylus axei.—Ross, Purcell, and Todd (1970b) found that, following infection, reduced fluid balance in the infected lamb was responsible for severe haemoconcentration. Dehydration of the host results and this masks hypoalbuminaemia which develops during the first 3 weeks. Four weeks after infection this process is reversed and the hypoalbuminaemia becomes obvious and is accompanied by severe weight-loss. Anorexia is shown at this time and is responsible for further weight-loss. The animal is now in a state of negative nitrogen balance. During the terminal phase prior to death haemodilution is seen and at autopsy there was evidence that oedema was developing.

Haemonchus contortus.—Silverman, Mansfield, and Scott (1970) showed that lambs 42 days old survived infection with 10,000 *Haemonchus contortus* larvae when maintained on high-protein levels. However, 2 of 5 lambs given 25,000 larvae died as did 4 of 5 given 50,000 larvae. Iron-deficiency anaemia was the most prominent sign of haemonchosis and deaths were apparently due to failure of the haemopoietic system.

Post-parturient Rise in Faecal Egg Count

Brunsdon (1970) demonstrated that in New Zealand the species responsible for the post-parturient rise in faecal egg count are *H. contortus* and *Ostertagia* spp. and to a lesser extent *T. axei* and *Cooperia curticei*. He considered that maturation of dormant larvae from the abomasal mucosa is not the only source of the increased worm burden which causes the rise. Another factor is the loss of resistance which occurs at the time of the rise in faecal egg count and which is species specific. The phenomenon which terminates the rise is also species specific. Salisbury and Arundel (1970) evaluated residual pasture larval infection and contamination from the post-parturient rise as sources of infection to the young lamb and concluded that the latter was more important. They recommended dosing ewes about 2 weeks before lambing to control the post-parturient rise and so lower the hazard to lambs.

Immunity

Ross (1970a) showed that a low level of initial infection produced stronger immunity in 7-month-old lambs than a high level. Removal of the patent infection at the time of challenge had no effect on the immunity stimulated by low initial infections but reduced that acquired following high initial infections. Ross (1970b) produced evidence that in lambs 2 weeks old a period of immune incompetence occurs but by 6 weeks a partial immune competence has developed. Between 10 weeks and 5 months of age complete immune competence develops. Ross (1970c) showed that the passage of *T. axei* in one host species produced strains which establish better in that species. He also showed (1970d) that a strain passaged in Scottish Blackface sheep became established less readily in Dorset lambs than in Blackface lambs.

Epidemiology and Control

Boag and Thomas (1970) showed that the larvae of *Ostertagia circumcincta* survive the winter better than those of *Trichostrongylus colubriformis*. Initial infections in young lambs tend, therefore, to be predominantly by *Ostertagia* spp. which are succeeded by *Trichostrongylus* spp. later in the season. Swan (1970) made a study of the epidemiology of haemonchosis and concluded that temperature records could be used to forecast the fluctuations in numbers of *H. contortus* larvae, but was unable to draw any conclusions as to the minimum amount of rainfall required before outbreaks occur. He used the mean maximum temperature in his predictions when diurnal fluctuation is small and the maximum temperature fluctuates about 63–65° F. The minimum temperature (critical value 50° F.) is used in environments where there is a wide diurnal fluctuation and maximum temperatures fluctuate about a mean higher than 63–65° F. Lindahl and others (1970) compared four management systems for the control of parasitic gastritis in lambs. When zero grazing was practised, the lambs remained parasite free and a change to clean pasture at biweekly intervals also controlled haemonchosis. Rotation on contaminated pasture at biweekly intervals accompanied by monthly therapeutic treatment and free choice phenothiazine was ineffective, whether the standard product or micronized purified phenothiazine was used. The investigation was repeated by Colglazier and others (1970) except that therapeutic treatment with pure micronized phenothiazine was used with one rotation group and with thiabendazole in the other. The results were similar. Smeal, Farleigh, and Major (1969) also evaluated rotational grazing for the control of parasitic gastritis in lambs using a system in which animals grazed a paddock for 4 days and did not return to graze it again for 60 days. During the first 2 years drought interrupted the rotation for 6 months and anthelmintic treatment was given before the animals were returned to the rotation. In these 2 years no clinical parasitism occurred but in the third year, in which rotation was practised throughout, clinical parasitism was seen. Pasture larval estimations showed that large numbers of trichostrongylid larvae were present on the paddocks after 60 days' rest and larvae continued to be present throughout the winter. There is accumulating evidence that rotational grazing is of little value in the control of gastro-intestinal parasitism.

Vaccination

Dhar and Singh (1970) investigated the effects of irradiation on infective larvae of *Oesophagostomum columbianum*. It was found that irradiation at 15,000–40,000 r caused fewer adults to develop but more intestinal nodules to be formed. The use of larvae irradiated at 40,000 r as a vaccine resulted in increased nodule formation and is therefore not of practical value. Irradiation at 80,000 r attenuated the larvae to such a degree that they failed to develop in the host.

Cysticercosis

Gemmell (1970) studied the distribution of the cysts of *Taenia ovis* in sheep and found that only about one-third of the cysticerci are found in the muscles of the heart, diaphragm, and head. In light infections the cysts may not be found in one or all of these sites. The number present in these sites does not provide accurate information of the number present in the carcass meat. This is contrary to the view of Sweatman (1962), who considered that meat from carcasses in which these sites were not affected could be safely fed to dogs.

Parasitic Diseases of Pigs

Gastro-intestinal Parasites

Hyostrongylus rubidus

Castelino and others (1970) surveyed the prevalence of *H. rubidus* in breeding pigs at two abattoirs in north Wales for 1 year and found that 792 of 1656 pigs were infected. The majority of infected pigs carried less than 100 worms and only 164 pigs harboured more than 500. Prevalence rose in the winter months but the reason for this was not ascertained. There was no correlation between carcass condition and the parasite burden. Pigs experimentally infected with 20,000 larvae of *H. rubidus* were found by Castelino, Herbert, and Lean (1970) to show no clinical signs. Infections of 200,000–500,000 caused mild fever, listlessness, inappetence, and diarrhoea, and a reduction in weight-gain which was most severe 3–4 weeks after infection. Baskerville and Ross (1970) also found that low doses of larvae did not produce clinical disease. An abattoir survey showed 60 per cent of sows to be carrying infection. Burden, Harding, and Kendall (1970) were unable to find any evidence of age resistance in pigs up to 4 years of age.

***Oesophagostomum* spp.**

Stockdale (1970a) investigated the role of *Oesophagostomum* spp. in the production of necrotic enteritis and found that the severity of the lesions varied with the number of infective larvae given. The mechanical damage to the mucosa produced by large numbers of larvae provides an environment conducive to the proliferation of organisms found in pigs showing necrotic enteritis.

Parasitic Diseases of Dogs and Cats

Dirofilaria immitis Infection

Diagnosis

Wylie (1970) described a filter technique for increasing the accuracy with which microfilariae may be recovered from the blood. Lysed blood is passed through a filter followed by methylene-blue solution. The filter membrane is then removed and placed on a glass slide and examined for the presence of microfilariae of *D. immitis.* Tashjian and others (1970) evaluated angiocardiography for the diagnosis of heartworm disease. They found it valuable for early diagnosis, and the severity of the disease can be estimated from the radiographic observations. The technique may be used preoperatively to locate the presence of the parasites and the extent of the damage and to evaluate the results of surgical removal of the parasites.

Treatment

Abadie and others (1970) devised a surgical procedure for the removal of heartworms from the dog. A pulmonary arteriotomy was performed in which the pulmonary artery was sutured to a vascular clamp, so ensuring maximum access to the site of infection and minimum (15–20 seconds) circulatory occlusion time.

Toxacariasis

Swerczek, Nielsen, and Helmbolt (1970) produced medial hyperplasia of the pulmonary arteries in cats by experimental infection with *Toxocara cati.* They consider this nematode to be the most important cause of this condition in cats. The severity of the medial hyperplasia produced by *T. cati* is greater than that induced by *Aelurostrongylus abstrusus*, *Toxocara canis*, and *Ascaris suum*, the other nematodes which have been implicated as causes of the condition.

Platynosomum fastosum Infection

The liver fluke, *P. fastosum*, was found in 73 per cent of 304 cats in a survey carried out by Retnasabapathy and Prathap (1971). The cats were clinically unaffected by the presence of the flukes. At autopsy the most prominent lesion was mottling and enlargement of the liver. Histological examination revealed fatty infiltration of the parenchymatous cells and fibrosis and epithelial proliferation of the bile-ducts.

Parasitic Diseases of Poultry

Raillietina tetragona.—Nadakal and others (1970b) observed no distinctive pattern of segment discharge in birds infected with *R. tetragona* and no correlation between feeding and segment discharge. Segment production per worm was greater in single than in multiple infections. The many variables relating to segment discharge suggest that segment counts could not be used as a measure of worm burden. Nadakal and others (1970a) report that *Tetramorium similimum* is a new intermediate host for *R. tetragona* in India.

Miscellaneous

Diplostomum spathaceum

Ashton, Brown, and Easty (1969) report that this trematode parasite of gulls is the cause of cataract in trout and other fresh-water fish. The ova of the parasite hatch to produce miricidia which invade water snails. Cercariae eventually leave the snails and swim until they are able to penetrate a fish, when they find their way to the lens of the eye.

Filaroides martis

The life cycle of this worm was studied by Stockdale and Anderson (1970). Third-stage larvae enter the gastric glands of the mink where they moult 3 or 4 days after infection. From the fifth to the eighth day the larvae were in the gastric submucosa often associated with blood-vessels. They were in the gastric subserosal fat 8 to 9 days after infection. The larvae arrive at the junction of the coeliac artery and dorsal aorta 10 days after infection. The fourth moult takes place on the eleventh day. The worms move forward through the diaphragm and reach the bronchial bifurcation. The worms then penetrate the lung substance, which they reach by the twenty-first day.

Perostrongylus pridhami

The infective larvae of this lungworm of mink were found by Stockdale (1970b) to penetrate the stomach wall, cross the peritoneal cavity, traverse the diaphragm, and enter the lungs within 24 hours of infection. The third moult occurs at about 3 days and the final moult 7 days after infection. The prepatent period is about 3 weeks. The discarded cuticles of the larvae provoke granuloma formation and cause bronchitis obliterans of the respiratory and terminal bronchioles. The adult worms cause a mild bronchiolitis of the respiratory and terminal bronchioles.

REFERENCES

ABADIE, S. H., BLACK, E., DUPUY, H. J., and GONZALEZ, R. (1970), *J. Am. vet. med. Ass.*, **156**, 884.

ALLEN, W. M., SWEASEY, D., BERRETT, S., HEBERT, C. N., and PATTERSON, D. S. P. (1970), *J. comp. Path. Ther.*, **80**, 441.

ASHTON, N., BROWN, N., and EASTY, D. (1969), *J. small Anim. Pract.*, **10**, 471.

BASKERVILLE, A., and ROSS, J. G. (1970), *Br. vet. J.*, **126**, 538.

BOAG, B., and THOMAS, R. J. (1970), *Res. vet. Sci.*, **11**, 380.

BREMNER, K. C. (1970), *Exptl Parasit.*, **27**, 236.

BRUNSDON, R. V. (1970), *N.Z. vet. J.*, **18**, 47.

BURDEN, D. J., HARDING, D. J. D., and KENDALL, S. B. (1970), *J. comp. Path. Ther.*, **80**, 601.

CASTELINO, J. B., HERBERT, I. V., and LEAN, I. J. (1970), *Br. vet. J.*, **126**, 579.

— — THOMAS, M., HERBERT, I. V., and LEAN, I. H. (1970), *Vet. Rec.*, **80**, 256.

COLGLAZIER, M. L., LINDAHL, I. H., ENZIE, F. D., WHITMORE, G. E., and WILSON, R. L. (1970), *Proc. helminth. Soc. Wash.*, **37**, 230.

CORNWELL, R. L., and JONES, R. M. (1970a), *Res. vet. Sci.*, **11**, 553.

— — — — (1970b), *Ibid.*, **11**, 560.

— — — — (1970c), *Ibid.*, **11**, 569.

DHAR, H., and SINGH, K. S. (1970), *J. Helminth.*, **44**, 11.

ENYENIHI, U. K. (1969), *Bull. épizoot. Dis. Afr.*, **17**, 171.

GEMMELL, M. A. (1970), *Aust. vet. J.*, **46**, 22.

GOLDBERG, A. (1970), *Proc. helminth. Soc. Wash.*, **37**, 166.

GUPTA, R. P., and GIBBS, M. C. (1970), *Can. vet. J.*, **11**, 149.

HUSSEIN, H., SAEED, A. A., and NELSON, G. S. (1970), *Bull. Wld Hlth Org.*, **42**, 745.

LINDAHL, I. L., COLGLAZIER, M. L., ENZIE, F. D., TURNER, J. M. WHITMORE, G. E., and WILSON, R. L. (1970), *J. Parasit.*, **56**, 991.

MICHEL, J. F., and LANCASTER, M. B. (1970), *J. Helminth.*, **44**, 107.

— — — — and HONG, C. (1970), *Res. vet. Sci.*, **11**, 25.

MURRAY, M., JENNINGS, F. W., and ARMOUR, J. (1970), *Ibid.*, **11**, 417.

NADAKAL, A. M., JOHN, K. O., MURALEEDHARAN, K., and MOHANDAS, A. (1970a), *Proc. Helminth. Soc. Wash.*, **37**, 141.

— — — — — — — — (1970b), *Ibid.*, **37**, 144.

RETNASABAPATHY, A., and PRATHAP, K. (1971), *Vet. Rec.*, **88**, 62.

ROSE, J. H. (1970), *Res. vet. Sci.*, **11**, 199.

ROSS, J. G. (1970a), *Br. vet. J.*, **125**, 648.

— — (1970b), *J. Helminth.*, **44**, 199.

— — (1970c), *Res. vet. Sci.*, **11**, 461.

— — (1970d), *Ibid.*, **11**, 465.

— — (1970e), *Br. vet. J.*, **126**, xxi.

— — PURCELL, D. A., and TODD, J. R. (1970a), *Ibid.*, **126**, 149.

— — — — — — (1970b), *Ibid.*, **126**, 159.

— — TODD, J. R., and PURCELL, D. A. (1970), *Ibid.*, **126**, 393.

SALISBURY, J. R., and ARUNDEL, J. H. (1970), *Aust. vet. J.*, **46**, 523.

SILVERMAN, P. H., MANSFIELD, M. E., and SCOTT, H. L. (1970), *Am. J. vet. Res.*, **31**, 841.

SMEAL, M. G., FARLEIGH, E. A., and MAJOR, G. W. (1969), *Aust. vet. J.*, **45**, 554.

SMITH, H. J. (1970), *Can. J. comp. Med.*, **34**, 303.

— — and STEVENSON, R. G. (1970), *Can. vet. J.*, **11**, 102.

STOCKDALE, P. H. G. (1970a), *Br. vet. J.*, **125**, 526.

— — (1970b), *J. Parasit.*, **56**, 559.

— — and ANDERSON, R. C. (1970), *Ibid.*, **56**, 550.

SWAN, R. A. (1970), *Aust. vet. J.*, **46**, 485.

SWEATMAN, G. K. (1962), *N.Z. vet. J.*, **10**, 93.

SWERCZEK, T. W., NIELSEN, S. W., and HELMBOLT, C. F. (1970), *Res. vet. Sci.*, **11**, 103.

TASHJIAN, R. J., LIU, S. K., YARNS, D. A., DAS, K. M., and STEIN, H. L. (1970), *Am. J. vet. Res.*, **31**, 415.
VAN ADRACHEM, P. W. M. (1970), *Vet. Rec.*, **87**, 675.
WINKS, R. (1970), *Aust. vet. J.*, **46**, 8.
WYLIE, J. P. (1970), *J. Am. vet. Med. Ass.*, **156**, 1403.

FASCIOLIASIS

S. B. Kendall, B.Sc., Ph.D., M.R.C.V.S., A.R.C.S., F.I.Biol.

Chemotherapy of fascioliasis is considered *in extensis* elsewhere (p. 207).

A very useful review by Fowler (1970) of the metabolism of carbon tetrachloride in sheep and in *Fasciola hepatica* discusses the possibility that activity against the parasite may depend on the production of toxic compounds in the damaged liver. In an earlier review (VETERINARY ANNUAL, 1970, 224) it was suggested that the work of Kendall and Sinclair (1969) indicated that unusual activity of hexachlorophane against very young parasites could be the result of an indirect effect of the drug. Later Kendall and Sinclair (1971) suggested that the interaction of a previous infection and a drug given immediately before challenge might be instrumental in affording 'protection' by adversely affecting the environment of the invading parasites. Serological changes observed during the course of this work lent support to the view that while a previous infection with *Fasciola* does not engender resistance in the ordinarily accepted sense it is possible to produce a transitory state which decreases the numbers of parasites.

All this reinforces the conclusion that the so-called 'resistance' to *F. hepatica* is no more than a rather non-specific reaction to less favourable conditions in the liver arising from overcrowding or from pathological change of various aetiology. The supporting serological work described by Sinclair and Kendall (1969) and Kendall and Sinclair (1971) utilized gel diffusion which gives specific and satisfactory results. It is of interest that Geyer (1969) has shown that *F. hepatica* antigen purified by gel filtration on Sephadex G-75 and disk electrophoresis in polyacrylamide gel fails to produce precipitins against seven other trematode species but does so against both *F. hepatica* and *F. gigantica*.

Owing to the special economic circumstances in those areas of Britain most subject to fascioliasis there has been a tendency to concentrate attention on the acute disease causing actual mortality in sheep. Roseby (1970), in Australia, has studied the effect on wool production in Merino sheep and has found up to 39 per cent reduction in yield from the sixth week after infection irrespective of the age of the sheep or the plane of nutrition. The liver remains, of course, the organ principally affected and very marked changes occur. Nisenbaum (1968) states that the changes are to an extent reversible. If effective treatment be instituted in sheep 50 days after infection hepatic tissue regenerates completely. If treatment is delayed to the hundredth day there is fragmentation of connective tissue around the bile-ducts and partial regeneration of the epithelial lining. If delayed to the one hundred and thirty-fifth day there is no regeneration.

In rabbits, according to Dodd and Nualláin (1969), the cellular response limits the damage caused by parasites migrating through the liver parenchyma and this may be suppressed by horse and sheep anti-rabbit lymphocyte serum. The rabbit appears normally to be a well-adapted host for *F. hepatica* and survives many years with a patent infection. By contrast, Tewari (1968) has found that the variable degree of infection in the guinea-pig plus the high rate of mortality makes it unsuitable as a test animal. Twenty-five metacercariae killed 80–100 per cent, although there was a lower mortality with 10 metacercariae.

Reports continue to appear implicating new 'species' of *Lymnaea* as vectors of *Fasciola*, but the criteria for the identification of the snails are rarely given. For this omission there are excellent reasons. Identification even at the specific level can be extremely difficult and in the past century very numerous subspecies and varieties were without doubt given unmerited specific rank, the basis for separation being the morphology of the shell, which is notoriously variable within a species according to, for instance, the circumstances of the environment. The classic monograph of Hubendick (1951) did much to clarify the position, did at least reduce the number of synonyms and could be consulted with advantage before more 'new vectors' are described. Not all such publication lacks merit. In New Zealand, Pullan (1969) has described the occurrence of *Lymnaea columella* (Say, 1817) acting as a host for *F. hepatica*. According to Hubendick *L. columella* is an easily recognized and distinct species which, originating in the eastern United States, has a history of artificial introduction into botanical gardens, parks, and aquaria in different parts of the world. In New Zealand it appears to have been introduced with tropical fish and in 1940 was identified as *L. tomentosa*, the recognized vector of *F. hepatica*. Pullan records natural and artificial infections and says that *L. columella* occupies the same niche as *L. tomentosa*. If in fact *L. columella* and *L. tomentosa* are morphologically and ecologically very similar not much harm will result from the introduction, but the observation does underline the dangers inherent in moving animals of whatever category from one country to another.

Control of fascioliasis by the use of molluscicides continues to be more the subject of precept rather than of practice largely because of basic weaknesses in the method. Apart from strategic application, i.e., to kill snails containing a mature infection, it is essential to produce an almost total kill and to prevent recolonization. Total kill is unlikely to be achieved because while it is true that at any moment in time the snail vector (*L. truncatula* at least) is likely to be occupying restricted and discontinuous habitats, there are large contiguous areas in which dormant populations remain until local conditions change. The snail is capable of very rapid multiplication indeed. Ross, Taylor, and Morphy (1970) have assessed the effect of *N*-tritylmorpholine, which in many ways is notably better than older molluscicides, in Northern Ireland. Snail populations were reduced by 70 per cent but rapidly repopulated. Kirsch (1970) reports more optimistically after using calcium cyanamide on cattle pastures for 2 successive years. Unless a treatment of the land produces dramatic changes in vegetation or soil structure it is difficult to visualize any chemical application being permanently successful.

Fasciola gigantica

This is a tropical species and in really tropical areas *F. hepatica* is likely to be found only at high altitudes. In Kenya a survey of 4190 bovine livers (Ogambo-Ongoma, 1969) indicated 618 infections with *F. gigantica* and 2 with *F. hepatica*. The pathology of infection with *F. gigantica* has been investigated by Bitakaramire and Bwangamoi (1970). Initially there was necrosis, inflammation, and thrombosis caused by the migrating parasites. This was followed by progressive development of biliary and portal cirrhosis as the parasites entered the bile-ducts. Finally there was local calcification. By contrast Alibasoğlu and Güralp (1969) showed that in fat-tailed sheep experimental infection, which was followed by death 72–113 days later with typical acute anaemia, was associated with haematomas in the liver 2–4 weeks after infection. Over 60 per cent developed a sero-fibrinous perihepatitis and peritonitis and parasites were found in the peritoneal exudate of 20 per cent. Haematomas were found in the lungs and these contained parasites. Some sheep had an acute haemorrhagic necrotic pneumonia.

It is a matter of observation, although not perhaps of scientific demonstration, that aberrant *F. hepatica* seem to appear in the lungs of cattle more often than in those of sheep, whereas the reverse seems to occur with *F. gigantica*.

Dicrocoelium

The reasons behind the distribution of the parasite remain a mystery. In Russia two of the four species of *Formica* identified as vectors appear commonly in the Moscow area but disease is rare. Incidence of suitable snails is not mentioned (Shumakovich and Sosipatrov, 1968). There are two new records of the tropical species *Dicrocoelium hospes* which has been found in Sierra Leone (Williams, 1969) and in the Iringa region of Tanzania (Mahlau, 1970). In the latter instance there was a 36 per cent incidence in 839 cattle together with a high rate of infection with *F. gigantica*.

REFERENCES

ALIBASOĞLU, M., and GÜRALP, N. (1969), *Vet. Pak. Derg. Ankars Univ.*, **16**, 110.
BITAKARAMIRE, P. K., and BWANGAMOI, O. (1970), *Bull. épizoot. Dis. Afr.*, **18**, 149.
DODD, K., and NUALLÁIN, T. O. (1969), *J. Path.*, **99**, 335.
FOWLER, J. S. L. (1970), *Br. J. Pharmac.*, **39**, 599.
GEYER, E. (1969), *Z. ParasitKde*, **33**, 135.
HUBENDICK, B. (1951), *K. svenska Vetensk. Akad. Handl.*, **3**, 1.
KENDALL, S. B., and SINCLAIR, I. J. (1969), *Res. vet. Sci.*, **10**, 481.
— — — — (1971), *Ibid.*, **12**, 74.
KIRSCH, H. (1970), *Tierärztl. Umsch.*, **25**, 299.
MAHLAU, E. A. (1970), *Bull. épizoot. Dis. Afr.*, **18**, 21.
NISENBAUM, I. A. (1968), *Mater. Konf. vses. Obsch. Gel'mint., Moskva*, 1967, **1**, 176.
OGAMBO-ONGOMA, A. H. (1969), *Bull. épizoot. Dis. Afr.*, **17**, 429.
PULLAN, N. B. (1969), *N.Z. vet. J.*, **17**, 255.
ROSEBY, F. B. (1970), *Aust. vet. J.*, **46**, 361.
ROSS, J. G., TAYLOR, S. M., and MORPHY, M. (1970), *Br. vet. J.*, **126**, 282.
SHUMAKOVICH, E. E., and SOSIPATROV, G. V. (1968), *Mater. Konf. vses. Obsch. Gel'mint., Moskva*, 1967, **2**, 360.
SINCLAIR, T. J., and KENDALL, S. B. (1969), *Res. Vet. Sci.*, **10**, 483.
TEWARI, H. C. (1968), *Ann. trop. Med. Parasit.*, **62**, 495.
WILLIAMS, M. O. (1969), *Bull. épizoot. Dis. Afr.*, **17**, 433.

REPRODUCTION AND REPRODUCTIVE DISORDERS

F. L. M. Dawson, M.A., B.Sc., Ph.D., M.R.C.V.S.

REPRODUCTION AND REPRODUCTIVE DISORDERS

PHYSIOLOGY AND PATHOLOGY OF REPRODUCTION

F. L. M. Dawson, M.A., B.Sc., Ph.D., M.R.C.V.S.

MALES

Male Physiology

Intermittent prolapse of the preputial lining has been recognized for many years as a tendency characteristic of certain foreign breeds of cattle; it has been claimed as the predisposing cause of serious cases of posthitis affecting bulls at free range. Long (1969) and Long and Hignett (1970) noted, in a study of 244 bulls standing in British cattle breeding centres, that most of the hornless bulls showed this eversion but that very few bulls of the horned dairy breeds did so. Dissection of sheaths obtained from 7 polled and 19 horned bulls revealed that the caudal preputial muscles, which are retractor in function, were absent from the polled bulls, all of which had been seen to evert their preputial membranes. Working on some of the same material, Meredith (1970) noted that the mean bacterial content of semen was 356,000 organisms per ml. for 7 everting bulls as against only 40,000 for 7 bulls which did not evert. The results of some earlier work on bacterial content of semen do suggest a slight prejudicial effect on fertility and sperm survival *in vitro*, when bacterial density exceeds 200,000–300,000 organisms per ml. Although these particular bulls had 'normal' conception rates, it may be that everting bulls are potentially at some disadvantage, apart from the risk of posthitis.

Goodwin (1970) reported that young Angus bulls were outstandingly good subjects for semen collection by the manual massage method carried out per rectum; in 173 of 200 such bulls an ejaculate averaging 3 ml. at a density of 700,000 sperms per c.mm. was obtained within 2 minutes. The response was markedly better in young than in old Angus bulls and in young Angus bulls than in young bulls of other breeds. Earlier work has indicated that samples thus obtained are highly fertile although the bacterial content also is high. Routine fertility assessment of young beef bulls is frequently requested; Goodwin's results suggest that the use of electro-ejaculation apparatus, which sometimes causes pain and always requires maintenance, may be entirely replaced by the trained hand.

Vasectomy in bulls is easy and is often required to provide teaser animals for heat detection in large dairy herds. Roberts (1970) mentioned reports that subsequent to the operation some cows had become pregnant to 'vasectomized' bulls. Therefore the operator should retain the sections of vasa deferentia removed and have them stained and mounted as evidence of correct operation. Roberts quoted an observation that in 5 of 432 men, in which such evidence of complete vasectomy had been obtained, spontaneous recanalization, with restored fertility, took place. This risk would appear slight in teaser bulls, which are seldom retained beyond the age of 2½ years.

Cooper (1969) summarized the advantages of meat production from entire male animals as contrasted with castrates. The risk of taint is unacceptable in pigs; milk fat entire lambs weigh 2–3 lb. more than castrates at the age of 3 months. In cattle entires have a great potential; the improvement in feed conversion averages 10–15 per cent, for a very small investment of capital. Cooper denied that entire carcass quality at 15 months would be inferior and protested against regulations which enforce castration on males not qualifying as sires.

Male Pathology

Testicular degeneration is probably the lesion most commonly found in the infertile bull's genital tract. To some extent this is simply an age change. Rao (1971) confirmed the effect of age; studying 23 infertile bulls clinically and after slaughter, he associated certain types of abnormal sperm head in the ejaculate with degeneration of the germinal epithelium; the proportion of these abnormal heads in fertile bulls rose from 5 per cent in young bulls to 11 per cent in those over 9 years old. The proportion of such abnormal heads was, however, higher in subfertile bulls and approached 25 per cent in the least fertile. Rao considered 19 of the infertile bulls to show degeneration; in 7 it was marked, at an average age for these 7 of less than 5 years.

We still know little about the causes of this degeneration, although the production of sperms showing an 'acrosome defect' in a high proportion is known to be a heritable trait. Wells and Awa (1970) described a new method of differential staining to identify such ejaculates—only the oil-immersion objective of a light microscope is needed. Specific infection remains an obvious possible cause of testicular degeneration. Larsen and Kopecky (1970) described the genital infection of bulls with *Mycobacterium paratuberculosis*, thus confirming that this organism has a predilection for genital sites (*see* VETERINARY ANNUAL, 1966–7, 327; 1968, 122, for its association with the female tract).

Carroll and Ball (1970) studied testicular changes in relation to extent of inbreeding; testicular hypoplasia appeared often to be determined by these genetic factors but not degeneration.

Bruere (1970), in the ram, described a variety of conditions in which the testicles and other genitalia were underdeveloped, and suggested that most of these had a genetic origin. Swift and Weyerts (1970), by means of a trial, proved that rams with lesions resulting from *Brucella ovis* infection on one side only of the tract and producing semen apparently of poor quality could nevertheless be quite fertile.

Dimigen and Schulze (1970) showed that cryptorchidism in pigs can be diagnosed by the palpation of Cowper's gland per rectum, using a single finger. The glands can each weigh up to 100 g. in a cryptorchid weighing 50–100 kg. and can be the size of a banana. Six weeks after total castration the glands always regress to less than half this diameter.

FEMALES

Pregnancy and Parturition

Pregnancy Diagnosis

Allen (1969) simplified the immunological assay for pregnant mare serum gonadotrophin (p.m.s.g.). By the use of turkeys instead of rabbits he avoided the need for previous reabsorption of the antisera prepared in them in order to remove non-specific antibodies. The concentrations of p.m.s.g. present were then plotted for 16 mares between the forty-first and eighty-seventh days of pregnancy, and it seemed that the genotype of the foetus determined the levels of p.m.s.g. produced. Mares carrying mule foetuses showed low levels; these pregnancies terminate in abortion more often than those involving horse foetuses, but the actual function of p.m.s.g. remains obscure. Allen (1970) removed the entire conceptus from 2 mares 40 and 54 days pregnant; they continued for further periods of 42 and 80 days to produce p.m.s.g. A similar continued production after embryonic death would explain the occasional false-positive pregnancy test. Hence the rectal method of diagnosis may be preferable, but even so, many existing pregnancies do not go to term (Cox and Galina, 1970).

Schilling and Cerne (1970) claimed success in applying a similar (immunological) method of pregnancy diagnosis to the pig. The test recognizes the presence of a 'luteinizing' gonadotrophin in the urine; drops of sow urine, specific antiserum, and sensitized sheep red cells are mixed on a black glass plate, when heavy agglutination of the red cells occurs within 3 minutes if the sow is empty. Intermediate reactions were obtained with afternoon urine but the morning urine of sows pregnant from 23 days onward completely inhibited agglutination. The reagents used are those in routine application for human testing and may be available as kits.

In sheep, the economic importance of differentiation at about mid-term between twin and single pregnancies is fully realized, but the practical problem is difficult to solve, although the use of ultrasonic instruments is promising. Stouffer and others (1969) correctly diagnosed 51 twin pregnancies by this means, but the remaining 27 in this batch of 136 heavy-pregnant ewes were diagnosed as singles. However, according to Fraser, Nagaratnam, and Callicott (1971) recent modifications in equipment suggest that an accuracy in twin diagnosis approaching 100 per cent may be in sight. Using older instruments on ewes 70–84 days pregnant this team has improved its accuracy from 53 to 82 per cent over 3 years' observations.

Helper (1970) used a Doppler ultrasonic instrument for pregnancy diagnosis in the dog; at 33 days he claimed 100 per cent accuracy; 25 bitches were correctly diagnosed pregnant by recognition of the foetal heart-beat, while 5 were found to be empty. In the 'earliest' bitch, foetal heart-beat at more than twice the maternal rate could be heard on the 29th day.

Elective Induction of Parturition

Following the successful use by Adams (*see* VETERINARY ANNUAL, 1970, 232) of 20 mg. dexamethasone for this purpose in the cow, Ficarelli, Vezzani, and Ballarini (1970) reported that 10 mg. flumethasone was equally effective. Eight of 11 cases treated were affected with reticuloperitonitis; they became very ill as pregnancy advanced but 7 recovered rapidly after calving. Most calves survived; placental retention occurred in half the cases but manual removal was easy. Grønborg-Pedersen (1969) used 10–25 mg. of oestradiol benzoate to induce parturition in cases of heart disease and hock arthritis. Ten of 12 cases treated calved within 48 hours, 7 retaining the placenta. Gindele, Buchegger, and Meyer (1971) recorded the *undesired* termination of pregnancy in 15 of 102 cattle, treated for mastitis with dexamethasone given by the intramammary route.

Management and Infertility

Heat Detection

Most cows have resumed cyclic ovarian activity by 30–35 days after calving; failure to notice behavioural oestrus by 75 days, when service has become due, is probably at least as often caused by a true failure in detection as by actually 'silent' heats. Georgiev and Iliev (1969) observed a population of 1800 cows to estimate the relative importance of 'lack of heat' and returning to service in losing breeding time; 'lack of heat' affected 30 per cent of all the cows which lost time. Ayalon and Weis (1970) produced data suggesting that the presence of a teaser bull enhances the expression of heat. In their experiment never more than 10 cows at one time were carefully watched for heat twice daily in an enclosed yard; alternate periods of 3 weeks were spent with and without a teaser bull incapable of natural service. The presence of the bull reduced the percentage of silent heats from 10 to 5: he was present throughout the 24 hours; this is not regarded as the best routine. The percentage of prolonged and anovulatory heats was also halved, thus confirming earlier observations by others on the effect of association by females with a bull.

General Management for Fertility

In the VETERINARY ANNUAL (1970, 234) the point was made that 2-year-old calving with management for high first lactation yields is not necessarily the most profitable system of dairy-herd management. Concern has since been expressed that working life (prejudiced by stress during immaturity) is too short. In future more British show classes will be related to *lifetime* production (Anon., 1970a); in Austria (Anon., 1969) a high official stated that the working life averaged only 3½ years (with infertility causing 40 per cent of discards), whereas seven lactations were necessary for a truly economic return. In Hungary, Hamori (1970) noted a mean working life of only 35 months, among 37,606 daughters of progeny-tested sires; animals not surviving to produce a fourth calf had poor reproductive histories, whereas the others bred regularly. Perhaps progeny testing on first lactations could be improved. Thus Dannenmann and Conrad (1969) considered the productive and reproductive histories of daughter groups by 12 Simmenthal bulls; there were at least 50 daughters for each bull and they were studied for four lactations unless they had to be discarded sooner. Only 13 per cent of the 'best' sire's progeny failed to complete four good lactations, whereas 47 per cent of the 'worst' sire's did not last so long; *the correlation between the discard rate during the first lactation (2–18 per cent) and the overall discard rate was very close*. The bull with the highest first lactation average (3573 kg.) was *not* the 'best'; he lost 35 per cent of his daughters within four lactations and thus came seventh in order of merit.

Koriath, Schüler, and Girschewski (1970) stated that, in their experience, when high-plane rearing of heifers is aimed at a calving age under 24 months, the incidence of genital disease becomes prohibitive. These workers reported a performance trial covering four lactations in which the control group first calved at 24 months and the experimental group, receiving only 70 per cent of the control group's daily ration, calved at 30 months. With 32 cows in each group the controls required means of 2·13 and 2·03 services for the second and third pregnancies as against 1·22 and 1·53 in the delayed calving group. The latter averaged only 76 days between first calving and conception (as against 101 in controls), and 79 days for all four calvings (controls 96). This reduction in calving interval more than compensated for reduced first lactations in the delayed group, while the control group exhibited 7 cases of cystic ovarian disease as against only 2 in the delayed group. 'Unforeseen fertility problems in the first lactation' were reported when a 250-cow dairy unit, based on 200 acres with zero grazing, was founded in Cheshire in 1968 (Anon., 1970b).

Part of the relative infertility following calving at unduly early ages is a sequel to dystocia. The percentage of heifers to develop dystocia may possibly be reduced by using only suitable bulls on heifers which have a narrow pelvic inlet. Bogner and others (1970) showed that foetal size was directly related, *inter alia*, to gestation length; bulls transmitting long gestation periods are thus less suitable for use on some heifers. Measurement of the pelvic inlet was carried out by Young (1970) and by Rice and Wiltbank (1970). Young recorded a mean inlet area of 219 cm.^{2} in 11 cases of dystocia against one of 235 in 22 heifers which calved normally. But he also noted that high-plane feeding increased the birth-weight of calves and thus independently contributed to the prevalence of difficult births. Young's heifers were of the Angus breed. Rice and Wiltbank (1970) were able to confirm, on Herefords, that a narrow pelvic inlet was an important cause of dystocia; at inlet areas under 200 cm.^{2} 69 per cent of heifers failed to calve normally; in animals with a greater area the figure was reduced to 28 per cent. These authors, however, unlike Young, could deduce no such relationship in Angus heifers although *83 per cent* were cases of dystocia.

Carbohydrate Metabolism: Failure to appreciate the very great differences existing between individuals in feed conversion ability is all too common. Lamb (1970), analysing results of feed measuring and milk recording trials in Friesian cow heifers, found the gross feed efficiency of individuals to vary from 13 to 35 per cent! For sire groups the variation was not much less, from 19 to 29 per cent. Gardner (1969) carried out a careful quantitative experiment on 'steaming-up'. The theory behind this practice is that since high yielders always 'milk off body-weight' during the early lactation period they should calve in relatively fat condition. Indeed, Broster and Gibbons (1970) noted that, after one high yield, some cows have not fully regained the lost weight by the time of the next calving. Gardner tried out high and low levels of 'steaming-up' in combination with two after-calving routines—feeding concentrates *ad lib.* and 'according to yield'. In the conditions of this experiment, steaming-up was shown to be useless; it increased after-calving weight-loss and predisposed to ketosis. The concentrates could be used far more economically by allowing *ad lib.* consumption during lactation, thus assisting the poorer feed converters. Reproductive efficiency did not significantly vary between the groups, probably because all had begun to regain weight before they were served.

Recent work by McClure (1970), a pioneer in the relation of carbohydrate metabolism to reproductive efficiency, did confirm that animals in the phase of body-weight loss were unlikely to conceive, but indicated that the blood-glucose level was a more accurate guide to fitness for service. The three infertile groups in this experiment consistently showed glucose levels below 30 mg. per cent. On the other hand, a total of five groups was losing weight during the service period; the three infertile groups, and two others which showed conception rates of 69 and 67 per cent with glucose levels of 38 and 41 mg. Determination of herd blood-glucose levels is being increasingly practised as a routine. Payne (1970) has observed means varying from 27 to 51 mg. per cent. Girou and Brochart (1970) fed 3 kg. of cake, for only 6 days after insemination, to half the cows on 400 farms in the Jura. This made no difference to conception rates except on 47 properties where feeding had been judged inadequate; on these farms a 12 per cent increase of conception rate resulted.

Interval between Parturition and Impregnation

Intensification has extended the importance of this interval's length, as a factor in fertility, to the sheep and pig, and recent work has emphasized that it is important in the horse. Stockbreeders should note the 'safety arrangements' provided in this respect by Nature for certain rodent species commonly used in the laboratory! Hamsters do not naturally ovulate at all during lactation, while if a mouse is impregnated during lactation, implantation of embryos, and thus normal pregnancy, is delayed for a period proportional to the number of mice being suckled (McLaren and Menke, 1971)!

Van Rensburg and van Niekerk (1969) studied the corpora lutea of pregnancy in the mare. Secondary ovulations occur around the fortieth day and after the ninetieth day the secondary luteal bodies which have resulted are producing more progesterone than the primary corpus luteum. These workers obtained evidence that, in mares conceiving *at the foal heat*, secondary ovulation and corpus luteum formation often do not occur; thus the increased incidence of pregnancy failure (at about 60 days) in such mares is due to progesterone deficiency and the conception of 'progesterone support' treatment can be justified scientifically.

Regarding cattle, Olds and Cooper (1970) made a vehement claim that service before 60 days from calving was often an economic practice and did not necessarily prejudice reproductive performance. The data advanced in support include no reference to yield levels, a factor which is highly relevant, or to first calving ages or longevity. They do suggest, as might be expected, a considerable increase in embryonic death following early service (mean return interval length of 31 days, as against 24 days with first service 90 days or more after calving). Moller (1970) mentioned that, in New Zealand, natural behavioural oestrus, not followed by ovulation, occurred in up to 40 per cent of cows within 60 days of calving, but very rarely after that interval.

Lees (1971) deprecated the tendency to assess too highly the economic potential of twice-yearly lambing, involving for the ewe a 30–40-day parturition–conception interval. He made out a good case for the view that sheep could most easily be made more profitable by improving lamb survival, ewe breeding life, and the use made of grass by concentrating lambing once yearly into the month of April.

Fertility in the Pig

Frobish and Steels (1970) and Scott and Thrasher (1969) studied the effects of differing energy input levels on the reproductive efficiency of gilts. Both teams agreed that fertility fell somewhat at maximum input levels (7–8·5 Mcal.); some of these gilts became lame as they were too heavy. At 3 Mcal. (the lowest input) the sole detrimental effect was lowered birth-weight of piglets.

The effects of microclimate as well as of feed levels appear to be important for pig reproduction. Temperature and humidity can rise markedly in conditions of crowded housing. Jensen and others (1970) demonstrated not only relative anoestrus in gilts kept in the high temperature of 35·4° C., but also reduced conception rates and litter sizes following their removal to housing at 20–30° C., 20 per cent becoming pregnant with 7 embryos only. Randall and Penny (1970) in a study on five enterprises revealed the converse effect of winter conditions on the stillbirth rate. The two farms using even-temperature farrowing houses maintained an even year-round minimum stillbirth rate of 4 per cent as against January–March rates of 9, 11, and 16 per cent on the other farms.

Preventive Contract Practice

Hahn (1970) stated that breeding control is now the main veterinary activity in connexion with dairy cattle in the U.S.A. As a source of information for dairy farmers a survey showed the practising veterinarian as the most popular; he scored '34' as against '26' by the agricultural adviser! Using results from 14 herds using the preventive routine and 13 others Hahn mentioned that each dollar paid to the practitioner for preventive work resulted in 5 dollars additional profit. On one British farm (Anon., 1970c) the corresponding (estimated) figures were £1 and £12. Sippell (1969) stressed the psychological value to the client—the adoption of a preventive contract system made the contracting parties in a sense partners instead of, as previously, rivals. Sippell claimed that under certain circumstances the contract system could obviate the need for afternoon work by the veterinarian on most days!

Specific Non-infectious Infertility

Genetic Aspects

In cattle, Stegenga (1970) established that very often a genetic component in the causation of structural anomalies was modified to a remarkable extent by variation in environment. For example, 166 per cent of amputate calves (based on genetic expectations) were born to dams less than 30 months old, and the incidence in all older dams was below expectation. Yet this condition has largely been controlled by the culling of transmitting sires. The month of the year determined the prevalence of spastic paresis, another heritable condition—little occurred in summer, so this may be conditioned by vitamin-A deficiency. Again, calves with double cervices are mainly born from June to September; Stegenga suggested an oestrogen deficiency at the time of their conception as a causal component. Similarly in the pig, Wijeratne, Crossman, and Gould (1970) observed 2 boars by the same sire; used on different farms the mortality of their progeny from *E. coli* scours was respectively 80 and 62 per cent as against only 6 and 3 per cent for 6 other boars used. Undue susceptibility was transmitted by both, but environmental factors lowered the death-rate on the better farm.

Bruere, Marshall, and Ward (1969) have reported the occurrence of testicular feminization in genetically male sheep. Dimmock and Bell (1970) described as a special case the development of haemolytic disease of the new-born in calves. This was only possible, in the authors' view, because the two dams had been repeatedly immunized over 4 years against babesiasis with preparations containing bovine blood-cells. The calves had inherited antigens from their sires which were lacking from the dams.

Mineral Deficiency

Moule (1970) had found that *selenium* deficiency, a cause of infertility in sheep, could be conditioned through the impairment of appetite resulting from cobalt deficiency, or else by inhibitors of selenium. For treatment Moule advocated injection of selenium 1 month before the admission of the rams, while others have advocated a selenium 'bullet' in the rumen. Wastell and others (1969) found that when gilts were deprived of selenium from their fourteenth day of life onward, no piglets of their first litter survived birth by more than a few days. When 0·5 p.p.m. of selenium was fed, up to 3 piglets per litter survived.

Interest in the importance of *zinc* for reproduction continues to mount. Neathery and others (1970) lowered libido and caused testicular regression in goats by feeding a zinc deficient diet for 5 months. There is also an indirect effect since the deficiency impairs feed-conversion ability. Abshagen and Beduhn (1970) analysed blood and forage samples from 7 large dairy herds (1 with 720 head of cattle). All these were regarded as herds with infertility problems, and in only one was the zinc intake sufficient. (Copper and manganese deficiencies were also conspicuous.) Miller (1970) reviewed the zinc nutrition of cattle; 9 p.p.m. suffice as a rule although 500 p.p.m. can be tolerated. Natural protein and lead water-pipes have in the past contained sufficient zinc for the requirements of cattle. With the substitution of urea and plastic pipes deficiencies are more likely to occur in the future.

All 7 of the infertile herds studied by Abshagen and Beduhn gave evidence of subnormal blood *copper* levels not exceeding 66 μg. per cent whereas 90 is normal. In one exceptional herd the forage copper content was normal though the blood levels were low. Bienfet, Binot, and Lomba (1969) encountered similar situations in Belgium, and these animals responded to copper injections, although the failure of assimilation was not explained. Mahadevan and Zubairy (1969), by the use of copper, reduced the calving interval in the treated half of an Indian herd to 468 days while the control half averaged 511 days. Copper sulphate 0·5 g. was fed daily for 6 years and this enabled the animals to 'retain' 114 mg. of elemental copper daily (controls only 14 mg.).

Mudd (1970) studied the effect on trace-element content of grass resulting from heavy application of nitrogenous manure; 500 kg. nitrogen per hectare did lower plant manganese content but several years' repetition would be needed before the effect became critical. Iodine uptake, however, was severely depressed at once. Cows on pastures thus treated are only kept going by the iodine content of the concentrates they receive.

Thyroid Dysfunction

In Austria the whole country tends to be iodine-deficient. Results by Stöckl and Günter (1969) showed that total bovine serum iodine was low—2·7–4·3 μg. per cent—in many areas, normal level being 5–8 μg. Leskova and Weiser (1969) found the Austrian average milk iodine content to be less than half the British values. Leskova (1969) studied the effect of supplementation with both protein-bound and inorganic iodine salts; the practice could be recommended using either source. Extensive forage analysis showed that leaves and roots contain more iodine than flowers or stem. Beet tops were rich in iodine. Leskova did not consider the possible effect of goitrogens in Austria. In Finland, also notorious for its human goitre areas, Arstila, Krusius, and Peltola (1969) demonstrated concentrations up to 100 μg. per litre of the goitrogen 'VTO'. These occurred in a majority of milk samples produced in the goitre districts, but also in the heavy growths of rape and cruciferous weeds occurring on the farms involved. VTO disappeared from the milk when these weeds were controlled by spraying. Reproductive impairment in cattle due to thyroid dysfunction has been a problem in Finland and this principle may help in its control. Wayman, Iwanaga, and Hugh (1970) were able to reduce litter sizes in sows to 6 from 10 by feeding the plant *Leucaena leucocephala* as 15 per cent of the ration. This plant contains the tyrosine analogue mimosine; the addition of 1 per cent ferrous sulphate, which forms a stable compound with mimosine, to the feed annulled the effect of *Leucaena* on reproduction in these experiments. Soya meal constitutes another source of undesired goitrogen in feed (Hemken, 1970).

Pasture Oestrogens

Lotthammer, Grunert, and Elghamry (1970) encountered an interesting oestrogen-caused reproductive disturbance in a 34-strong cattle herd near Hamburg. Heats were prolonged, return intervals short, all cattle showed some degree of ovarian cyst formation, vulval oedema, and chronic slime production. Both the clover silage and the maize silage contained oestrogens, equivalent to 16 and 5 μg. of oestradiol per kg. silage, and revealed by chromatography as including genistein, formononetin, and biochanin A. The silage ration was halved and the cattle eventually bred following treatment with an androgen.

Lotthammer and Rigelnik (1970) quoted evidence that beet tops possessed an oestrogen content and that a breakdown product of DDT, used for spraying beet, was oestrogenic also. In their own work they showed that the incidence of ovarian cysts in heifers rose from zero, at an intake rate of less than 30 kg. of beet tops daily, to 14 per cent when over 35 kg. was fed. As the intake rate went up, conception rate also fell and culling rate for infertility rose. These effects were noted in a population of 300 cattle on thirteen farms under breeding control, but there was no direct demonstration of oestrogenic content. Bauminger and others (1969) were able to produce genistein-specific antibodies in rabbits, using as antigen genistein-2-carboxylic acid coupled to a co-polymer of three amino-acids. The presence of biochanin A blocked this antigen–antibody reaction but it is possible that, as a result of this work, a 'vaccination' technique could be developed to protect animals against the effects of phytoestrogen, and this might be valuable as well as of theoretical interest.

Special Pathology of Female Genitalia

Ovary

Prachov, Doichev, and Hadjiiski (1970) claimed that skin reactions to 1 per cent adrenaline injected in the perineal area of cattle produced separate characteristic reactions for four stages of the ovarian cycle and four stages of pregnancy, thus obviating much of the need for examination of the tract per rectum.

Trommer and Scheffler (1970) treated 35 fairly well-nourished Friesian cattle, in which serial rectal examinations had established that the ovaries were quiescent, with combined gonadotrophins, 400 I.U. of a follicle stimulating and 2000 I.U. of a luteinizing preparation. Two or 3 days later follicles were palpable and vaginal mucus was being secreted; 23 were on heat by the fourth day and 8 more within 8 days. Eighteen of the 31 conceived at the induced heat.

Grunert (1969) assayed a number of cystic corpora lutea for progesterone content and concentration. He concluded generally that cystic corpora of normal tissue mass had about half the progesterone concentration of normal corpora lutea (15–36 μg. per g. as against 50–70 μg.). This is pioneer work and requires a wider-scale follow-up. Follicular cystic ovarian disease is a commoner disorder and continues prominent in reports on abnormal ovaries. Thus Betteridge (1970) criticized the organization of a computerized data programme designed to indicate the relative frequency of the more important disease conditions. 'Endocrine pathology' was allegedly involved in only 1·3 diagnoses per thousand sick cattle, whereas 'cystic ovaries' were diagnosed in over 29 per thousand (and metritis and retained placenta in 170 per thousand—both often of endocrine origin)!

Signorini (1970) gave interesting figures on the occurrence of cystic disease in one practice over 10 years. During this period 2069 cases were encountered; in 80 per cent the disease appeared 35–40 days after calving, 47 per cent of the total following second and third calvings. These data certainly support the concept of cystic disease as a reaction to lactation stress; furthermore, the dams of 73 per cent of Signorini's cases were known to have had the disease at some time—and at a higher average age than their daughters, which suggests either an effect of increasing yield during immaturity in the last generation, or of 'genetic regress' through injudicious selection of breeding stock. Petkov, Antonov, and Dzourova (1969) reported on the zinc and copper content of normal follicles and of ovarian cysts. Zinc content rose in step with the volume of the cyst fluid in nymphomanic cases, whereas copper fell; hence zinc metabolism may be involved in the disease process.

Fiebiger (1969) treated cystic disease using luteinizing hormone, 5000 I.U. injected into the peritoneal cavity. The effects were compared with those from treatment by two other routes and also with another drug, a synthetic progestin. The results from intraperitoneal therapy appeared to be better than from the other methods, 22 of 25 well-established cases conceiving. As the method is easy to apply its sole drawback is the large dose. Strobel (1970) accordingly used dose-rates of 1000–3000 I.U. by the same route. He concluded that 3000 I.U. might be adequate but smaller doses were not. Surve (1969) endeavoured to monitor the results of effective intravenous treatment, with luteinizing hormone, of chronic nymphomanic cases. Blood and urine were analysed respectively for progesterone and oestrogens; this was done before treatment and repeatedly for up to 29 days afterwards. Urinary oestrogen fell after treatment and with the highest dose-rates there was, within 24 hours, a transient but significant increase in plasma progesterone levels.

Gurdan (1969) worked on the relationship between the occurrence of cysts in the ovaries of the pig and the condition of the vaginal epithelium. He considered that six types of ovarian cyst could all be provisionally diagnosed from vaginal biopsies, but this work is also of interest for its data on the numbers and types of cystic ovary found.

Arthur (1970) studied the induction of oestrus in pony mares by the uterine infusion of warm saline solution (250 ml.). Mares with quiescent ovaries were included, as were also cyclic mares and oestrous mares. 'Primary' cases of ovarian quiescence did not ovulate as a result of treatment, but all 3 mares in which quiescence followed early embryonic death came on heat (within 3, 6, and 9 days) and ovulated. When cyclic mares were treated between the fifth and ninth days they came on sooner than expected with punctual ovulation and good fertility. The treatment can thus also be recommended for silent heat, which is not uncommon.

Oviduct

Carlson, Black, and Howe (1970) collected the oviduct secretion from 2 normal bovine subjects over three entire ovarian cycles; the cyclic variations in volume resembled those which others have reported for the sheep. Individuals differed appreciably in the protein and glucose content.

Harrasser (1970) followed up the work of Berchtold and Brummer (VETERINARY ANNUAL, 1970, 241) on the diagnosis of tubal obstruction in cattle by the intra-uterine injection of phenol sulphonphthalein and its recognition later in the urine of normal cases. Whereas the earlier work on 25 cows had indicated that the application of this test could within its limitations be straightforward, Harrasser found on 102 slaughter cattle and 14 field cases that this was only so if the test was done during the luteal phase of the cycle. There was a strong tendency for normal oviducts not to transmit fluid during other phases (El Banna and Hafez, 1970, confirmed the presence of an isthmic sphincter which was relatively closed during the fourth to seventh days of the cycle).

Uterus

Brandt and Manning (1969) described two new instruments for the clinical investigation of endometritis in the mare; both may be used for the removal of endometrial samples and the more elaborate of the two enables the user to inspect the living endometrial surface. Solomon and others (1970) described in detail the performance of uterine curettage which they first attempted on 5 normal mares; the procedure led to active hyperaemia but not to inflammation or accidental infection. Of 16 infertile mares so treated, all were served after treatment; though only 5 conceived, 1 was pregnant for the first time at 22 years of age. Bacteriological culture before and after curettage suggested that the treatment, unsupported by drugs, worked well in about half the cases.

In cattle, Migaki and others (1970) recorded the diagnosis in the abattoir of 192 cases of malignant disease—uterine adenocarcinoma in 192 animals over a 6-year period. Metastatic lesions were evident in the lungs and lymph-nodes and some cows had shown dyspnoea. Lamothe and Guya (1970) investigated the content of endometrial secretion in sodium, potassium, calcium, magnesium, and phosphorus at all stages of the cycle in groups of normal and infertile animals. Only the infertile animals showed no cyclic variation in levels of potassium, magnesium, and phosphorus; the concentrations present were higher than those in the blood.

Endometritis: Priester (1970) mentioned that uterine inflammation was the commonest diagnosis of all in 6059 cattle submitted to a group of twelve veterinary school clinics in North America. Zafrakas (1969) reported that of 842 sets of bovine genitalia inspected, 401 had histories or lesions of infertility and among these the commonest individual finding was chronic endometritis (in 72 cases).

Nunn (1970) studied the bacterial flora in 118 clinical cases of 'symptomless infertility'. Positive cultures were obtained in only 36 per cent but these animals had all been calved at least 120 days before the samples were collected. Thus the evidence of this work was negative as regards the role of bacteria, but Nunn, Griffiths, and Hartigan (1970) found in normal cattle studied from 10–90 days after calving, local agglutinating antibody in discharge and endometrial tissue. Antibody to *Corynebacterium pyogenes* was found in 20 per cent of the cases and to *Staphylococcus aureus* in 21 per cent. Overall 80 per cent yielded antibody up to 28 days after calving; by 90 days the effect had faded, antibody being then evident in only 10 per cent. These results confirm the value of a routine veterinary examination at 3 weeks after calving to detect and treat cases of incipient 'post-puerperal' endometritis.

A quite new approach to the treatment of endometritis was described in Rumania by Oeriu and others (1969, 1970). In the earlier work double the control levels of oxidized glutathione were found in infertile cattle; this was considered evidence of disturbed endocrine balance and treatment designed to liberate disulphate (thiol) groups was advocated. Accordingly this was attempted, using folcystein on 18 cases of chronic endometritis, some receiving the preparation orally and others by intramuscular injection in doses of 1·5 g. The oxidized glutathione blood levels returned to normal and 11 cases conceived. It is a pity that no untreated controls were left; the statement by the authors that 'each animal served as its own control' cannot be accepted as it assumes no possible effect from simple lapse of time.

More orthodox treatment of this condition has been aimed either at stimulating the protective function of the endometrium (as with Lugol's iodine) or at destroying invasive micro-organisms as with antibiotics or disinfectants.

Djourova and Dimitrov (1970) applied the principle of endometrial stimulation to the drastic extent of uterine irrigation with 0·5 per cent silver nitrate solution. In healthy cows the effect of this treatment simulated a mucopurulent endometritis with a high density of lymphocytes and histiocytes. The recovery was slower than after treatment with Lugol's solution, taking 29 or more days instead of 19–21. In cases of natural endometritis silver nitrate treatment, which increases the extravasation of polymorphs, was recommended by these authors, with the proviso that insemination be delayed until the epithelium has had time to regenerate.

It is not widely enough appreciated that antibacterial drugs introduced into the uterus during oestrus do not remain there, but are in great measure passed into the peritoneal cavity by action of the uterine muscle. Thus it is no great saving of money or time to give treatment for endometritis at or too near the time of insemination. Zoller and Zoller (1970) treated 278 cows with an antibiotic (Tardomyocel L suspension) *immediately* following the third insemination. The conception rate was 72 per cent, whereas in 214 cows in which treatment was delayed for a further 24–48 hours this rate was 84 per cent, probably because more of the drug remained in the uterus. Hermans (1970) observed conception rates of 49 per cent to third insemination when an antibiotic was given within 24 hours of insemination time, and a similar rate, 51 per cent, when no treatment was given. But the treated animals showed an improved rate of 60 per cent to the fourth insemination and the final pregnancy rate of such animals was 76 per cent, whereas it was only 64 per cent for the untreated controls. It is possible that in these animals just enough antibiotic remained in the uterus to produce an effect, provided it received time to act.

Specific Infections

Salmonella dublin infection of sheep with enteritis and abortion continues to increase in frequency in Britain. Gitter and Sojka (1970) purchased 7 surviving ewes from an acute field outbreak, in which 30 ewes aborted and 23 subsequently died. These did not transmit the infection to clean animals placed in contact with them but, although no organisms could be recovered at slaughter 32 months or more after the acute phase, high agglutination titres persisted in the blood of all these ewes. Such titres are thus no indication that infection is still present.

Hirth, Nielsen, and Tourtellotte (1970) determined the comparative pathogenicity for the genital tract of ten separate isolates of *Mycoplasma*; strains from prepuce and from aborted foetuses were used for the experimental intra-uterine infection of heifers but there was no 'take' at all. Apart from one strain 'Donetta', originally isolated from cases of mastitis, which was pathogenic (VETERINARY ANNUAL, 1968, 123), the strains appeared relatively harmless. Ernø and Philipsen (1969) carried out similar work with strains of *Mycoplasma* recovered from Danish bulls. Again no effect could be induced on the uterus of heifers although these strains made calves ill and caused vesiculitis in bulls and a mild mastitis in cows.

Schliesser and Schmidt (1970) recorded that infection with *Coxiella burneti* had become endemic in the bulls of one cattle breeding centre in Germany. Sixty-five bulls gave positive complement-fixation tests up to a titre of 1 : 320—not all were bulls standing at this centre.

Storz and McKercher (1970) investigated the antibody response in complement fixation before and after abortion in cows and ewes artificially infected with *Bedsonia* organisms. They mentioned a decision made in 1966 to name this organism *Chlamydia* but acceptance of this term is not general. These workers were able to detect two types of antibody, and concluded that titres are low just before abortion and then rise steeply so that paired samples collected soon after abortion and again 2 weeks later are satisfactory for purposes of diagnosis, even if the animals had been in contact with infection before becoming pregnant. Work by Danieli and Ayalon (1970) showed that *Bedsonia* infection in one Israeli dairy herd complicated cases of placental retention and leucorrhoea in cows which had not aborted, and was present in other, normal cows. Both types of cow were sampled within 14 days of calving and in each series 30–40 per cent yielded positive stamp smears for elementary bodies; culture on chick allantoic membrane was successful in 1 of 2 cases tried. The prognosis proved to be distinctly worse in those leucorrhoea cases which yielded *Bedsonia*.

Virus Infections: Ward and others (1969) infected 11 cows 5–7½ months pregnant with a strain of bovine virus diarrhoea–mucosal disease agent recovered from a field case of abortion; the calves were all born alive at full term but 3 showed pronounced lesions of the disease and high serum titres.

Probably infection earlier in pregnancy is necessary to cause abortion. Kahrs, Scott, and de Lahunta (1970) described a field outbreak of this disease in which all 40 cows in the herd were ill, 2 died, and 8 aborted up to 175 days following the introduction of infection.

BVD virus has been successful in immunizing pigs against swine fever. Similarly, McKercher, Saito, and Mathis (1969) mentioned that infectious bovine rhinotracheitis and equine rhinopneumonitis viruses have a common antigen, and that in the guinea-pig IBR virus can be used to boost immunity to ER virus. These authors attempted to boost immunity in ponies in the same way, but there was no antibody response in this case. Equine immunity is best achieved according to Kendrick (1969) by controlled infection using living virus, at first early in pregnancy before the foetus and placenta are susceptible. Eight months later there is enough immunity established to prevent the second injection of vaccine from causing abortion; this second injection strongly boosts the immunity sufficiently to resist almost any field challenge.

Petzoldt (1970) described his work with the virus of horse pox. Electron microscopy showed it to be a herpes virus closely related to that of ER, on the evidence of cross-neutralization tests, but not to the IBR virus. One pregnant mare experimentally infected with this virus aborted, possibly as a result, but this is not made clear.

Dunne and others (1969) compared the effects on pregnancy in the pig of porcine picorna viruses, which have been recovered from field outbreaks of infertility and abortion, with those resulting from swine fever vaccinal virus. The latter appeared the more virulent, causing up to 40 per cent of embryonic death and proving capable of invading foetuses in the latter half of gestation, whereas picorna virus could rarely do so after the first 30 days of pregnancy.

Experimental Physiology

The bulk of work in this field which has a veterinary application has continued to involve attempts at controlled breeding, by the induction of synchronized heat periods at predetermined times in groups of animals. Interest has by now spread from sheep and beef cattle to dairy cattle. One reason may be connected with the claim (Anon., 1970d) that the most profitable way to run a British dairy herd is to have all the cows calve in the first 3 weeks of April for completely efficient summer milk production.

Attempts have been made with a variety of progestogens to synchronize the cycles both of heifers and cows. When de Bois and Bierschwal (1970) used melengoestrol acetate in 19 Friesian heifers all were on heat on the sixth day after withdrawal and 9 held to service then with another 8 at the second heat. Kordts (1970), using chlormadinone acetate, delayed service for all 26 of his heifers until the second heat; synchronization was still good and 23 held then with 2 by second service. Results in cows have not been anywhere near as good (though in some trials the untreated controls have also been relatively infertile). Synchronization of large groups is only possible to within 14 days, according to Schmidt and others (1970); thus with silent heat in a fair proportion, timing of insemination is a problem. These workers obtained a fair conception rate using chlormadinone in cows, 38 per cent to service during the induced heat only 39–49 days after calving. Another promising result was obtained by Spahr, Hays, and Graves (1970);

using medroxyprogesterone, with service withheld to the second heat, 52 per cent conceived to first service, as against 57 per cent in controls which were served at slightly shorter intervals from calving, namely 63–75 days. Wagner and others (VETERINARY ANNUAL, 1970, 245) claimed excellent conception rates at the induced heat if the course of progestogen was begun during the last 7 days of an ovarian cycle. This observation was confirmed by de Bois and Bierschwal (1970), who found a rate of 88 per cent in those heifers whose courses began while mature dioestrous corpora lutea were present. However, van Niekerk, Belonje, and Spreath (1970) found it worked the other way! They claimed normal rates only when the course began during the first 11 days of the cycle; the technique, of course, demands a partial synchronization before the start (perhaps achievable by corpus luteum expulsion). This team achieved a 79 per cent pregnancy rate to service at the well-synchronized induced heat in 19 cows using medroxyprogesterone. All 19 were in the first half of the cycle when the course began.

In the sheep, Roche and Crowley (1971) claimed that one easy way to improve the low conception rate at the induced heat was to control ovulation with luteinizing hormone. By this means with mating 12 hours before ovulation, they were able to raise the percentage pregnant from 50 to 80. Moseley and Lamming (1969) preferred manipulation of day length to control ovine reproduction; they exposed ewes to a 16-hour 'day length' in December, decreasing to 8 hours in June. Following March lambing, 22 of 28 were served within 6–10 weeks of parturition and 20 lambed again the following autumn.

Clomiphene, a non-steroidal 'oestrogen' not very unlike stilboestrol in structure, inhibits ovulation in laboratory animals but induces it in human cases of ovarian quiescence. Lindsay and Robinson (1970) attempted by its use to induce ovulation in sheep during the three spring months. The ewes came on heat fairly well, but did not ovulate, and in half the ewes treatment was followed by the uterus swelling and filling with clear fluid.

Following the deep freezing of boar semen, motility is well recovered on thawing but no pregnancies result following its use for insemination in the normal way. Polge, Salamon, and Wilmut (1970) made the important observation that such thawed semen inseminated into the isthmus of the oviduct resulted in a normal conception rate, 6 of 9 gilts thus treated conceiving with an average of over 7 embryos, better than in the controls.

Although successful egg transfer in the pig is not a new achievement, it may be a fresh application of the technique, that Wrathall and others (1970) obtained a litter of 3 piglets by transferring to a British recipient sow fertilized eggs obtained from donors slaughtered in Canada and flown over in plastic tubing 'packets'. This method of importing pigs minimizes the risk of importing infectious disease along with them.

Anti-androgens: Chlormadinone acetate reduces sex drive in the male to some extent. Cyproterone and its acetate are chemically very similar compounds and, like chlormadinone, cyproterone (not the acetate) is also gestagenic. Cyproterone appears to be a more powerful anti-androgen and has been applied for this purpose in human penology; it is known to decrease libido in the pig and has been used successfully in cases of prostatic hypertrophy, a common condition in the dog. Although cyproterone has been used in canine practice, Ficus and Jöchle (1970) concluded that chlormadinone had strong enough anti-androgenic properties to make it a very useful means of controlling both excessive sex drive and aggressive behaviour in dogs, even in black Alsatians. 'Itch of uncertain origin' and circum-anal tumour also respond to chlormadinone. A single dose of 2 mg. may be enough.

REFERENCES

ABSHAGEN, H., and BEDUHN, M. (1970), *Mh. VetMed.*, **25**, 489.
ALLEN, W. R. (1969), *J. Endocr.*, **43**, 581, 593.
— — (1970), *Equine vet. J.*, **2**, 64.
ANON. (1969), *Dt. tierärztl. Wschr.*, **76**, 676.
— (1970a), *Br. Farmer*, N.S., No. 674, 34.
— (1970b), *Ibid.*, 6–26 June, 42.
— (1970c), *Ibid.*, N.S., No. 658, 42.
— (1970d), *Fmr Stk Breed.*, 20 Oct. (Abstr. in *Vet. Rec.*, **87**, 551.)
ARSTILA, A., KRUSIUS, F.-E., and PELTOLA, P. (1969), *Acta endocr., Copenh.*, **60**, 712.
ARTHUR, G. H. (1970), *Vet. Rec.*, **86**, 584.
AYALON, N., and WEIS, J. (1970), *Refuah Vet.*, **27**, 22.
BAUMINGER, S., LINDNER, H. R., PEREL, E., and ARNON, R. (1969), *J. Endocr.*, **44**, 567.
BETTERIDGE, K. J. (1970), *Vet. Rec.*, **87**, 600 (letter).
BIENFET, V., BINOT, H., and LOMBA, F. (1969), *Annls Med. vet.*, **113**, 399.
BOGNER, H., VAN BAER, H., AVERDUNK, G., SCHMITTER, W., and MATZKE, P. (1970), *Berl. Münch. tierärztl. Wschr.*, **83**, 208.
DE BOIS, C. H. W., and BIERSCHWAL, C. J. (1970), *Am. J. vet. Res.*, **31**, 1545.
BRANDT, G. W., and MANNING, J. P. (1969), *Vet. Med. small Anim. Clin.*, **64**, 977.
BROSTER, W. H., and GIBBONS, J. P. L. (1970), *M.M.B. Handbook*, Article 92.
BRUERE, A. N. (1970), *N.Z. vet. J.*, **18**, 189.
— — MARSHALL, R. B., and WARD, D. P. J. (1969), *J. Reprod. Fert.*, **19**, 103.
CARLSON, D., BLACK, D. L., and HOWE, G. R. (1970), *Ibid.*, **22**, 549.
CARROLL, E. J., and BALL, L. (1970), *Am. J. vet. Res.*, **31**, 241.
COOPER, M. M. (1969), 'Meat Production from Entire Male Animals', in *Proceedings of a Symposium held at the Meat Research Institute, April 1969* (ed. RHODES, D. N.). London: Churchill.
COX, J. E., and GALINA, C. S. (1970), *Vet. Rec.*, **86**, 97.
DANIELI, Y., and AYALON, N. (1970), *Refuah Vet.*, **27**, 63.
DANNENMANN, H.-V., and CONRAD, R. (1969), *Dt. tierärztl. Wschr.*, **76**, 604.
DIMIGEN, J., and SCHULZE, W. (1970), *Ibid.*, **77**, 529.
DIMMOCK, C. K., and BELL, K. (1970), *Aust. vet. J.*, **46**, 44.
DJOUROVA, Y., and DIMITROV, D. (1970), *Vet. Med. Nauki, Sof.*, **7** (1), 27.
DUNNE, H. W., WANG, J. T., CLARK, C. D., HOKANSON, J. F., MORIMOTO, T., and BUBASH, G. R. (1969), *Can. J. comp. Med.*. **33**, 244.
EL BANNA, A. A., and HAFEZ, E. S. E. (1970), *Anat. Rec.*, **166**, 469.
ERNØ, H., and PHILIPSEN, H. (1969), *Aarsberetn. Inst. Sterilitetsforsk, Copenhagen*, p. 91.
FICARELLI, R., VEZZANI, E., and BALLARINI, G. (1970), *Nuova vet.*, **46**, 340.
FICUS, H. J., and JÖCHLE, W. (1970), *Kleintier-Prax.*, **15**, 32.
FIEBIGER, K. (1969), Dissertation, Free University, Berlin.
FRASER, A. F., NAGARATNAM, V., and CALLICOTT, R. B. (1971), *Vet. Rec.*, **88**, 202.
FROBISH, L. T., and STEELS, N. C. (1970), *J. Anim. Sci.*, **31**, 200.
GARDNER, R. W. (1969), *J. Dairy Sci.*, **52**, 1973.
GEORGIEV, G., and ILIEV, I. (1969), *Vet. Med. Nauki, Sof.*, **6** (9), 57.
GINDELE, H. R., BUCHEGGER, O., and MEYER, J. (1971), *Tierärztl. Umsch.*, **26**, 76.
GIROU, R., and BROCHART, M. (1970), *Annls Zootech.*, **19**, 67.
GITTER, M., and SOJKA, W. J. (1970), *Vet. Rec.*, **87**, 775.
GOODWIN, D. E. (1970), *J. Am. vet. med. Ass.*, **157**, 831.
GRØNBORG-PEDERSEN, H. (1969), *Nord. VetMed.*, **21**, 591.
GRUNERT, E. (1969), *Dt. tierärztl. Wschr.*, **76**, 668.
GURDAN, P. (1969), Dissertation, Munich University.
HAHN, J. (1970), *Dt. tierärztl. Wschr.*, **77**, 448.
HAMORI, D. (1970), *Mag. Allatorv. Lap.*, **25**, 266.
HARRASSER, D. (1970), Dissertation, Munich University.
HELPER, L. C. (1970), *J. Am. vet. med. Ass.*, **156**, 60.

HEMKEN, R. W. (1970), *J. Dairy Sci.*, **53**, 1138.
HERMANS, J. (1970), *Vlaams diergeneesk. Tijdschr.*, **39**, 156.
HIRTH, R. S., NIELSEN, S. W., and TOURTELLOTTE, M. E. (1970), *Infect. Immun.*, **2**, 101.
JENSEN, A. H., YEN, J. T., GEHRING, M. M., BAKER, D. H., BECKER, D. E., and HARMON, B. G. (1970), *J. Anim. Sci.*, **31**, 745.
KAHRS, R. F., SCOTT, F. W., and DE LAHUNTA, A. (1970), *J. Am. vet. med. Ass.*, **156**, 851.
KENDRICK, J. W. (1969), *Ibid.*, **155**, 306.
KORDTS, E. (1970), *Dt. tierärztl. Wschr.*, **77**, 287.
KORIATH, G., SCHÜLER, W., and GIRSCHEWSKI, H. (1970), *Mh. VetMed.*, **25**, 492.
LAMB, R. C. (1970), *J. Anim. Sci.*, **30**, 1043.
LAMOTHE, P., and GUYA, P. (1970), *Can. J. comp. Med.*, **34**, 167.
LARSEN, A. B., and KOPECKY, K. E. (1970), *Am. J. vet. Res.*, **31**, 255.
LEES, J. L. (1971), *Outl. Agric.*, **6**, 82.
LESKOVA, R. (1969), *Wien. tierärztl. Mschr.*, **56**, 369.
— — and WEISER, M. (1969), *Ibid.*, **56**, 89.
LINDSAY, D. R., and ROBINSON, T. J. (1970), *J. Reprod. Fert.*, **23**, 277.
LONG, S. (1969), *Vet. Rec.*, **84**, 495.
— — and HIGNETT, P. G. (1970), *Ibid.*, **86**, 161.
LOTTHAMMER, K. H., GRUNERT, E., and ELGHAMRY, M. I. (1970), *Berl. Münch. tierärztl. Wschr.*, **83**, 353.
— — and RIGELNIK, L. (1970), *Dt. tierärztl. Wschr.*, **77**, 445.
MCCLURE, T. J. (1970), *Res. vet. Sci.*, **11**, 247.
MCKERCHER, D. G., SAITO, J. K., and MATHIS, R. M. (1969), *J. Am. vet. med. Ass.*, **155**, 300.
MCLAREN, A., and MENKE, T. M. (1971), in 'Experiments on Mammalian Eggs and Embryos'. *9th Symposium of the Society for the Study of Fertility* (ed. PERRY, J. S.). *J. Reprod. Fert.*, Suppl. 14.
MAHADEVAN, V., and ZUBAIRY, A. W. (1969), *Indian vet. J.*, **46**, 892.
MEREDITH, M. J. (1970), *Vet. Rec.*, **87**, 122.
MIGAKI, G., CAREY, A. M., TURNQUEST, R. U., and GARNER, F. M. (1970), *J. Am. vet. med. Ass.*, **157**, 1577.
MILLER, W. J. (1970), *J. Dairy Sci.*, **53**, 1123.
MOLLER, K. (1970), *N.Z. vet. J.*, **18**, 140.
MOSELEY, S. R., and LAMMING, G. E. (1969), *Anim. Prod.*, **11**, 283.
MOULE, G. R. (1970), *Aust. vet. J.*, **46**, 428.
MUDD, A. J. (1970), *Br. vet. J.*, **126**, 38.
NEATHERY, M. W., MILLER, W. J., BLACKMON, D. M., PATE, F. M., and GENTRY, R. P. (1970), *J. Dairy Sci.*, **53**, 682.
NUNN, W. R. (1970), *Irish vet. J.*, **24**, 181.
— — GRIFFITHS, J. F. T., and HARTIGAN, D. J. (1970), *Vet. Rec.*, **87**, 380.
OERIU, I., TIMARIU, S., PETCO, D., SERBAN, D., and OERIU, S. (1970), *Zentbl. VetMed. Reihe A.*, **17**, 34.
OERIU, S., MARZA, E., CIMPEANU, R., DUMITRASC, N., and BAGEACU, V. (1969), *Ibid.*, **16**, 927.
OLDS, D., and COOPER, T. (1970), *J. Am. Vet. med. Ass.*, **157**, 92.
PAYNE, J. M. (1970), B.V.A. Congress paper, Abstr. in *Vet. Rec.*, **87**, 205.
PETKOV, K., ANTONOV, S., and DZOUROVA, I. (1969), *Vet. Med. Nauki, Sof.*, **6** (6), 91.
PETZOLDT, K. (1970), *Dt. tierärztl. Wschr.*, **77**, 162.
POLGE, C., SALAMON, S., and WILMUT, I. (1970), *Vet. Rec.*, **87**, 424.
PRACHOV, R., DOICHEV, S., and HADJIISKI, D. (1970), *Vet. Med. Nauki, Sof.*, **7** (1), 17.
PRIESTER, W. A. (1970), *Vet. Rec.*, **86**, 654.
RANDALL, G. D. B., and PENNY, R. H. C. (1970), *Br. vet. J.*, **126**, 593.
RAO, A. R. (1971), Thesis, Stockholm University.
RICE, L. E., and WILTBANK, J. N. (1970), *J. Anim. Sci.*, **30**, 1043.
ROBERTS, S. J. (1970), *J. Am. vet. med. Ass.*, **157**, 8 (letter).
ROCHE, J. F., and CROWLEY, J. P. (1971), *J. Reprod. Fert.*, **24**, 307.
SCHILLING, E., and CERNE, F. (1970), *Berl. Münch. tierärztl. Wschr.*, **83**, 46.
SCHLIESSER, T., and SCHMIDT, U. (1970), *Zentbl. VetMed., Reihe B.*, **17**, 238.
SCHMIDT, H., HUBER, E., GÜNZLER, O., JÖCHLE, W., and SMIDT, D. (1970), *Zuchthyg.*, **5**, 11.
SCOTT, V. B., and THRASHER, D. M. (1969), *J. Anim. Sci.*, **29**, 143.

SIGNORINI, G. (1970), *Atti Soc. ital. Sci. vet.*, **23**, 357.
SIPPELL, W. L. (1969), *J. Am. vet. med. Ass.*, **155**, 1493.
SOLOMON, W. J., RAKER, C. W., McFEELEY, R. A., and PETERSON, F. B. (1970), *Ibid.*, **156**, 333.
SPAHR, S. L., HAYS, R. L., and GRAVES, C. N. (1970), *J. Anim. Sci.*, **31**, 231.
STEGENGA, T. (1970), *Zuchthyg.*, **5**, 4.
STÖCKL, W., and GÜNTER, G. (1969), *Wien. tierärztl. Mschr.*, **56**, 325.
STORZ, J., and McKERCHER, D. G. (1970), *Cornell Vet.*, **60**, 192.
STOUFFER, J. R., WHITE, W. R. C., HOGUE, D. E., and HUNT, G. L. (1969), *J. Anim. Sci.*, **29**, 104.
STROBEL, K. (1970), Dissertation, Free University, Berlin.
SURVE, A. H. (1969), *Diss. Abstr. int.*, **30B**, 2390.
SWIFT, B. L., and WEYERTS, P. R. (1970), *Cornell Vet.*, **60**, 204.
TROMMER, F., and SCHEFFLER, K. H. (1970), *Mh. VetMed.*, **25**, 339.
VAN NIEKERK, C. H., BELONJE, P. C., and SPREATH, E. B. (1970), *Jl S. Afr. vet. med. Ass.*, **41**, 39.
VAN RENSBURG, S. J., and VAN NIEKERK, C. H. (1969), *Onderstepoort J. vet. Res.*, **35**, 301.
WARD, G. M., ROBERTS, S. J., McENTEE, K., and GILLESPIE, J. (1969), *Cornell Vet.*, **59**, 525.
WASTELL, M. E., EWAN, R. C., BICKNELL, E. J., and SPEER, V. C. (1969), *J. Anim. Sci.*, **29**, 149.
WAYMAN, O., IWANAGA, I., and HUGH, W. (1970), *Ibid.*, **30**, 583.
WELLS, M. E., and AWA, O. A. (1970), *J. Dairy Sci.*, **53**, 227.
WIJERATNE, W. V. S., CROSSMAN, P. J., and GOULD, C. M. (1970), *Br. vet. J.*, **126**, 94.
WRATHALL, A. E., DONE, J. T., STUART, P., MITCHELL, D., BETTERIDGE, K. L., and RANDALL, G. C. B. (1970), *Vet. Rec.*, **87**, 226.
YOUNG, J. S. (1970), *Aust. vet. J.*, **46**, 1.
ZAFRAKAS, A. M. (1969), *Hellen. Kten., Thessalonika*, **12**, 74.
ZOLLER, K., and ZOLLER, A. (1970), *Vet. med. Rev., Leverkusen* (3), 194.

PHARMACOLOGY AND THERAPEUTICS

T. E. Gibson, D.V.Sc., F.R.C.V.S., F.I.Biol.

L. P. Joyner, B.Sc., Ph.D., F.I.Biol.

J. Donnelly, B.Sc.

Olga Uvarov, M.R.C.V.S.

PHARMACOLOGY AND THERAPEUTICS

ANTHELMINTICS

T. E. Gibson, D.V.Sc., F.R.C.V.S., F.I.Biol.

PARASITIC DISEASES OF CATTLE

Gastro-intestinal Nematodes

Cambendazole

Egerton, Eary, Lanza, Wombolt, and Campbell (1970) tested the anthelmintic efficacy of cambendazole in naturally infected cattle using dose rates varying from 11 to 44 mg. per kg. A dose of 22 mg. per kg. removed almost 100 per cent of the mature forms of *Haemonchus*, *Ostertagia*, *Trichostrongylus*, *Cooperia*, and *Oesophagostomum* and also of the immature forms of *Trichostrongylus.* Virtually no activity was recorded against the fourth-stage larvae of *Ostertagia* and *Bunostomum.* Increasing the dose to 33 mg. per kg. improved activity against these species but it was still inadequate. Action against *Nematodirus* was variable and inadequate at all dose levels.

PARASITIC DISEASES OF SHEEP

Gastro-intestinal Nematodes

Haloxon

A comparison of the effect of haloxon on sheep in which esterase A was present with that on sheep in which the esterase was absent was made by Baker and others (1970). Seven of 8 sheep which were esterase negative developed ataxia or posterior paresis 21–35 days after a dose of haloxon at the rate of 353 mg. per kg. None of the esterase-positive sheep was affected. Neurotoxicosis following haloxon treatment is determined by the absence of esterase A and this trait is inherited. The protective effect of esterase A in preventing neurotoxicosis appears to result from its action in hydrolysing haloxon.

Benzimidazole Anthelmintics

The occurrence of strains of *Haemonchus contortus* resistant to the action of thiabendazole was reported in the VETERINARY ANNUAL (1969, 258). Further evidence of this phenomenon has now become available. Colglazier, Kates, and Enzie (1970) demonstrated that a strain of *H. contortus* which was derived from a flock of sheep which had been treated frequently with thiabendazole over a period of 3 years was markedly less responsive to a dose of 50 mg. per kg. of thiabendazole than a strain which had no known previous exposure to the drug. The response of fourth-stage worms was the same as that of adult worms in both cases. Taking all their trials together, Colglazier and others (1970) found that 67 per cent of the susceptible worms were removed but only 39 per cent of the resistant ones. With both strains it was found that a proportion of the worms were inhibited in the fourth stage and that the drug removed only 30 per cent of these. An earlier isolate of *H. contortus* from the flock which provided the strain resistant to thiabendazole was markedly resistant to the action of technical phenothiazine and also possessed considerable resistance to a similar purified product. Theodorides, Scott, and Laderman (1970) demonstrated that five strains of *H. contortus* resistant to the action of thiabendazole were also resistant to the related benzimidazole anthelmintic parbendazole. A test with one of the resistant strains showed that three times the therapeutic dose of both products successfully removed the resistant worms. Hotson, Campbell, and Smeal (1970) reported the isolation of two strains of *Trichostrongylus colubriformis* resistant to the action of thiabendazole. These strains were derived from flocks on research farms where frequent treatment with thiabendazole had been given. The two strains showed different degrees of resistance, one having an LD_{50} dose of 70 mg. per kg. and the other one of 125 mg. per kg. compared with 10 mg. per kg. for susceptible strains. One of these strains was found also to be resistant to the action of parbendazole but tetramisole was fully effective against it.

Rafoxanide

This compound was first developed as a fasciolicide, but Egerton, Yakstis, and Campbell (1970) have shown it also to be active against *H. contortus*. A dose of 10 mg. per kg. was 99 per cent effective against both 8-day-old and 22-day-old worms. When 5 or 10 mg. per kg. was administered along with 44 mg. per kg. of thiabendazole to sheep infected with a strain resistant to the action of thiabendazole over 95 per cent of the worms were removed. Combination with rafoxanide may be a solution to the problem of strains of *H. contortus* resistant to the effects of thiabendazole, which have occurred in several locations throughout the world.

Lungworms

Tetramisole

Sahai (1970) gave doses of 12·5 mg. per kg. to sheep carrying natural infections of *Protostrongylus rufescens* and *Muellerius capillaris*. Action against *P. rufescens* was good, but the treatment was ineffective against *M. capillaris*. The drug also removed the strongylid worm burden. The treated animals gained an average of 3 kg. more than untreated controls during the 4 weeks following dosing.

Fascioliasis

Hexachlorophene

Czipri (1970) used a paste formulation of hexachlorophene which is administered by means of a special dosing pistol. Using a dose of 10 mg. per kg., 67, 71, and 73 per cent of 6-, 8- and 10-week-old flukes, respectively, were removed. With 15 mg. per kg. 69 and 81 per cent of 6- and 8-week-old flukes were removed. There was no action against 4-week-old flukes. In naturally infected animals 10 mg. per kg of the paste removed over 96 per cent of the adult flukes and 78–99 per cent of the immature forms.

Niclofolan

Dimitrov and Käntscher (1970) gave 3 mg. per kg. in the form of tablets to 80 naturally infected sheep and 93·8 per cent of the animals ceased to pass fluke eggs. In a second trial in which the results were assessed at autopsy over 90 per cent of the flukes were removed. After treatment, a few animals refused food and water for 2–3 days but this effect is transient.

Clioxanide

Pearson and others (1970) used clioxanide under field conditions in 14,063 sheep, kept under a variety of climatic and husbandry conditions. The drug was found to be well tolerated by pregnant sheep and treatment had no effect on the subsequent lamb flock. A dose of 20 mg. per kg. is recommended for the treatment of sheep affected with mature *Fasciola hepatica* and *H. contortus*. Forty mg. per kg. is used in acute fascioliasis. The LD_{50} is over 400 mg. per kg.

Rafoxonide

Campbell, Ostlind, and Yakstis (1970) showed that doses of 11–15 mg. per kg. of rafoxonide removed almost 100 per cent of 6-week-old flukes. Efficacy is related to the formulation of the drug. In solution high efficacy was achieved but in suspension only one of three formulations was effective. Ross (1970) using a commercial formulation found 5 mg. per kg. to be almost 100 per cent active against mature flukes. Ten mg. per kg. removed 67 per cent of 4-week-old flukes and 97 per cent of 6-week-old flukes. With a dose of 7·5 mg. per kg. the corresponding percentages were 45 and 87. Armour and Corba (1970) obtained a similar order of efficacy when using 7·5 and 10 mg. per kg. In addition they also gave 15 mg. per kg. to sheep carrying 2-, 4-, or 6-week-old flukes and removed 36, 98, and 96 per cent respectively. Rafoxonide shows great promise for the treatment of acute fascioliasis.

Tapeworms

Resorcantel

Gaenssler and Reinecke (1970) gave doses of 65 mg. per kg. to lambs carrying natural infections of *Moniezia expansa* and 13 of 14 animals were completely cleared of infection.

Paramphistomiasis

Resorcantel

Gaenssler and Reinecke (1970) used doses of 65 mg. per kg. in sheep carrying natural infections of *Paramphistomum microbothrium*. A 75 per cent reduction in the burden of mature flukes was observed. A similar efficacy was observed against immature worms in 11 artificially infected sheep.

Parasitic Diseases of Pigs

Gastro-intestinal Nematodes

Dichlorvos

Jacobs and others (1970) administered dichlorvos in the food at the rate of 35 mg. per kg. to pigs artificially infected with *Hyostrongylus rubidus*. Treatment failed to remove 5-day-old worms but removed 26·8 per cent of 15-day-old worms and 99·4 per cent of 26-day-old worms. Jacobs, Curran, and Taffs (1971) carried out a similar test with pigs artificially infected with *Oesophagostomum* spp. and 0·7 per cent of 5-day-old worms were removed and an average of 57 per cent of 14-day-old worms. Against these immature stages the drug was more active against *O. quadrispinulatum* than against *O. dentatum*; 99 per cent of mature (42-day-old) worms were removed with no difference in efficacy between the two species.

Parbendazole

Taffs (1970) carried out a critical test of parbendazole using naturally infected pigs. A dose of 30 mg. per kg. completely removed *Ascaris suum*, and removed 99·9 per cent of *Oesophagostomum* spp. and 88·3 per cent of *Trichuris suis*. There was indirect evidence that the drug is also effective against *Hyostrongylus rubidus*.

Cambendazole

Egerton, Di Netta, Neu, Walther, and Campbell (1970) administered cambendazole in the food at the rate of 0·01 per cent and 0·03 per cent for 12 days to pigs given artificial infections of *A. suum*; 0·01 per cent was effective in controlling a moderate infection but not a severe one. The higher dose gave almost complete protection against moderate and severe infection. Given as a single dose of 7·5 or 15 mg. per kg. to pigs carrying artificial infections of *Strongyloides ransomi*, over 99 per cent of the worms were removed by treatment given 9 days after infection.

Fascioliasis

Niclofolan

Flücke and Günther (1970) treated 24 sows naturally infected with *F. hepatica* at doses of 3 or 5 mg. per kg. Counts of fluke eggs in the faeces fell to zero and 2 animals examined post mortem were found to be free from flukes. The treatment was well tolerated both in lactating and pregnant sows.

Parasitic Diseases of Horses

Gastro-intestinal Nematodes

Tetramisole

Critical tests were carried out on 9 naturally infected horses by Lyons and Drudge (1970). Tetramisole was administered subcutaneously at doses of 2·2, 5, and 10 mg. per kg. or orally at 20 or 30 mg. per kg. All dose levels were effective against *Parascaris equorum*; 98 per cent of *Strongylus vulgaris* was removed by 20 and 30 mg. per kg. but only about 50 per cent of *S. edentatus* was eliminated; 74 per cent of the small strongyles were removed and there was some evidence of action against *Oxyuris equi*, although the numbers present were too small for an accurate assessment of efficacy. About 1 hour after the administration of the largest dose the animal showed sweating, lacrimation, and hyperexcitability. The severity of the reaction decreased after 3 hours and had disappeared after 6 hours.

Parasitic Diseases of Dogs and Cats

Ancylostomiasis

Morantel pamoate

Cornwell and Jones (1970) carried out critical tests on dogs artificially infected with *Ancylostoma caninum*. A dose of 6 mg. per kg. removed 91 per cent of the adult worms and a dose of 12·5 mg. per kg. removed 97 per cent.

Tapeworms

Bunamidine Hydrochloride

Cook (1970) used bunamidine in a field trial for the eradication of *Echinococcus granulosus*, *Taenia hydatigena*, and *Taenia ovis*. Using dose rates of

25 or 50 mg. per kg., the incidence of *E. granulosus* fell from 7·9 to 0·1 per cent in a 12-month trial. Taking all tapeworms together incidence fell from 15·6 to 0·4 per cent. The incidence of *Dipylidium caninum* fell from 4·5 to 0·1 per cent. In discussing these results the author expresses the view that treatment alone will not result in the eradication of hydatid cysts but that it is a useful supplement to hygienic procedures.

Parasitic Diseases of Birds

Gastro-intestinal Nematodes

Tetramisole

Clarkson and Beg (1970) tested tetramisole in chickens artificially infected with *Ascardia galli* and *Capillaria obsignata*, administering the medicament either directly into the crop or into the drinking water. Given at 25 mg. per kg., 94·5 per cent of 5-day-old *A. galli* were removed, 91·9 per cent of 12-day-old worms, 93·8 per cent of 17-day-old worms, and 91·7 per cent of 30-day-old worms. Against *C. obsignata* 25 mg. per kg. was 96 per cent efficient against adult worms and 89 per cent against 16-day-old worms. Negligible effects were observed against 3- and 10-day-old worms. Bennejean, Meurier, and Mevel (1970), using both experimentally and naturally infected birds, found that a dose of 40 mg. per kg. removed the adult forms of *A. galli*, *C. obsignata*, and *Heterakis gallinae*. Action against immature forms was less satisfactory. Doses of 40 mg. per kg. cause no ill effects except a slight decrease in the hatchability of the eggs. Froyd (1970) treated naturally infected goslings with 25 mg. per kg. of levamisole in the drinking water; 99 per cent of *Amidostomum anseris* were removed and 50 per cent of *Heterakis* spp. but no effect was observed on *Capillaria* sp.

Echinostomiasis

Niclosamide

Krehmer (1970) used niclosamide in the treatment of pigeons infected with *Echinoparyphium paraulum*. Doses of 50–1200 mg. per kg. were given orally. Only the highest dose was consistently effective in removing the worms.

REFERENCES

Armour, J., and Corba, J. (1970), *Vet. Rec.*, **87**, 213.
Baker, N. F., Tucker, E. M., Stormont, C., and Fisk, R. A. (1970), *Am. J. vet. Res.*, **31**, 865.
Bennejean, G., Meurier, C., and Mevel, M. (1970), *Cah. Méd. vét.*, **39**, 3.
Campbell, W. C., Ostlind, D. A., and Yakstis, J. J. (1970), *Res. vet. Sci.*, **11**, 99.
Clarkson, M. J., and Beg, M. K. (1970), *Vet. Rec.*, **86**, 652.
Colglazier, M. L., Kates, K. C., and Enzie, F. D. (1970), *J. Parasit.*, **56**, 768.
Cook, B. R. (1970), *N.Z. vet. J.*, **18**, 152.
Cornwell, R. L., and Jones, R. M. (1970), *Res. vet. Sci.*, **11**, 485.
Czipri, D. A. (1970), *Vet. Rec.*, **87**, 531.
Dimitrov, G., and Käntscher, L. (1970), *Vet. med. Rev., Leverkusen* (1), 13.
Egerton, J. R., Di Netta, J., Neu, D. C., Walther, R. J., and Campbell, W. C. (1970), *Res. vet. Sci.*, **11**, 590.
— — Eary, C. H., Lanza, G. R., Wombolt, T. H., and Campbell, W. C. (1970), *Ibid.*, **11**, 495.
— — Yakstis, J. J., and Campbell, W. C. (1970), *Ibid.*, **11**, 382.
Flücke, W., and Günther, W. (1970), *Vet. med. Rev., Leverkusen* (1), 3.
Froyd, G. (1970), *Vet. Rec.*, **86**, 788.
Gaenssler, J. G., and Reinecke, R. K. (1970), *Jl S. Afr. vet. med. Ass.*, **41**, 211.

HOTSON, I. K., CAMPBELL, N. J., and SMEAL, M. G. (1970), *Aust. vet. J.*, **46**, 356.
JACOBS, D. E., CURRAN, M. K., and TAFFS, L. F. (1971), *Res. vet. Sci.*, **12**, 189.
— — TAFFS, L. F., LEAN, I. J., and CURRAN, M. K. (1970), *Br. vet. J.*, **126**, xliii.
KREHMER, E. (1970), *Vet. med. Rev., Leverkusen* (1), 27.
LYONS, E. T., and DRUDGE, J. H. (1970), *Am. J. vet. Res.*, **31**, 1477.
PEARSON, I. G., WHITLOCK, H. V., DE GOOSH, C. P., FARRINGTON, K. J., JONES, R. C., and HAIGH, J. H. (1970), *Aust. vet. J.*, **46**, 480.
ROSS, D. B. (1970), *Vet. Rec.*, **87**, 110.
SAHAI, B. N. (1970), *Indian J. Anim. Hlth*, **9**, 25.
TAFFS, L. F. (1970), *Res. vet. Sci.*, **11**, 515.
THEODORIDES, V. J., SCOTT, G. C., and LADERMAN, M. (1970), *Am. J. vet. Res.*, **31**, 859.

CHEMOTHERAPY OF PROTOZOAL INFECTIONS

L. P. Joyner, B.Sc., Ph.D., F.I.Biol.

BABESIASIS

Cattle

Quinuronium, 5,5′methylene-*bis*-salicylate, administered as a 20 per cent suspension in arachis oil and given in 1-g. doses subcutaneously, was found by Newton and O'Sullivan (1969) to have marked prophylactic effects against *Babesia argentina* infections in young calves. A dose of 2·0 g. proved toxic producing nephritis which was fatal in some calves, but the recovered animals were protected. None of the 31 calves treated 7–35 days previously developed clinical babesiasis following the inoculation of infective blood or exposure to infected ticks. *B. argentina* became established and clinical signs with fever, reduced haemoglobin, and haematocrit levels developed in the untreated control calves.

Similar tests conducted by Klinger (1969) with amicarbalide in doses of 10 or 20 mg. per kg. detected little or no prophylactic activity.

In screening tests with a series of substituted carbanilides, imidocarb [3,3′-*bis*-(2-imidazolin-2-yl) carbanilide dihydrochloride] was found to be the most active against *B. rodhaini* infections in mice and rats (Beveridge, 1969; Schmidt, Hirt and Fischer, 1969). The compound proved to be less toxic and more effective than amicarbalide diisethionate, diminazine diaceturate, and quinuronium sulphate.

Trials of imidocarb in cattle in Australia were conducted by Callow and McGregor (1970). The activity against *B. argentina* was tested in 47 splenectomized calves and 18 intact steers in which it readily controlled very severe infections at dose rates of 1 mg. per kg. to 20 mg. per kg. The compound completely cured (sterilized) the infections in clinically recovered steers treated subcutaneously with 2 mg. per kg. to 10 mg. per kg. but not with 1 mg. per kg. Prophylactic activity was evident in a group of steers treated subcutaneously with 2 mg. imidocarb per kg. 33 days before infection with *B. argentina* and was pronounced in groups treated 24, 23, and 13 days before inoculation. Prophylaxis did not interfere with the normal development of acquired immunity to *B. argentina*.

The activity of imidocarb against *B. bigemina* was tested in 19 splenectomized calves. Treatment was successful with dose rates from 0·4 to 20 mg. per kg. Two of 6 splenectomized calves given the lowest dose showed relapses of parasitaemia. The drug was effective by both subcutaneous and intravenous routes. Acute toxicity followed intravenous injection of 20 or 10 mg. per kg. although the animals survived. Toxic signs were mild or absent for subcutaneous dosage of 10 mg. or less. Calves with acute *B. bigemina* infections were sterilized with subcutaneous dosage at 0·4 and 0·6 mg. per kg. In prophylactic tests against *B. bigemina* 2 animals given 2 mg. imidocarb per kg. were strongly protected 12 weeks after treatment and 3 others given higher dosages were refractory to infection up to 10 weeks after treatment.

Neitz (1969) showed that imidocarb injected subcutaneously protected cattle for 3 months against artificial infection with *B. bovis* or *B. bigemina.*

Horses

Kirkham (1969) found that both phenamidine isethionate and diminazine were effective against *Babesia caballi* and *B. equi* in horses but amicarbalide was effective in clearing *B. caballi* only. Symptomatic and supportive therapy was beneficial, but old horses and those with damaged livers were considered poor risks with these treatments.

Dogs

The activity of phenamidine against experimental and natural infections with *Babesia gibsoni* in dogs was recorded by Groves and Vanniasingham (1970). The drug was effective in treating clinical infections because all dogs showed a definite and continuous decrease in parasitaemia 72 hours or less after treatment. Complete elimination of the parasites was not obtained. The best dosage was 7·5 mg. per lb. (16 mg. per kg.) on two consecutive days.

Coccidiosis

Poultry

Although nicarbazin was in current use a number of years ago, it has now been largely superseded by other types of drugs partly because of supposed limitations in its activity. Its activity against *Eimeria mivati*, *E. hagani*, and *E. praecox* has recently been demonstrated by McManus (1970). The latter two species are not generally associated with high pathogenicity while *E. mivati* had not been recognized when the drug was first evaluated. The usually recommended level of 0·0125 per cent in the food was highly active against these three species.

Clopidol is a widely used pyridone coccidiostatic drug. Its possible use for replacement pullets was studied by Siegmann and Hoeck (1969). It was found that the normal concentration of 0·0125 per cent in the food arrested *E. tenella* at an early endogenous stage but after removal of the drug the infection recurred in a milder form. Sulphadimidine (0·1 per cent) in the drinking water for 3 days, beginning 72–96 hours after withdrawal of the drug, controlled the infection but permitted the immunogenic stages to develop.

The effects of this drug on laying birds was studied by Bucek (1969). Clopidol was administered in the food to laying hens for three generations at levels of 0, 125, 250, and 500 parts per million (p.p.m.). There were no significant differences in egg production, fertility, or hatchability. Egg size was not significantly different in the first and second generations but in the third generation the eggs of birds receiving 125 or 250 p.p.m. clopidol in the food were significantly smaller than those of the controls.

The problem of drug resistance in strains of coccidia has attracted considerable attention recently. Williams (1969) isolated a series of strains from flocks receiving decoquinate having been reared in houses where chemically unrelated coccidiostats had been used. It was concluded that the parasites were still incompletely controlled by the coccidiostats which had been used in the same houses up to 90 weeks previously. Unfortunately it was not possible to compare this response with the initial activity of the drugs concerned.

3,5-Dinitrotoluamide (zoalene) has been widely used for many years. Burow and Hartwigk (1969) attempted to induce resistance to this drug by passaging a field strain of *E. tenella* in chicks receiving 60, 80, or 100 p.p.m. of zoalene in the drinking water. As the number of passages increased the growth-rate of the chicks diminished and the mortality and oocyst counts increased both in the medicated groups and in the untreated controls. At the twenty-fifth passage, however, when the strains were tested in chicks receiving 100 or 120 p.p.m. of zoalene, they appeared to be fully susceptible to the drug. It was suggested that the results could be explained by an increase in the virulence of the organisms rather than a manifestation of drug resistance.

Millard (1970) found a field strain of *E. tenella* which was resistant to methyl benzoquate in that levels of 0·005 and 0·025 per cent in the food appeared to be ineffective. In comparative experiments decoquinate (another quinoline drug) failed to control both haemorrhage and mortality. Clopidol (a pyridone compound) prevented mortality but not haemorrhage, while robenidene (a new guanidine derivative, q.v.) was completely effective.

Robenidene [1,3-*bis*(*p*-chlorobenzylideneamino)guanidine hydrochloride] is a new type of coccidiostatic drug with a wide spectrum of activity against all the major pathogenic species in the chicken. In experiments described by Kantor and others (1970) 66 p.p.m. of the drug in the food prevented coccidiosis in experimentally infected birds. Up to 200 p.p.m. had no toxic effects although 330 p.p.m. reduced the weight of the birds by 7 per cent when administered in the food for 8 weeks.

Reid and Davis (1969) reported on an interesting case in which heavy losses from coccidiosis occurred in a flock given high-level medication for the eradication of mycoplasma infection. Tylosin, chlortetracyline, and 3,5-dinitro-*o*-toluamide (zoalene) were given from 1 day of age until 3, 3–6, and 10 weeks respectively and then withdrawn. No anticoccidial immunity had been acquired and *E. tenella*, *E. necatrix*, *E. acervulina*, and *E. brunetti* were found at 16 weeks. The programme was successfully modified by eliminating the 3,5-dinitro-*o*-toluamide and reducing the chlortetracycline (both of which have coccidiostatic activity). Tests showed that tylosin was only partially active against *E. tenella*, *E. maxima*, and *E. mivati*.

Joyner and Norton (1970) reported on three strains of *E. meleagrimitis* which were isolated from outbreaks of coccidiosis in turkeys in Sussex, Yorkshire, and Carmarthenshire respectively. All three strains failed to respond to the normal preventive levels of sulphaquinoxaline (0·0125 per cent) and amprolium (0·0125 per cent) which are the most commonly used coccidiostats for turkeys. Clopidol, decoquinate, and 3,5-dinitro-*o*-toluamide (zoalene) at the dosages normally active in chickens were equally ineffective against these strains.

Ruminants

Amprolium was used by Horak, Raymond, and Louw (1969) to treat naturally acquired coccidial infections in sheep, goats, and calves. The sheep and calves were given 50 mg. per kg. for four consecutive days and the goats were given 100 mg. per kg. for the same period. Coccidiostatic activity was deduced from the rapid decrease in faecal oocyst counts.

From the U.S.S.R. Gobzem (1970) has published a review of experiences in the prevention and control of coccidiosis in calves using a wide range of different drugs and antibiotics. Among the conventional coccidiostats, 3,5-dinitrotoluamide (Zoalene, 80 mg. per kg.), sulphathiazole (50 mg. per kg.), and amprolium (70–90 mg. per kg.) were all found to be effective, controlling the gametogony cycle. Chloramphenicol (20 mg. per kg.) was among the drugs reported to control schizogony.

Rabbits

Lämmler and Dürr (1969) found that a potentiated mixture of sulphadimethoxine and diaveridine given in the food for 3 days (125 mg. per kg. food) or for 8 days in either the food or drinking water (100 mg. per kg. food or 1 litre of water) prevented hepatic coccidiosis following a single infection with oocysts of *Eimeria stiedae*. This species is generally considered to be very sensitive to sulphonamides and although low doses of the above mixture prevented coccidiosis from repeated challenges over a period of 35 days a good immunity did not develop. It would appear from this that the potentiated sulphonamide formulation is best used for therapy.

Dürr (1969) pointed out that drugs which are highly effective against avian coccidiosis are not always effective in rabbits. Hepatic coccidiosis may be controlled by strict attention to hygiene but it is not always possible to achieve optimum conditions. It was suggested that the oral administration of a suitable sulphonamide mixed with the food and given once every 10–14 days may be the only practicable form of treatment for commercial rabbit farms.

Pellérdy (1969) considered the possibility of inducing immunity to coccidiosis by exposing young rabbits to repeated infection with a mixture of oocysts of known pathogenic species simultaneously with sulphonamide prophylaxis. He described experiments in which young rabbits were given doses of 10–20,000 oocysts eight times at intervals of 2 or 3 days using one of three sulphonamides to provide prophylaxis (sulphadimidine, 0·1 per cent in the drinking water; sulphaquinoxaline, 0·5 ml. of a 10 per cent solution subcutaneously; sulphachloropyridazine, 0·01 per cent in the drinking water). An almost complete immunity was demonstrated. Pellérdy (1969) concluded that in rabbitries where conditions permitted a continuous coccidial population, intermittent sulphonamide prophylaxis would give adequate protection and permit the development of immunity, but only to those species of *Eimeria* which were present in the stock.

Metronidazole has been reported by Reshetnyak, Bartenev, and Rubanov (1970) to be effective in the treatment of hepatic and intestinal coccidiosis in rabbits. In field trials spontaneous infections were successfully treated with daily oral doses of 40 mg. per kg. for 3 days with subcutaneous injections of 20 mg. per kg.

Histomoniasis

Poultry

Ipronidazole (1-methyl-2-isopropyl-5-nitroimidazole) was selected from a series of related compounds as the most effective against *Histomonas meleagridis*. Studies on its efficacy and toxicity have been reported by Mitrovic and Schildknecht (1970) and by Marusich, Ogrinz, and Mitrovic (1970a, b). A dose of 0·00625 per cent in the food enabled experimental turkeys to withstand challenge infections. The drug has therapeutic activity and 0·025 per cent in the food or 0·0125 per cent in the drinking water were recommended for short-term treatment.

The maximum tolerated level in turkeys was estimated to be 0·12 per cent in the food. In growth experiments over 8-week periods 0·003125 per cent and 0·00625 per cent ipronidazole in the food improved the growth rate of turkeys by 4·9 and 4·4 per cent and the food conversion by 4·2 and 4·1 per cent respectively.

Theileriasis

Cattle

Theileria annulata infections were reported from India in 4 Danish Red bulls, 3 Jersey bulls, and a Holstein yearling. Repeated intramuscular injections of diminazine (Berenil) in doses of 10 to 15 mg. per kg. were reported by Gautam, Sharma, and Kalra (1970) to be an effective treatment. Doses below 7 mg. did not reduce the pyrexia or parasitaemia.

Against the same infection Narasimhamurty, Rajulu, and Reddy (1970) reported a response to treatment with amodiaquine hydrochloride (Camoquin) given in doses of 4·0–4·8 mg. orally daily for 5–8 days. The treatment, however, was coupled with the intramuscular injection of oxytetracycline which itself is active against parasites of this group.

Toxoplasmosis

Dapsone (2-sulphamoyl-4,4′-diaminodiphenylsulphone) has been shown to be active against experimental infections with *Toxoplasma gondii*. Its efficacy against the infection in pigs has been demonstrated by Ohshima, Inami, and Tanaka (1969). The animals were infected with a strain of porcine origin and treatment started the day after the appearance of obvious symptoms. The minimal effective dosage required to eliminate all the organisms was about 10 mg. per kg. given once daily for 7 days. When treatment was delayed or the dosage reduced, symptoms were still effectively reduced but the organisms were not entirely eliminated.

Trichomoniasis

Cattle

McLoughlin had published a number of reports on the activity of demetridazole in the treatment of bulls infected with *Trichomonas foetus* (*see* Veterinary Annual, 1970, 269). In trials with experimentally infected cows the author succeeded in eliminating the infection from 2 out of 3 animals by oral administration of dimetridazole (50 mg. per kg. body-weight daily for 5 days) and from 7 out of 8 cows by a single intravenous injection of 50 mg. per kg. Repeated treatment of the 2 cows which were not cured failed to eliminate the parasites even when larger doses were used (McLoughlin, 1970).

Pigeons

Ronidazole (1-methyl-2-carbamoyl-oxymethyl-5-nitroimidazole) has been introduced for the control of histomoniasis in poultry (*see* VETERINARY ANNUAL, 1970, 267). Its activity appears to be comparable with that of other imidazole compounds. The latter drugs (e.g., metronidazole) are effective in controlling infections with *T. gallinae* in pigeons, and Devos, Viaene, and Devriese (1969) included the new drug in their tests with this parasite. Ronidazole added to the drinking water (0·6 g. per litre) for 5 days was as effective as metronidazole (1 g. per litre). Carbarsone (1 g. per litre) was less effective. Some pigeons given three times the normal concentration of metronidazole for 5 days developed locomotory disorders from which they recovered after removal of the drug.

TRYPANOSOMIASIS

Cattle

Little general research on the chemotherapy of trypanosomiasis seems to be in progress. Most of the recent reports concern field experience of existing drugs.

In an attempt to assess the prophylactic efficacy of isometamidium (Samorin) Na'isa (1969) observed the progress of 80 cattle trekked along a trade route of 575 miles in Northern Nigeria in 28 days. The route passed through three *Glossina morsitans* belts interspersed with *G. tachinoides*. Thirty animals were treated initially with 0·25 mg. isometamidium chloride per kg. A further 30 were given 0·5 mg. per kg., while 20 were untreated. Heavy casualties occurred in all groups which in some instances in the untreated group were due to trypanosomiasis. Both treatment doses appeared to give equal protection against trypanosome infection although parasites were detected in small numbers.

Ford (1969) has made a plea for a wider view of the control of African trypanosomiasis, advocating that efficient control of the disease in man and animals at a tolerable level is more important at present than large-scale eradication. A new control policy would require a more detailed analysis of the epidemiology of the disease, the natural foci of infection, the land-use potential of fly belts, etc.

Dogs

Although it is general experience that diminazine may be used effectively in dogs, Oppong (1969) has drawn attention to a type of toxicity which followed the treatment of 3 dogs acutely infected with *Trypanosoma evansi*. The symptoms and infection responded to treatment with 3·5 mg. per kg. and subsequent inoculations of blood into mice confirmed the absence of parasites. The three dogs died during the third and fourth weeks after treatment and post-mortem examination showed swollen kidneys, liver damage, and jaundice. It was suggested that liver damage during the infection left the animals unable fully to detoxify the drug.

REFERENCES

BEVERIDGE, E. (1969), *Res. vet. Sci.*, **10**, 534.
BUCEK, O. C. (1969), *Poult. Sci.*, **48**, 2173.
BUROW, H., and HARTWIGK, H. (1969), *Berl. Münch. tierärztl. Wschr.*, **82**, 288.

CALLOW, L. L., and MCGREGOR, W. (1970), *Aust. vet. J.*, **46**, 195.
DEVOS, A., VIAENE, N., and DEVRIESE, L. (1969), *Vlaams diergeneesk. Tijdschr.*, **38**, 297.
DÜRR, U. (1969), *Parasit. hung.*, **2**, 187.
FORD, J. (1969), *Bull. Wld Hlth Org.*, **40**, 879.
GAUTAM, O. P., SHARMA, R. D., and KALRA, D. S. (1970), *Indian vet. J.*, **47**, 78.
GOBZEM, V. R. (1970), *Veterinariya, Moscow* 1970, No. 3, 71. (Abstr. *Vet. Bull., Weybridge*, **40**, 901.)
GROVES, M. G., and VANNIASINGHAM, J. A. (1970), *Vet. Rec.*, **86**, 8.
HORAK, I. G., RAYMOND, S. M., and LOUW, J. P. (1969), *Jl S. Afr. vet. med. Ass.*, **40**, 293.
JOYNER, L. P., and NORTON, C. C. (1970), *Res. vet. Sci.*, **11**, 349.
KANTOR, S., KENNETT, R. L., jun., WALETZKY, E., and TOMCUFCIK, A. S. (1970), *Science, N.Y.*, **168**, 373.
KIRKHAM, W. W. (1969), *J. Am. vet. med. Ass.*, **155**, 457.
KLINGER, I. (1969), *Refuah Vet.*, **26**, 149.
LÄMMLER, G., and DÜRR, U. (1969), *Berl. Münch. Tierärztl. Wschr.*, **82**, 480.
MCLOUGHLIN, D. K. (1970), *J. Parasit.*, **56**, 39.
MCMANUS, E. C. (1970), *Res. vet. Sci.*, **11**, 101.
MARUSICH, W. I., OGRINZ, E. F., and MITROVIC, M. (1970a), *Poult. Sci.*, **49**, 92.
— — — — — — (1970b), *Ibid.*, **49**, 98.
MILLARD, B. J. (1970), *Res. vet. Sci.*, **11**, 394.
MITROVIC, M., and SCHILDKNECHT, E. G. (1970), *Poult. Sci.*, **49**, 86.
NA'ISA, B. K. (1969), *Bull. épizoot. Dis. Afr.*, **17**, 45.
NARASIMHAMURTY, G., RAJULU, P. S., and REDDY, J. S. (1970), *Indian vet. J.*, **47**, 357.
NEITZ, W. O. (1969), *Jl S. Afr. vet. med. Ass.*, **40**, 419.
NEWTON, L. G., and O'SULLIVAN, P. J. (1969), *Aust. vet. J.*, **45**, 404.
OHSHIMA, S., INAMI, Y., and TANAKA, H. (1969), *J. Japan vet. med. Ass.*, **22**, 239.
OPPONG, E. N. W. (1969), *Vet. Rec.*, **85**, 370.
PELLÉRDY, L. (1969), *Magy. Allatorv. Lap.*, **24**, 546.
REID, W. M., and DAVIS, R. B. (1969), *Avian Dis.*, **13**, 447.
RESHETNYAK, V. Z., BARTENEV, V. S. and RUBANOV, A. A. (1970), *Veterinariya, Moscow* 1970, No. 3, 75. (Abstr. *Vet. Bull., Weybridge*, **40**, 901.)
SCHMIDT, G., HIRT, R., and FISCHER, R. (1969), *Res. vet. Sci.*, **10**, 530.
SIEGMANN, O., and HOECK, P. (1969), *Poult. Sci.*, **48**, 1236.
WILLIAMS, R. B. (1969), *Res. vet. Sci.*, **10**, 490.

INSECTICIDES AND CONTROL OF ARTHROPOD PARASITES

J. Donnelly, B.Sc.

General

The collected papers of a recent three-day symposium on Veterinary Pesticides have been published (Society of Chemical Industry, 1969). Two of the five sessions of this symposium were concerned with control of arthropod parasites; one was devoted to control of ticks and another to mites, sheep scab, blowflies, and warble-fly.

Cattle Parasites

Various strategies for the control of cattle tick in Australia were compared by Wharton and his colleagues (1969). These were: planned dipping, which involved dipping every 21 days until the pasture was nearly free of larvae; conventional dipping, where dipping was done whenever the infestation of the pasture reached a standard level; spelling of pastures. It was found that planned dipping gave better results than conventional dipping and that pasture spelling involved less dipping which was only required when stock were moving on to freshly spelled pastures. Zebu cross cattle required less frequent dipping than did British breeds.

A new broad spectrum organophosphorus compound, oxinothiophos, is reported by Stendel (1969) as being effective against normal and resistant strains of ticks of the genera *Boophilus*, *Rhipicephalus*, *Amblyomma*, and *Hyalomma*. The field strength applications were well tolerated by sheep and calves. Russian trials of four compounds have been reported by Badalov (1970). Applications of aqueous suspensions (0·75–1 per cent) of dimethoate, imidan, carbaryl, and trichlormetaphos-3 reduced tick populations on infested cattle. Trichlormetaphos-3 was not recommended because of toxicity. Simetskii (1969) has reported on 1 per cent carbaryl, at doses of 200–350 ml. per head for young cattle, and 600–800 ml. per head for old cattle, as giving control of *B. calcaratus*, *H. scupense*, and *H. anatolicum*. Control of *Ixodes ricinus* on cattle was achieved by 0·25–0·5 per cent aqueous suspension of coumithioat according to Nepoklonov and others (Nepoklonov, Nepoklonova, and Pavlova, 1969). Bromophos ethyl at a concentration of 0·01 per cent gave 95 per cent of ticks and 0·005 per cent gave 75 per cent control of ticks, in Central America, when applied three times at monthly intervals (Rueda and Mateus), 1968). Another report from the same area (Parra, 1969) records 100 per cent control of *Boophilus* spp. following three applications, at monthly intervals, of Dursban at a concentration of 0·0125 per cent and a dose rate of 3 litre per head. This was compared with 85–93 per cent control achieved using 0·0065 per cent Dursban and 93–98 per cent using 0·015 per cent coumaphos similarly applied.

Chorioptic mange of cattle was successfully treated with 0·25 per cent ciodrin administered as a spray (Smith, 1967). Treated cattle remained free of mites for 6 weeks. Psoroptic mange of cattle was successfully controlled, according to Ilyashchenko (1969a), by means of a single, scrubbed-in application of 1·5 per cent fenchlorphos or three washes with 0·5 per cent dicresyl-*N*-methylcarbamate given 7–10 days apart. One treatment with 0·5 per cent propoxur successfully controlled mites of the genus *Sarcoptes* and *Chorioptes* on cattle (Ballarini and others, 1969) but a second treatment was necessary to treat the mange caused by these in some cases. Orally administered famophos at a rate of 2·5 mg. per kg. body-weight over a minimum period of 30 days eliminated cattle lice, *Haematopinus eurysternus* (Roberts, Meleney, and Apodaca, 1969). Lower doses or shorter periods of administration were only partially effective. Infestations of *H. eurysternus*, *Linognathus vituli*, and *H. tuberculatus* on calves were only incompletely controlled by application of 0·1 per cent fenitrothion, according to Mohanty and Pat (1970). Some effect was seen on the adult lice, but in all cases examined the nymphs were seen to survive and develop normally. It was suggested that higher concentrations would be needed for eradication. Treatment of the backs of cattle with a 12 per cent alcoholic solution of trichlorphon was a simple, effective, and well-tolerated method of controlling warbles, as reported by the German workers Rosenberger, Hempel, and West (1969). Russian workers (Podobedov and others, 1967) used an 8 per cent aqueous solution of trichlorphon as a pour-on application at a rate of 200 ml. per animal during the months September–November. Warble numbers were reduced thereby. Another Russian worker (Pakhlevanyan, 1969) claimed 99–100 per cent effectiveness using the same insecticide. Delić, Muftić, and Čanković (1969), working in Sarajevo, got

88–94 per cent control of *Hypoderma* using 2 per cent fenthion as a pour-on application.

Lee (1969) urges that more attention be paid to research results which show the possibility of good control of tsetse by means of low volume aerial applications of pyrethrum. Recent improvements in spray equipment permit sprays of very fine droplet size to be produced at low cost. Research into ways of increasing effective spray paths and methods of determining tsetse populations in woodland and savannah would allow the proved eradication possibilities by aerial sprays to be exploited.

American workers also have been turning their attention to low volume aerial spraying for the control of horn fly, *Haematobia irritans*. Kinzer (1969) reports on trials with malathion at 6·8 oz. per acre, fenthion at 1·97 oz. per acre, and trichlorphon at 4·3 oz. per acre. When these were applied to open range by ultra low volume aerial spray they gave 74, 66, and 74 per cent control respectively 2 days after treatment and 46, 34, and 55 per cent 7 days after treatment. However, it was concluded that the method was impractical, and uneconomic for such a short duration of control.

Ciodrin gave better control of horn fly when applied by rubbing the back of cattle with wax bars impregnated with the insecticide than when applied by spray of emulsion (Harvey and Ely, 1969).

Sheep Parasites

Indian workers (Devi and Sisodia, 1969; Strivastava and Sisodia, 1969) have claimed that an ether extract of Juniper berries in linseed oil was highly effective in controlling sarcoptic mange in sheep. Even in the case of a flock of 44, where there was no response to benzyl benzoate, complete cure was reported after application of the Juniper extract to the lesions for 12 days. The extract gave no skin reaction and was also reported as being effective against *Trichophyton* and *Microsporium* infections in cattle.

Ilyashchenko (1969b), in Russia, found fenchlorphos to be effective in control of sheep scab mites, *Psoroptes ovis*, in both *in vitro* and *in vivo* tests. A dip strength of 1·5 per cent was recommended.

Thermo mechanical aerosols of trichlorphon eliminated the sheep nostril fly, *Oestrus ovis*, from 94 per cent of a flock of 1200 sheep (Nepoklonov and Bukshtynov, 1969). Forty litres of warm 10 per cent trichlorphon were mechanically dispersed in a 1000 $m.^3$ space and the sheep were exposed for 1 hour to the aerosol. There were no apparent toxic effects.

Surveys of sheep dipping in Britain by Leech and Macrae (1970) confirmed that, from the end of 1965, organophosphorus compounds began to replace organochlorine compounds in sheep dipping.

Fleece characteristics were shown by O'Neill and Hebden (1968) to govern the amount of diazinon stripped from dipping fluid by different breeds of sheep which were shower-dipped. All the breeds which were tested (Merino, Dorset Horn, Romney Marsh, and Border Leicester) stripped diazinon from the dipping fluid. In Merinos there was more insecticide deposited towards the wool tips, whereas in the British breeds deposition was greatest nearest the skin. *In vitro* experiments suggested that wax was responsible for attracting the diazinon emulsion to the fleece. Wax concentrations were greatest in the areas of diazinon deposition near the skin in British breeds. The compactness of the Merino fleece probably impeded inward passage of the insecticide.

Pig Parasites

Trichlorphon at a rate of 40 mg. per kg., applied by the pour-on method to pigs, controlled *H. suis* as reported by Hiepe and his German colleagues (Hiepe and others, 1969). Breeding animals remained free of lice for 28 days and fattening animals were clear for 70 days after one application. Two treatments with a 10-day interval gave control in all animals for 70 days. The treatment was well tolerated locally and systemically by the pigs.

Poultry Parasites

The use of metriphonate for control of poultry ectoparasites is elaborated in a paper by Plate (1969). It is claimed as effective against red mite, *Dermanyssus gallinae*, northern fowl mite, *Ornithonyssus sylviarum*, and feather lice, *Mallophaga*, when used as a dip or spray at a concentration of 0·1–0·15 per cent. Treatments should be repeated after an interval of 5–8 days and more permanent results are obtained where buildings and equipment are also sprayed. Oral application is effective in controlling red mite and scaly mite but the substance tends to be toxic at even low oral doses. External applications up to 3 per cent are well tolerated and do not affect egg production nor lead to residues in eggs.

Rabond when sprayed as a 1 per cent emulsion in occupied hen houses did not adversely affect birds, according to Lamina, Lucas, and Schoop (1969), and any red mites which escaped the spray died within 14 days. There was no recurrence of the mites several months after treatment. Both Rabond and carbaryl gave control of *O. sylviarum* as 0·5 per cent sprays applied at a rate of 1 gal. per 100 birds. At this concentration the action of carbaryl was improved by the addition of 1 per cent Ro5-1923 as a synergist (Furman and Lee, 1969). Infestations of *D. gallinae* were also controlled by bromophos sprays at a concentration of 0·125 or 0·25 per cent and a rate of 1·0–1·5 litre per $m.^2$ in work reported by Sander (1969). Infestations on birds and in buildings had disappeared within 5 days and did not recur for 16 weeks. No taint or toxicity was reported.

The use of resin which has been impregnated with dichlorvos is currently being used for a growing range of pest control purposes. Kunz and Hogan (1970) have described a variety of ways in which the substance has been used for the control of poultry lice, *Menopon gallinae* and *Lipeurus caponis*. Resin strips containing 10 per cent dichlorvos, worn as leg bands by the hens or attached to the bottoms of cages, gave control of lice for 147 days. A single strand of impregnated resin, woven through the floor of the cage, gave control for 28 days.

A feedmix containing a mixture of sulphonamides (sulphaquinoxaline, sulphadimidine, sulphamerazine, and sulphathiazole at 0·0125–0·02 per cent expressed as total sulphonamides), when given in feed to poultry for periods from 18 to 42 days, eliminated feather mites from 14 out of 15 treated flocks (Goldhaft, 1969).

Parasites of Cats and Dogs

In a previous issue (VETERINARY ANNUAL, 1970, 274) mention was made of the use of dog collars made of resin strip impregnated with dichlorvos as described by Kibble (1969). Two other Australian workers (Parkinson and Ketterer, 1969), commenting on the same paper, drew attention to the fact that the wearing of these collars had caused severe and persistent dermatitis in some animals. In reply Kibble (1969) acknowledged this and suggested possible causes of the skin reaction.

Fox and his fellow American workers have reported success in controlling cat fleas, *Ctenocephalides felis*, by means of dichlorovs impregnated collars. After 3 months there was good control of fleas on the cat but there was evidence that there were still some breeding fleas active in the cat's environment (Fox, Rivera, and Bayona, 1969). These authors considered that continuous elimination of adult fleas on the host would eventually bring about complete control. Seven out of twenty treated animals showed skin irritation arising from the wearing of such collars. Control of ear mite, *Otodectes cynotis*, in cats wearing such collars was not very good (Fox, Bayona, and Armstrong, 1969). Of 11 infested cats fitted with collars, 4 still had ear mites a month later and a fifth showed clinical symptoms of infestation.

Control of demodectic mange was good in 31 dogs out of 47 given oral doses of cyothioate at 3 mg. per kg. body-weight every 3 days. A satisfactory level of control was obtained in a further 8 of the animals (Manson and Malynicz, 1969). Trichlorphon at 1·5 mg. per kg. twice weekly for a month controlled demodectic mange in 4 out of 6 Boxer dogs. Lindane was successful in only 2 out of 6 cases (Scheffler and Schultz, 1969).

Farmyard Fly Control

The size and species composition of fly populations, arising from poultry manure heaps, and of the predators of these flies is greatly influenced by the physical conditions within the manure. Peck and Anderson (1970) examined the effect of weekly or monthly removal and non-removal of poultry manure on the resulting entomofauna. In general, larvae of the nuisance flies were commonest in week-old manure; predators were more numerous in two- to three-week-old manure. Non-removal of manure thus favoured build-up of the predator population, whereas monthly or bi-weekly removal kept down predator population whilst allowing development of the pest flies.

Control of house flies breeding in piggeries can be achieved by improvements in methods of waste disposal. Dobson and Kutz (1970) studied the effects of waste disposal methods such as septic tanks, spreading of liquid manure over adjacent fields, and slotted floor housing. Known numbers of fly pupae were introduced into fly-proof houses which varied in their method of waste removal. All the methods had some effect in reducing fly numbers.

Yeoman and Warren (1970) have reported some success with butyl methylcinchonate as a repellent for the stable fly, *Stomoxys calcitrans*.

Insecticidal Action

In tests on insecticidal activity of 25 compounds topically applied to the back of the soft tick *Argas persicus*, Frolov and Talonov (1969) found that between 1 and 8 per cent of ticks recovered from the effects of 8 of the 15 organophosphorus compounds being tested. The dose applied in all cases was the minimum one which induced paralysis in more than 50 per cent of the ticks. Recovery from this paralysis occurred after applications of dibrom, dichlorvos, the orthocresyl ester of *N*-methyl carbamate, and carbaryl among others.

H. bovis larvae were removed at slaughter from animals recently dosed with coumaphos, crufomate, and trichlorphon by Steward (1969). These larvae were then tested histochemically for the presence of cholinesterase.

Virtually complete inhibition of the enzyme was found to have occurred in larvae as a result of all three insecticides, whereas no evidence of inhibition was found in larvae from untreated animals. This is offered as histochemical evidence that these insecticides act by inhibiting the cholinesterase enzymes, causing the larvae to die in the body of the host.

Insecticidal Toxicity

During the period 1964–8 there were 563 deaths from insecticide poisoning, in New South Wales, out of 17½ million cattle being dipped to control *B. microplus* (Roe, 1969). Three compounds which were each used in the dipping of more than 1 million of these sheep were: coumaphos, responsible for 6·1 deaths per million dipped; dioxathion, 34·2 deaths per million; and ethion, 34·9 deaths per million.

Dieldrin levels in the tissues of sheep treated for infestations of the ked, *Melophagus ovinus*, were examined by Fearn (1969) after each animal had received the equivalent of 0·3 g. dieldrin either as a tip spray or as a shower dip. Residues of insecticide rose to 0·2–0·7 p.p.m. by the fifth week after treatment and remained at that level for a further 6 weeks at least. McLaughlin (1968), in a similar study on cattle using 0·1 per cent fenchlorphos, found that the highest level of insecticide residue (2·63 p.p.m.) was in the omental fat on the fourth day after treatment. Residues were consistently higher in the omental than in the perirenal fat.

Maximum detectable residues in poultry and egg tissues when Gardona dust was incorporated in floor litter and dusting boxes were: skin 0·058 p.p.m., body fat 0·048 p.p.m., egg white 0·002–0·003 p.p.m. (Ivey and others, 1969). No residues were detectable 2 weeks after treatment was discontinued and no ill effects on the birds were observed.

Control by Means other than Insecticides

It is usually impossible or impractical to sex immature insects so that only males are released in control programmes using sterile males. Whitten and Taylor (1970) have studied the mating biology of *Lucilia cuprina* and conclude that females released along with the sterile males have a part to play in the control programme. Since each normal male can mate about ten times, these sterile females, unavoidably released, will absorb one-tenth of the mating potential of the normal males in the population being controlled.

Two independent studies on radiation sterilization of *B. microplus* have been reported. Eggs of this tick were irradiated at a ^{60}Co source by Guisasola (1969), in South America, and the minimum lethal dose found to be 708 rad. After 150 rad there was no detectable loss in oviposition in the resulting females, but after 500 rad the viability of the eggs was halved. Kitoaka and Morii (1967), in Japan, irradiated engorged females. Doses of 1000–1500 rad inhibited oviposition, 500 rad reduced the fertility of resulting eggs to half. They also found that thiotepa was the most effective of four chemosterilants they tested and this had a 50 per cent sterilizing dose of 1·5 μg. per g. body-weight.

Wright (1970) tested some synthetic compounds for a juvenile hormone effect on the stable fly, *S. calcitrans*. Synthetic juvenile hormone I and Synthetic juvenile hormone II were highly active as were four insecticide synergists: piperonyl butoxide, sesamex, sulfoxide, and Niagara N1A-16388. Topical applications of these produced pupal intermediate forms when applied to prepupae but application to pupae produced no effect.

Insecticide Resistance

Resistance to dieldrin has been detected in *L. sericata* in Ireland (Shaw, Page, and Blackman, 1968). Breakdown of protection from dieldrin and γ-BHC was noted on sheep in Dublin County. Adults were bred from larvae surviving on these sheep and subjected to topical applications of insecticides. It was found that the resistance to dieldrin was 50 times that of normal susceptible blowflies. Evidence of low level resistance to γ-BHC, aldrin, and DDT was also found. Uilenberg (1967) has reported that BHC resistant ticks showed a cross resistance to other organochlorine insecticides such as: dieldrin, toxaphene, endrin, and isobenzan. Another resistant strain showed resistance to these four insecticides but not to BHC.

Schnitzerling and his fellow Australian workers (Schnitzerling, Roulston, and Schunter, 1970) followed the absorption and metabolism of ^{14}C-labelled DDT in resistant and susceptible *B. microplus*. They could find no causal relationship between DDT absorption or metabolism and resistance to the compound.

Cholinesterase activity levels were lower in organophosphorus resistant *B. decoloratus* than in susceptible strains (Hart and Batham, 1969). The enzyme in the resistant ticks differed from that in the susceptibles in three enzyme types which showed differences in their reaction with organophosphorus compounds.

Roulston and associates (Roulston and others, 1969) studied the MacKay strain of organophosphorus resistant *B. microplus* and found that it differed from either the Biarra or Ridgelands strain in its spectrum of compounds to which it was resistant. The cholinesterase activity resembled that of the Biarra strain but its sensitivity to inhibition was similar to that of susceptible strains. Metabolic studies using labelled insecticide suggested the presence of a detoxification or degradation mechanism in the MacKay strain. This mechanism of resistance does not appear to operate in other known resistant strains of this tick.

Host Resistance

As the number of resistant strains of *B. microplus* in Australia seems to grow so too does the number of reports of work on natural host resistance to this tick. Some of the work of Roberts has already been reported on (VETERINARY ANNUAL, 1969, 170), in which the resistance was shown to be due to innate host factors including an immune response. Wharton, Utech, and Turner (1970) have found that resistance to *B. microplus* in Illawara Shorthorns was a heritable character, and have suggested that this fact provides encouragement for selecting breeding animals on the basis of tick resistance. O'Kelly and Seifert (1969) demonstrated an effect of diet on tick resistance. Animals with deficient diets can show a breakdown of acquired tick resistance.

REFERENCES

BADALOV, E. T. (1970), *Veterinariya*, No. 3, 68.

BALLARINI, G., FICARELLI, R., VEZZANI, E., and SCANDIANI, O. (1969), *Atti Soc. Ital. Buiatria*, **1**, 383.

DELIČ, S., MUFTIĆ, R., and ČANKOVIĆ, M. (1969), *Vet. Glasn.*, **23**, 659.

DEVI, G., and SISODIA, C. S. (1969), *Indian J. anim. Sci.*, **39**, 345.

DOBSON, R. C., and KUTZ, F. W. (1970), *J. econ. Ent.*, **63**, 171.

FEARN, J. T. (1969), *Exptl Rec. Dep. Agric. S. Aust.*, No. 3, 5.

FOX, I., BAYONA, I. G., and ARMSTRONG, J. L. (1969), *J. econ. Ent.*, **62**, 1503.
— — RIVERA, G. A., and BAYONA, I. G. (1969), *Ibid.*, **62**, 1246.
FROLOV, B. A., and TALONOV, G. A. (1969), *Trudy vses. Inst. vet. Sanit.*, **33**, 164.
FURMAN, D. P., and LEE, D. (1969), *J. econ. Ent.*, **62**, 1246.
GOLDHART, T. M. (1969), *Refuah Vet.*, **26**, 167.
GUISASOLA, A. A. (1969), *Revta Med. vet., B. Aires*, **50**, 475.
HART, R. J., and BATHAM, P. (1969), *Jl S. Afr. vet. med. Ass.*, **40**, 284.
HARVEY, T. L., and ELY, D. G. (1969), *J. econ. Ent.*, **62**, 1386.
HIEPE, T., STIMMLER, L., RIBBECK, R., and KÖHLING, M. (1969), *Mh. VetMed.*, **24**, 334.
ILYASHCHENKO, V. I. (1969a), *Trudy vses. Inst. vet. Sanit.*, **34**, 389.
— — (1969b), *Ibid.*, **33**, 170.
IVEY, M. C., HOFFMAN, R. A., CLABORN, H. V., and HOGAN, B. F. (1969), *J. econ. Ent.*, **62**, 1003.
KIBBLE, R. M. (1969), *Aust. vet. J.*, **45**, 36.
KINZER, H. G. (1969), *J. econ. Ent.*, **62**, 1515.
KITOAKA, S., and MORII, T. (1967), *Jap. J. Sanit. Zool.*, **18**, 126.
KUNZ, S. E., and HOGAN, B. F. (1970), *J. econ. Ent.*, **63**, 263.
LAMINA, J., LUCAS, H., and SCHOOP, G. (1969), *Berl. Münch. tierärztl. Wschr.*, **82**, 272.
LEE, C. W. (1969), *Bull. Wld Hlth Org.*, **41**, 261.
LEECH, F. B., and MACRAE, W. D. (1970), *Pesticide Sci.*, **1**, 53.
MCLAUGHLIN, J. E. (1968), *Qd J. agric. anim. Sci.*, **25**, 1.
MANSON, E. R., and MALYNICZ, G. L. (1969), *Aust. vet. J.*, **45**, 533.
MOHANTY, R. K., and PAT, K. B. (1970), *Orissa vet. J.*, **5**, 19.
NEPOKLONOV, A. A., and BUKSHTYNOV, V. I. (1969), *Veterinariya*, 49.
— — NEPOKLONOVA, M. I., and PAVLOVA, N. V. (1969), *Trudy vses. Inst. vet. Sanit.*, **34**, 380.
O'KELLY, J. C., and SEIFERT, G. W. (1969), *Aust. J. biol. Sci.*, **22**, 1497.
O'NEILL, D. K., and HEBDEN, S. P. (1968), *Aust. vet. J.*, **44**, 344.
PAKHLEVANYAN, A. SH. (1969), *Veterinariya*, No. 1, 65.
PARKINSON, K. D., and KETTERER, P. J. (1969), *Aust. vet. J.*, **45**, 36.
PARRA, G. D. (1969), *Revta Inst. Colomb. agropec.*, **4**, 73.
PECK, J. H., and ANDERSON, J. R. (1970), *J. econ. Ent.*, **63**, 82.
PLATE, G. (1969), *Vet. med. Rev. Leverkusen*, No. 2, 115.
PODOBEDOV, A. I., NEPOKLONOV, A. A., TALANOV, G. A., and IVASHKOV, I. S. (1967), *Veterinariya*, No. 3, 50.
ROBERTS, I. H., MELENEY, W. P., and APODACA, S. A. (1969), *J. Am. vet. med. Ass.*, **155**, 504.
ROE, R. T. (1969), *Aust. vet. J.*, **45**, 332.
ROSENBERGER, G., HEMPEL, E., and WEST, G. (1969), *Dt. tierärztl. Wschr.*, **76**, 551.
ROULSTON, W. J., SCHUNTER, C. A., SCHNITZERLING, H. J., and WILSON, J. T. (1969), *Aust. J. biol. Sci.*, **22**, 1585.
RUEDA, H. C., and MATEUS, V. G. (1968), *Revta Inst. Colomb. agropec.*, **3**, 103.
SANDER, H. (1969), *Tierärztl. Umsch.*, **24**, 338.
SCHEFFLER, M., and SCHULTZ, W. (1969), *Mh. VetMed.*, **24**, 429.
SCHNITZERLING, H. J., ROULSTON, W. J., and SCHUNTER, C. A. (1970), *Aust. J. biol. Sci.*, **23**, 219.
SHAW, R. D., PAGE, K. W., and BLACKMAN, G. G. (1968), *Vet. Rec.*, **81**, 755.
SIMETSKII, M. A. (1969), *Trudy vses. Inst. vet. Sanit.*, **34**, 327.
SMITH, H. J. (1967), *Can. vet. J.*, **8**, 88.
SOCIETY OF CHEMICAL INDUSTRY (1969), Monograph, No. 33, London.
STENDEL, W. (1969), in SOCIETY OF CHEMICAL INDUSTRY (1969).
STEWARD, C. C. (1969), *Can. Ent.*, **101**, 463.
STRIVASTAVA, S. C., and SISODIA, C. S. (1969), *Indian vet. J.*, **46**, 826.
UILENBERG, G. (1967), *Revue Élev. Méd. vét. Pays trop.*, **20**, 301.
WHARTON, R. H., HARLEY, K. L. S., WILKINSON, P. R., UTECH, K. B., and KELLEY, B. M. (1969), *Aust. J. agric. Res.*, **20**, 783.
— — UTECH, K. B., and TURNER, H. G. (1970), *Ibid.*, **21**, 163.
WHITTEN, M. J., and TAYLOR, W. C. (1970), *J. econ. Ent.*, **63**, 269.
WRIGHT, J. E. (1970), *Ibid.*, **63**, 878.
YEOMAN, G. H., and WARREN, B. C. (1970), *Bull. ent. Res.*, **59**, 563.

RECENT TRENDS IN ANTIBACTERIAL THERAPY

Olga Uvarov, M.R.C.V.S.

The discovery of the therapeutic value of sulphonamides triggered off what is known as the 'therapeutic explosion'.

The discovery of penicillin arose from a careful observation by Flemming, but subsequent discoveries resulted from intensive searches for antibiotic activity in organisms recovered from soil samples from many parts of the world. Garrod and O'Grady (1971) summarized some of these developments which took place up to 1963.

Although many hundreds of antibiotics have been discovered, comparatively few have been introduced for clinical use. Many formulations, for one reason or another, of well-established antibiotics, singly or in combination with newer ones, are now marketed. At times this makes it difficult to choose the most suitable preparation for use, having regard to safety and efficacy. The Medicines Act (1968), when in full operation, should remedy this in that all new preparations will require to be tested in the field before becoming freely available. Uvarov (1968, 1971) stressed the importance of clinical pharmacology and the need for clinical trials of new therapeutics. Although some standardized methods of evaluation of drugs are now accepted, difficulties may arise with powerful new agents in achieving a balance between therapeutics and side-effects. Sanford (1971) emphasized the need to describe the disease for which the drug is to be tested and to include a control drug for comparison purposes in such trials. Alexander (1969) gives advice as to the choice of antibiotic and its method of selection in practice. Thus it is evident that more information is now available on veterinary therapeutics. In addition, the Report of the Swann Committee on the *Use of Antibiotics in Animal Husbandry and Veterinary Medicine* makes recommendations regarding the use of antibiotics therapeutically and as food additives in farm animals.

Currently Available Antibacterial Agents

Of the twelve available antibiotics described by Uvarov (1955), ten are still in use: penicillin singly or in combination, streptomycin, chlortetracycline, oxytetracycline, chloramphenicol, tetracycline, bacitracin, neomycin, polymixin, and erythromycin. The newer ones have been classified as follows:—

1. The Semi-synthetic Penicillins and the Cephalosporins

The latter have not been introduced for veterinary use. The semi-synthetic penicillins (developed from the penicillin nucleus) are similar in spectrum to the parent compound, but are resistant to staphylococcal penicillinase and are used where these staphylococci are resistant to penicillin. The main members of this group are cloxacillin, used in mastitis in cattle, and ampicillin, which is active against both Gram-positive and Gram-negative organisms and is used systemically in a number of conditions, such as enteritis, pneumonia, etc.

2. The Macrolide Antibiotics

These are so called because they possess the large macrolide lactone ring (Alexander, 1969). Their spectrum closely resembles that of penicillin. In veterinary practice erythromycin, spiramycin, oleandomycin, and tylocin are used.

3. Polypeptide Antibiotics

This group is chiefly known as a result of work on polymixins which are regarded as too toxic for parenteral use. Like bacitracin, polymixins are used for topical application for skin conditions and ear diseases in dogs.

4. Nitrofurans

This group includes nitrofurazone, furazolidone, and nitrofurantoin. These preparations have a marked activity against both Gram-positive and Gram-negative organisms. They are used to treat infections of the alimentary and respiratory tracts. Nitrofurazone and furazolidone are also used in the control of some coccidiosis.

5. Trimethoprim

This synthetic agent combined with sulphadiazine or sulfadoxine has become available for treatment of a number of alimentary, respiratory, and urinary-tract infections. Extension studies are still being carried out on this compound which is active against many pathogenic bacteria, but it is predominantly bacteriostatic in action.

The work on the sulphonamide drugs was, for a time, superseded by that on antibiotics, but the introduction of trimethoprim may well stimulate interest again in some of the sulphonamides, especially if other compounds of trimethoprim are found to be of value.

6. Antibiotics in Feedstuffs

Following the recommendations of the Swann Committee (1969), prescribing of antibiotics for medication of livestock has been accepted. Only veterinary surgeons are able to issue prescriptions for these preparations as food additives. This will apply to penicillin, chlortetracycline, and oxytetracycline as from March, 1971, and to nitrofurazone, furazolidone, nitrofurantoin, and furaltadone as from September, 1971. Flavomycin and virginamycin will be allowed as food additives without prescription, and zinc bacitracin will be supplied as a feed antibiotic as at present. The Regulations under the Therapeutic Substance Act (1956) will come into force on the dates indicated. Future regulations will be made so that sulphaquinoxaline and sulphanitran can be used as coccidiostats without prescription (*Veterinary Record*, 1971).

The Swann Committee also recommended voluntary control for the use of chloramphenicol (the drug of choice in the treatment of typhoid in man), so that it is only prescribed in special situations.

According to the *Index of Veterinary Specialities* (1971) there has been a trend towards the introduction of chloramphenicol-containing products for systemic as opposed to topical use. Oxytetracyclines, some sulphonamides, combinations of penicillin and streptomycin, and some other products are frequently quoted in the *Index*.

Principles of Chemotherapy

The widespread use of antibiotics makes it necessary, from time to time, to consider some of the fundamental principles of chemotherapy, especially in the light of new knowledge. Parker and Paterson (1968) and Crofton (1969) have discussed some of these principles which also are applicable in veterinary medicine. Among the main points to consider are:—

1. Antibiotic Activity

This may be:—

a. Bactericidal, where the antibiotic affects the cell wall or membrane, and exerts a lethal effect on protein synthesis, so killing the organisms outright; or

b. Bacteriostatic, where there is interference with manufacture of protein—preventing the growth and proliferation of organisms without actually destroying them (Crofton, 1969).

In addition, the activity of some antibiotics can be bacteriostatic in low and bactericidal in high concentrations.

2. Synergism and Antagonism between Drugs

Synergism can be achieved by combining two drugs with similar properties to produce a greater effect than that produced by the single drug. This effect is not easy to determine, but Uvarov (1971) showed that it can be obtained with a combination of penicillin and streptomycin when used against staphylococci of mastitic origin. Garrod and O'Grady (1971) quote the law postulated by Jowetz and Gunnison that a combination of:—

a. Bacteriostatic+bacteriostatic is simply additive.

b. Bactericidal+bacteriostatic may be antagonistic.

c. Bactericidal+bactericidal may be synergistic.

3. Drug Resistance

This is now recognized as:—

a. Natural—in which the bacterial population is resistant to the drug whether the bacteria have been exposed to the drug or not.

b. Acquired—arising as the result of exposure to the drug or drugs.

c. Transferable or Infectious—this phenomenon was first noted in enterobacteria in Japan by Watanabe, and later investigated by several other workers. Here resistance is transferred from one species to another, even after a short exposure between the susceptible and non-susceptible organisms.

Therapeutic Failure and Bacterial Persistence

Any study of a drug should take into account its failures as well as its successes in practice. Therapeutic failures are not widely reported, but Platnow and Blobel (1963), Waite and Blackburn (1963), and Kingwill and others (1968) have reported some such failures in the treatment of mastitis.

Recently Wilson, Little, and Roberts (1970) reported a severe outbreak of mastitis in a herd treated with benzathine penicillin at the 'drying-off' period. He isolated L forms of *Streptococcus agalactiae* from the milk of affected cows and suggests that if emergence of L forms amongst staphylococci and streptococci were to become more widely encountered, then the treatment of dry cows with penicillin-type antibiotics may have to be reconsidered. The survival of fully sensitive bacteria in the presence of antibiotic has been known for some time (Bigger, 1944). It is probable that persistent bacteria may be dormant during initial exposure to the antibiotic, but subsequently become pathogenic. It would appear that the most satisfactory therapy should aim at a high concentration of a suitable bactericidal antibiotic given early in the course of the disease. If large groups of animals are to be treated regularly with antibacterial drugs, the possibility of bacterial repopulation or the emergence of L forms of organisms should not be discounted.

Variations in antimicrobial therapy will continue to emerge in the light of new knowledge and experience with these substances. Garrod and O'Grady

(1971), however, suggest that it is unlikely that new antibiotics remain to be discovered. It is wise, therefore, to use the currently available therapeutics in such a way as to safeguard their use for the future.

REFERENCES

ALEXANDER, F. (1969), *An Introduction to Veterinary Pharmacology*, 2nd ed. Edinburgh: Livingstone.

BIGGER, J. W. (1944), *Lancet*, **2**, 497.

CROFTON, J. (1969), *Br. med. J.*, **2**, 209.

GARROD, L. P., and O'GRADY, F. (1971), *Antibiotic and Chemotherapy*. Edinburgh: Livingstone.

Index of Veterinary Specialities (1971), Ewell, Surrey: M.C. Magazines.

KINGWILL, R. G., NEAVE, F. K., DODD, F. H., MEEK, A. M., WESTGARTH, D. R., and GRIFFIN, T. K. (1968), in *Annual Report*, p. 56. Reading: National Institute for Research in Dairying.

PARKER, H., and PATERSON, P. (1968), *J. chron. Dis.*, **21**, 719.

PLATNOW, I., and BLOBEL, H. (1963), *J. Am. vet. med. Ass.*, **142**, 1097.

SANFORD, J. (1971), *Vet. Rec.*, **88**, 82.

SWANN COMMITTEE (1969), *Report of the Joint Committee on the Use of Antibiotics in Animal Husbandry and Veterinary Medicine*. London: H.M.S.O.

UVAROV, O. (1955), *Vet. Rec.*, **67**, 67.

— — (1968), *Proc. R. Soc. Med.*, **5**, 569.

— — (1971), *N.Z. vet. J.*, **19**, 127.

Veterinary Record (1971), **88**, 218.

WAITE, R., and BLACKBURN, P. S. (1963), *J. Dairy Res.*, **30**, 209.

WILSON, C. D., LITTLE, T. W., and ROBERTS, D. H. (1970), *Vet. Rec.*, **87**, 300.

APPENDIX

SYNONYMS OF THE DRUGS MENTIONED IN THE THERAPEUTICS SECTION

Most drugs are sold under a variety of trade names and many of the newer compounds have one or more common names. In the text the approved common name or the most widely used common name is employed, but to assist field workers who may wish to purchase any of the drugs referred to a list of synonyms is given below. The first of these is usually the chemical name. No claim is made that the list is exhaustive but all names which have come to the notice of the contributors are included.

The list has been compiled by Dr. T. E. Gibson from information supplied by the authors concerned.

Name in Text	*Synonyms*
Aldrin	1,2,3,4,10,10-Hexachloro-1,4,4a,5,8,8a-hexahydro-1,4-*exo*-5,8*endo*-dimethanonaphthalene
Amicarbalide	3,3′-Diamidinocarbanilide. Diampron
Amodiaquine	4-(7-Chloro-4-quinolylamino)-α-diethylamino-*O*-cresol. Camoquin
Amprolium	1-(4-Amino-2- propylpyrimidin-5-ylmethyl)-2-picolinium chloride, hydrochloride. Amprolmix. (One component of Pancoxin and Amprol-plus.)
Bromophos	*O,O*-dimethyl *O*-2,5-dichloro-4-bromphenyl phosphorothionate. SD 1942. Nexion
Bromophos ethyl	*O,O*-diethyl *O*-2,5-dichloro-4-bromophenyl phosphorothionate. Nexagon
Bunamidine hydrochloride	*N,N*-di-*n*-butyl-4-hexyloxy-1-naphthamidine-HCl. Scolaban

Name in Text	*Synonyms*
Cambendazole	5-Isopropoxycarbonylamino-2-(4-thiazolyl) benzimidazole
Carbarsone	4-Carbamidophenylarsenic acid
Carbaryl	1-Naphthyl *N*-methyl carbamate. Sevin
Chloramphenicol	Chloromycetin. Alficetyn. Animycetin
Chlortetracycline	Aureomycin
Ciodrin	α-Methylbenzyl-3-hydroxy-*cis*-crotonate dimethyl phosphate. SD 4294
Clioxanide	2-Acetoxy-4′chloro-3,5-diidobenzanilide. Tremerad SYD 230. CI 633
Clopidol	3,5-Dichloro-2,6-dimethyl-4-pyridinol
Coumaphos	3-Chloro-4-methyl-7-coumarinyl diethyl phosphorothionate. Co-Ral. Asuntol. Muscatox. Resitox
Coumithioate	*O,O*-diethyl *O*-(7,8,9,10-tetrahydro-6-oxodibenzo-[*C*]-chroman-3-yl) phosphorothioate
Crufomate	4-*tert*-Butyl-2-chlorophenyl methyl-*N*-methylphosphoroamidate. Ruelene. Dowco 132
Cyothioate	*O,O*-dimethyl-*O*-*p*-sulphamoyl-phenyl phosphorothionate
Dapsone	2-Sulphamoyl-4,4′-diaminodiphenyl sulphone
DDT	1,1,1-Trichloro-2,2-di-(4-chloromethyl)-ethane. Neocid Gesarol
Decoquinate	Ethyl 6-*n*-decyloxy-7-ethoxy-4-hydroxyquinoline-3-carboxylate. Deccox
Diaveridine	2,4-Diamino-5-(3,4-dimethoxybenzyl) pyrimidine
Diazinon	Diethyl 2-isopropyl-6-methyl-4-pyrimidinyl phosphorothionate. Basodin
Dibrom	1,2-Dibromo-2,2-dichloroethyl dimethyl phosphate
Dichlorvos	2,2-Dichlorovinyl dimethyl phosphate. DDVP. Nogos. Nuvan. Vapona. Atgard. Task. Equigard
Dieldrin	1,2,3,4,10,10-Hexachloro-6,7-epoxy-1,4,4a,5,6,7,8,8a-octa-hydro-1,4-*exo*-5,8-*endo*-dimethanonaphthalene. Betalox. Octalox
Dimethoate	*O,O*-dimethyl S-methylcarbamoylmethyl phosphorodithionate. Rogor. Am. Cyanamid 2880
Diminazene	4,4′-Diamidinodiazoaminobenzene diaceturate. Berenil. Ganaseg
Dioxathion	1,4-Dioxane-2,3-ylidene *bis*-(*O,O*-diethyl phosphorothiolothionate). Delnav. Navodil
Dursban	*O,O*-diethyl *O*-3,5,6-trichloro-2-pyridyl phosphorothionate. Dowco 179
Endrin	1,2,3,4,10,10-Hexachloro-6,7-epoxy-1,4,4a,5,6,7,8,8a-octahydro-5,8-*exo*-dimethanonaphthalene
Ethion	Tetraethyl *SS′*-methylene-*bis*-(phosphorothiolothionate)
Famophos	*O*-[*p*-(dimethyl sulphamoyl) phenyl]-*O,O*-dimethyl phosphorothionate. Famphur. Warbex
Fenchlorphos	Dimethyl 2,4,5-trichlorophenyl phosphorothionate. Ronnel. Nankor. Trolene. Korlan
Fenitrothion	Dimethyl 3-methyl-4-nitrophenyl-phosphorothionate
Fenthion	Dimethyl 3-methyl-4-methylthiophenyl phosphorothionate. Tiguvon. Baytex. Lebaycid
Gamma-BHC	1,2,3,4,5,6-Hexachlorocyclohexane. Lindane
Haloxon	*O,O*-di-(2-Chloroethyl)-*O*-(3-chloro-4-methylcoumarin-7-yl) phosphate. Loxon. Helmiron. Eustidil. Galloxon
Hexachlorophane	2,2′-Methylene-*bis*-(3,4,6-trichlorophenol). Hexachlorophene. G11. Distocid. Hisohex. Bisophene. Coopaphene. Fascophene
Imidocarb	3,3′-*bis*-(2-Imidazolin-2-yl) carbanilide dihydrochloride
Ipronidazole	1-Methyl-2-isopropyl-5-nitroimidazole

Name in Text	*Synonyms*
Isobenzan	1,3,4,5,6,7,8,8a-Octachloro-1,3,3a,4,7,7a-hexahydro-4,7 methanophthalon. Telodrin. WL-1650
Isometamidium	7-*m*-Amidinophenyldiazoamino-2-amino-10-ethyl-9-phenylphenanthridinium chloride hydrochloride. Samorin
Malathion	*S*-[1,2-di(ethoxycarbonyl) ethyl] dimethyl phorothiolothionate. Carbofos. Hercaptothion
Methyl benzoquate	Methyl-7-benzyloxy-6-*n*-butyl-1,4-dehydro-4-oxoquinoline-3-carboxylate. Statyl
Metronidazole	1-β-Hydroxyethyl-2-methyl-5-nitro-imidazole. Flagyl
Niclofolan	2,2′-Dehydroxy-3,3′-dinitro-5,5′-dichlorodiphenyl. Bilevon M. Bilevon R. Meniclopholan. Bayer 9015. Bayer 9015A. Distlan Me 3625
Oxinothiophos	*O*-ethyl *O*-quinolyl-8-benzenephosphorothionate
Parbendazole	Methyl 5-(6)-butyl-2-benzimidazole carbamate Helmatac. SKF 29044. Worm Guard 33. Verminum
Phenamidine	4,4′-Diamidinodiphenyl ether
Propoxur	2-Isopropoxyphenyl-*N*-methyl carbonate. Aprocarb. Baygon
Quinuronium	6,6′-di-(*N*-methylquinolyl) urea. Acapron. Acaprin
Rabond	2-Chloro-1-(2,4,5-trichlorophenyl) vinyl dimethyl phosphate. Rabon. Gardona
Rafoxanide	3,5-Diiodo-3′-chloro-4′-(*p*-chlorophen-oxy) salicylanilide. Flukanide
Resorcantel	4-Bromo-2,6-dihydroxybenzanilide. Terenol. Hoechst 296V
Robenidene	1,3-*bis*-(*p*-Chlorobenzylideneamino) guanidine hydrochloride. Cycostat
Ro 5-1923	2-Nitrophenyl 2 propynyl ether
Ronidazole	1-Methyl-2-carbamoyloxymethyl-5 nitroimidazole
Sulphachloropyridazine	Sodium 3-*p*-aminobenzene sulphonamido-5-chloropyridazine
Sulphadimethoxine	*N*-2,6-dimethoxy-4-pyrimidinylsulphanilamide. Madribon
Sulphadimidine	Sulphadimethylpyrimidine. Sulphamezathine
Sulphamerazine	2-Sulphanilamido-4-methylpyrimidine
Sulphaquinoxaline	2-Sulphanilamidoquinoxaline—a constituent of Pancoxin
Sulphathiazole	*N*′-2-thiazolysulphanilamide
Tetramisole	DL-2,3,5,6-tetrahydro-6-phenyl-imidazo (2,1-b) thiazole hydrochloride. Nilverm. R 8299. Citarin. Nemicide Ripercol. Bayer 9051. Decaris. Galanid. Concurat
Thiabendazole	2-(Thiazol-4-yl)-benzimidazole. MK360. Thibenzole. Hyozole. Equizole. Bovizole. Omnizole
Toxaphene	Polychlorocamphone
Trichlormetaphos	*O*-ethyl *O*-methyl-*O*-2,4,5-trichlorophenyl phosphorothionate
Trichlorphon	Dimethyl 2,2,2-trichloro-1-hydroxyethylphosphonate. Neguvon. Dipterex. Metriphonate. Chlorplus. Bayer L13/50. Dryex. Bubalin
Tylosin	Antibiotic of erythromycin group
Zoalene	3,5-Dimitro-*O*-toluamide. Zoamix

POISONS AND POISONING

E. G. C. Clarke, M.A., Ph.D., D.Sc., F.R.I.C.
Myra L. Clarke, F.R.C.V.S.

POISONS AND POISONING

E. G. C. Clarke, M.A., Ph.D., D.Sc., F.R.I.C., and Myra L. Clarke, F.R.C.V.S.

Inorganic Compounds

It is only during the past few years that man has realized that he is slowly but surely poisoning the world he lives in, and taken steps to prevent the continuous pollution of his environment. So far little that is effective has been done. Lead is a case in point. Most of the environmental contamination with lead comes from additives to petrol and is particularly heavy near highways. In Germany it has been found that there may be 35–50 p.p.m. of lead in the grass growing by the roadside (Kloke and Leh, 1969), while in Holland this figure is given as 135–150 p.p.m. (Tesink, 1969) with 400 p.p.m. in the underlying soil. The lead is not entirely deposited on the ground. Part of it remains suspended in the atmosphere, and it has been found that up to 5 per cent of the particulate matter in the air near a large city may consist of lead (Chow and Earl, 1970); this seems to be increasing at about 5 per cent a year.

Petrol, however, is only one source of lead. Paint, car batteries, and so on are well known, but Buck (1970) considers that used crank-case oil is the most common cause of lead poisoning in cattle; it appears to be more toxic than the common salts of lead and the animals seem to relish it.

Careless disposal of toxic material is another frequent cause of trouble. Rybolt (1970) records a case in which 7 calves died as the result of eating lead arsenate carelessly abandoned in paper sacks in an old building. All species are susceptible to lead poisoning, and cases have recently been quoted in bats (Zook, Sayer, and Garner, 1970) and a Rhesus monkey (Houser and Frank, 1970). Poultry become at first sluggish, then excitable. They lose condition, egg production falls, fertility and hatchability are low, and mortality high (Cristea and others, 1970). Chicks fed 10,000 p.p.m. of lead in the diet showed ataxia and decrease in body-weight and food intake. The lead content of the livers was 82·5 p.p.m. against 0·5 p.p.m. of controls. Rüssel (1970) finds that lead is absorbed by iron in the livers and kidneys of cattle. This has the effect of reducing the availability of iron in the body as only 7 per cent of liver iron is in soluble form in poisoned cattle compared with 70 per cent in normal animals. Christian and Tryphonas (1971) note that gross brain lesions (cerebrocortical softening, yellowish discoloration, and cavitation) are only seen in cattle with prolonged clinical illness.

Mercury is another substance which has recently been causing concern on account of its widespread environmental distribution. Inorganic mercury or phenyl mercury is converted in the bottom mud of lakes and rivers to soluble methyl mercury which is concentrated in living things, notably fish and birds, that have difficulty in excreting mercury. The concentration factor from water to pike, for example, is over 3000; this constitutes a great risk to people and animals living largely on fish (Bäckström, 1969; Abelson, 1970). Platonow and Funnell (1970) have shown that even low levels of inorganic mercury will accumulate in the tissues of chickens until a toxic level is reached. This may well give rise to secondary poisoning. Hanko and others (1970) fed methyl mercury dicyandiamide to chickens for 35–44 days and then killed them and fed their flesh to ferrets. The birds showed no toxic symptoms, but the ferrets died of mercury poisoning in about 7 weeks. Borg and others (1970) carried out a somewhat similar experiment, feeding the flesh of mercury-fed chickens to goshawks, which died in 5–7 weeks. A high level of mercury was found in brain and gonads of both hawks and ferrets. In pigs, 20 mg. per kg. of methyl mercury dicyandiamide is lethal while 5 mg. per kg. will produce symptoms of poisoning. Three weeks may sometimes elapse before onset of symptoms (Piper, Miller, and Dickinson, 1971). In mice it was found that methyl mercury is stable in the body and slowly excreted, mainly in the faeces, but that dimethyl mercury is excreted rapidly, about 80–90 per cent being exhaled within 16 hours and the rest converted to methyl mercury (Östlund, 1969). Prior administration of spironolactone not only protects rats from death from mercuric chloride but also from the tubular necrosis and calcification which it causes (Selye, 1970). Ascorbic acid supplements will protect young quail against the growth retardation and anaemia caused by cadmium (Fox and Fry, 1970).

Tait and others (1971) report the deaths of 19 of 55 lambs after consuming a concentrate containing 27 p.p.m. of copper for 4 months. The liver copper averaged 1300 p.p.m. of dry matter. Ross (1970) treated lambs with a similar liver copper concentration with 100 mg. of ammonium molybdate and 1 g. anhydrous sodium sulphate daily. The copper level fell to two-thirds of its value in 6 weeks, and to half in a further 7 weeks. The connexion between molybdenum and copper is further emphasized by the development of hypocuprosis by cattle grazing near an industrial plant producing molybdenum oxide (Verwey, 1969). Copper sulphate given by mouth at a level of 0·13 g. per kg. produced fatal copper poisoning in 2 sheep out of 5, but half this amount had no permanent effect (Cabadaj and Gdovin, 1970). The copper content of the livers of sheep suffering from chronic copper poisoning varies considerably between different breeds (Lüke and Wiemann, 1970); Olsen (1969) has shown that copper in the livers of poisoned sheep may be demonstrated histochemically. Fish have been poisoned by copper particles released into a river from a copper plant (Jara, 1970).

Arsenilic acid fed at a level of 0·0375 per cent of diet caused blindness in pigs in about a month. It is interesting to note that the levels of arsenic found in the hair by neutron activation analysis were not high enough to support a definite diagnosis of arsenic poisoning (Menges and others, 1970). Robison (1970) found that the LD_{50} of fluoracetate was 0·393 mg. per kg. in cows and 0·221 mg. per kg. in calves—figures that emphasize the care that must be taken in using this compound as a rodenticide. After feeding nitrate to calves, Dollahite and Holt (1969) concluded that the rate at which the nitrate was consumed was of more importance than the total amount, and also the level of haemoglobin remaining in the blood was of greater significance than the amount of methaemoglobin formed. Pigs inhaling silo gas, a mixture of varying proportions of carbon dioxide, nitric oxide, and nitrogen dioxide, died in 21–72 minutes. A concentration of nitrogen dioxide of 100–150 p.p.m. is dangerous, one of 250–300 p.p.m. lethal. The gas combines with the aqueous film lining the respiratory passages to produce a mixture of nitric and nitrous acids, resulting in plumonary oedema, haemorrhage, and anoxaemia (Giddens, Whitehair, and Sleight, 1970). A 5 per cent solution of sodium chlorate killed a quarter of the cattle that drank it. Acute cases died in 12–24 hours, but animals that survived 5 days recovered (Mustaffa-Babjee, Lee Chin Hua, and Nazarddin, 1970). In lambs the lethal dose by mouth of sodium selenite was found to vary from 0·7 to 3·1 mg. per kg. The intramuscular dose was 0·453 mg. per kg. (Caravaggi, Clark, and Jackson, 1970). Gabbedy (1970) has noted that lambs are sometimes poisoned by doses of selenium well below the level usually assumed to be toxic, and suggests that stress and cobalt deficiency may be contributory factors. Rats fed with 5–15 p.p.m. of sodium selenite develop haemolytic anaemia, but the effect may be reduced by the administration of sodium arsenite (Halverson and others, 1970). Superphosphate has been shown to be without toxic effect in sheep (Labadie and others, 1970).

Organic Compounds

The pollution is no less urgent when we come to consider organic substances, the most important of these being the persistent organochlorine compounds such as DDT and the polychlorinated biphenyls (PCB). In spite of the fact that the use of DDT in the U.S.A. is decreasing, the DDT content of phytoplankton samples collected off the coast of California increased threefold between 1955 and 1969 (Cox, 1970). From the plankton the compounds spread to fish (Bjerk and Sundby, 1970) and fish-eating predators such as birds and men (Prestt, Jefferies, and Moore, 1970). The toxicity of different commercial samples of PCB seems to vary, and may be due to the presence of varying quantities of impurities such as the chick-oedema factors (Vos and Koeman, 1970). The sea is not the only reservoir for organochlorine compounds. DDT applied to pasture as a top dressing to control soil pests may remain in the top layer of soil for years and can thus continue to be ingested by stock and accumulate in the body fat (Harrison, Mol, and Healy, 1970). Various methods for the removal of chlorinated pesticides from poultry and dairy cattle have been suggested (Liska and Stadelman, 1969).

Organophosphorus compounds, being less stable than organochlorine, do not present so large a pollution problem. Trouble usually arises from their careless use or disposal. This may be on the grand scale, as when 4500 sheep were killed as the result of a chemical warfare exercise in Utah (Van Kampen, Shupe, and others, 1970; Van Kampen and others, 1969), or on a purely local level as when 4 cattle died through the careless disposal of a bag of phorate (Kitto, 1970). The correct method of getting rid of unwanted pesticides is not easy to find. It has been suggested that manufacturers of toxic sheep dips, for example, should supply some compound to render the residues harmless (Sinclair, 1970). This is easier to suggest than to accomplish. To be of value the dip must be comparatively stable and thus not easy to break down. Any antidote must be cheap, easy to use, non-toxic, and able to form a non-toxic end-product. And how many farmers would use it correctly? (Lane, 1970; Womack, 1971). The filling of eggs with highly toxic pesticides as bait for vermin (Kelsey, 1971) is a habit greatly to be deprecated, as it produces a very real hazard to farm stock and household pets. The writers know of several cases in which dogs have been poisoned in this way. The selective herbicides 2,4-D and 2,3,5-T have usually been assumed to be relatively non-toxic. Certainly, all the controlled experiments carried out credit them with only mild toxicity (Milhaud and Riet Alvariza, 1970), though it is perhaps worth noting that Kutches, Church, and Duryee (1970), investigating the action of 12 pesticides on rumen flora, found 2,4,5-T to be most toxic. Recently Pinsent and Lane (1970) have described a case of poisoning in horses that may very well have been due to these compounds. There have also been persistent stories in the popular press about their teratogenic effects in man when used as defoliating agents in Vietnam, but the facts have been so distorted by the fog of war and the miasma of propaganda that it is difficult to make any critical assessment of their value. The toxicity of paraquat has been highlighted by several cases of poisoning in man, but the 'fibrosing pneumonitis' recorded is not found in all species. It occurs in pigs and guinea-pigs, but hamsters and sheep show pulmonary congestion and oedema (Smalley and Radeleff, 1970).

The acrid smell of 'burning fat' is familiar to everyone, but the toxicity of acrolein, the compound responsible for it, is not so well known, although it was in fact used as a war gas ('Papite') in 1916; and accidental cases of poisoning in man have been reported (von Oettingen, 1958). We have recently heard of a case in a dog (Stuckey, 1971). A poodle was shut up for half an hour in a small unventilated kitchen with a chip-pan of boiling fat. When seen next day it had a temperature of 103° F. with swollen tonsils and blood from the nostrils. The eyes and breathing were normal. Twenty-four hours later there was slight dyspnoea, the pulse faint and the tongue cyanosed, the eyes congested and discharging pus. It collapsed and died shortly afterwards.

Banerjee, Miller, and Stowe (1969) found that amidopyrine caused excitement, incoordination, and muscular weakness in cattle, and they make the interesting suggestion that the toxicity is due to the formaldehyde liberated as the drug is metabolized. The damage done by aspirin to gastric mucosa is well known but Brodie, Tate, and Hooke (1970) have shown by experiments in rats that the intestinal mucosa is also damaged, although in this case it is the animal which has been fed that is more susceptible than the fasting animal; with the gastric mucosa the opposite is true. A new syndrome in cats, characterized by loss of balance, weakness, intermittent blindness, and a change of temperament—the animals becoming so savage that they cannot be examined—has recently been described (Brockis and others, 1970; Kydd, Boswood, and Watts, 1970). Various suggestions have been put forward as to its cause. In a case recorded by White and Vonesch (1970), zinc phosphide was found in the body of a cat that died. Stopforth (1970) noted a sudden change in temperament in a kitten that had eaten alphachloralose. Bedford and Clarke (1971a), however, consider that the cause is benzoic acid used as a food preservative. In a case in which 17 cats in a cattery died after showing typical symptoms, no less than 2·38 per cent of this compound was found in the pet food which they had eaten. The condition has since been produced experimentally (Bedford and Clarke, 1971b). A single meal containing 1 per cent of benzoic acid may be fatal, or 0·5 per cent fed repeatedly. This emphasizes the importance of thorough mixing of any additive substance. Tutt (1970) records 2 cases in which domestic animals were poisoned by carbon monoxide in fumes given off by stoves burning solid fuel in inadequate draught. A cat which eventually recovered was blind and deaf for 3 weeks. A dog had a concentration of 15 per cent of CO in the blood. Wray and

Mathieson (1970) record the death of 4 calves after receiving a mixture of glucose and milk substitute in a ratio of 2 : 1. They showed depression and diarrhoea with very fluid faeces; 0·5 per cent of glucose was found in the urine. The toxic effect is probably caused by the hypertonic solution in the intestine.

As motoring increases, so does the use of anti-freeze solution and accordingly poisoning by ethylene glycol. Durham and Sharman (1970) report 2 cases of dogs that drank the fluid drained from a car radiator and died in 26 and 32 hours after exhibiting ataxia, spasms, and coma. Oxalate crystals were found in cortical and medullary tubules. The kidneys of one contained 6·2 per cent of calcium oxalate on a dry-weight basis. In experimental poisoning in dogs, Dobos Kovács (1970) found that 5–10 ml. of ethylene glycol was fatal in 36 hours. Crystals of calcium oxalate were found in the walls of the cerebral vessels as well as in the renal tubules. Berg and others (1971) performed a kidney transfer on an Alsatian which had drunk almost a quart of anti-freeze. The dog appeared to improve, but died on the eleventh day of generalized mycotic infection. Beckett and Shields (1971) have successfully treated dogs experimentally poisoned with glycol with intraperitoneal injections of ethanol and sodium bicarbonate, a 20 per cent solution of the former and 5 per cent of the latter, the amount injected being equivalent to 1·1 ml. of ethanol and 0·44 g. of bicarbonate. The treatment was repeated six times at 6-hour intervals. Out of 10 dogs that had ingested 4·4 g. of glycol per kg. of body-weight only 1 died, whereas none of the untreated control dogs survived.

Baird, Hutchins, and Lepherd (1970) report a case of poisoning in a horse which showed depression, anorexia, weakness, and haemoglobinuria after being dosed with 30 g. of micronized phenothiazine, although 8 other horses receiving a similar dose showed no clinical illness. It made a slow recovery after receiving blood transfusion, fluids, antibiotics, and corticosteroids. A horse that had eaten oats mixed with 0·025 per cent of strychnine died in convulsions after 2 hours. A second horse recovered after treatment with sodium pentobarbitone (Meek and Keatts, 1971). Fountain (1970) recommends the use of methocarbamol for the treatment of strychnine poisoning in dogs. The solution is rapidly injected intravenously until muscle spasms no longer occur in answer to stimuli. The average dose used is 67 mg. per lb., followed, if the convulsions recur, by a second dose of 41 mg. per lb. an hour or so later.

Poisonous Plants

Camp (1970) considers that the effects of the sympathomimetic amines *N*-methyltyramine and *N*-methyl-*beta*-phenethylamine, present in *Acacia berlandieri* (guajillo), a bush responsible for 'limberleg' among sheep and goats in periods of drought in Texas, can be largely counteracted by dietary factors capable of maintaining the detoxicating mechanisms of the rumen flora and the liver. Basson and others (1970) have described an outbreak of poisoning in cattle by *Albizia tanganyicensis* and record feeding experiments on sheep with this plant. The chief characteristics, which develop in a few hours, are hyperthermia (temperature 109–111° F.), hypersensitivity, convulsions, and dyspnoea. The toxic principle is unknown, and is evidently different from that of *A. stipulata* (syn. *A. chinensis*) which after several weeks caused grunting, spasmodic bleats, icteric conjunctivitis, and blood-stained faeces in rams (Sharma, Chander, and Negi, 1969). Wild onion (*Allium validum*), a plant which abounds on some western ranges in America, gave rise to haemoglobinuria and mild icterus in sheep. The toxic principle is *n*-propyl disulphide (Van Kampen, James, and Johnson, 1970). Rowe, Ohlenbusch, and Dollahite (1970) have found that 0·5 per cent of body-weight of *Asclepias brachystephana* is lethal to sheep. James, Van Kampen, and Johnson (1970) fed *Astragalus lentiginosus* and other 'locoweeds' to sheep, cattle, and horses and noted depression, stiffness, anorexia, and loss of body-weight. They describe the physiopathologic changes caused. James and Van Kampen (1971) note that in horses fed *A. lentiginosus* the renal lesions disappear rapidly but that the damage to Purkinje's cells of the cerebellum persists for a considerable time. Horses that have suffered from locoweed poisoning are unsuitable for draught or riding owing to their unpredictable behaviour, but mares can be used for breeding. On incubation in ruminal fluid miserotoxin, the active factor in timber milk vetch (*A. miser*), is metabolized to 3-nitro-1-propanol (Williams, Norris, and Van Kampen, 1970). Rosca and Pavel (1969) record that sedges of the *Carex* spp., which were found to contain 1140–1580 p.p.m. of HCN, affected 90 per cent of the cattle feeding on them, between 6 and 18 per cent having to be destroyed.

Yellow star thistle (*Centaurea solstitialis*) is well known to cause nigro-pallidal encephalomalacia in horses, and it has recently been shown that Russian knapweed (*C. picris*) has the same effect (Larson and Young, 1970). The condition has been produced experimentally. *C. picris* appears to be the more toxic of the two plants (Young, Brown, and Klinger, 1970). Rams bedded on wood shavings, probably of *Entandrophragma utile*, a member of the Meliceae (mahogany) family, developed balanoposthitis with inflammation of the preputial mucosa and the glans penis. They returned to normal after bedding on straw (Jackson, 1969). Calves bedded on wood shavings (species not stated) or peat developed hypomagnesaemia (Ivins and Allcroft, 1970).

Mouldy sweet potatoes (*Ipomoea batatas*), which had caused fatal poisoning in cattle, were found to contain three toxins. Somewhat alarmingly, these were all found in sweet potatoes with slight blemishes offered for sale for human consumption (Wilson, Yang, and Boyd, 1970).

James and Johnson (1970) found that calcium chloride was effective in preventing poisoning in sheep by *Halogeton glomeratus*; even when given 4 hours later, 50 per cent of the sheep recovered. Slow introduction to halogeton, in order to allow time for the rumen flora to become habituated, and avoidance of the plant at times of stress were also important. Poisoning occurs most widely when sheep are watered and then allowed to graze the plant (James, Butcher, and Van Kampen, 1970). Cattle which had consumed halogeton showed stiffness and recumbency after being driven. Convulsions and haematuria were also observed in calves (James, 1970). Lanigan and Whittem (1970) found that cobalt pellets were of no value in reducing morbidity or mortality due to *Heliotropium europaeum*. Jago (1970) considers that the lesions caused in the livers of young rats can be used as a means of assessment of the hepatotoxicity of the pyrrolizidine alkaloids. The metabolism of these compounds in the rumen of sheep has been described by Lanigan (1970) and Lanigan and Smith (1970). Charlton and Pierce (1969) have described the lesions in the peripheral nerves of goats poisoned with coyotillo (*Karwinskia humboldtiana*).

Poisoning by laburnum (*Laburnum anagyroides*) in farm stock is well known, but does not appear to have been noted previously in the dog. Clarke, Clarke, and King (1971) record a case in which a fox terrier died an hour after chewing the bark of a laburnum branch with which it had been playing. Symptoms were vomiting, incoordination, and mild epileptiform convulsions. Cytisine was found in the stomach, liver, and kidney. Calves poisoned by ganskweek (*Lasiospermum bipinnatum*) showed abdominal pain and photosensitivity. Necrosis of the liver was found post mortem (Fair, Tustin, and Adelaar, 1970).

It looks as if, after nearly a century, the lupinosis problem has been solved at last. Van Warmelo and others (1970) have produced the condition in sheep fed a pure culture of the fungus *Phomopsis leptostromiformis* isolated from the pods and seeds of *Lupinus albus* plants which had caused a severe outbreak in South Africa. They note the similarity of the lesions to those of aflatoxicosis, but show that the hepatotoxin elaborated by the fungus is not aflatoxin. It has not as yet been characterized, although Petterson and Parr (1970) have shown that a similar substance, isolated from lupin roughage, is non-alkaloidal, and contains phenolic and acidic groups. Peterson and Butler (1971) have shown that the selenium in *Morinda reticulata* is present as the amino-acid selenocystothionine. Horses that had eaten Iceland poppies (*Papaver nudicaule*) showed ataxia and convulsions, but recovered (de Malmanche, 1970). Calves and sheep fed with fresh leaves and roots of *Phytolacca dodecandra* died in 4–5 days after showing salivation, muscular spasms, coughing, and blood-stained diarrhoea (Mugera, 1970).

Cattle fed with desert rice flower (*Pimelea simplex*) developed a syndrome indistinguishable from St. George disease, with typical liver lesions (McClure and Farrow, 1971; Roberts and Healy, 1971). A similar syndrome was caused by the forced inhalation of the dried plant *P. trichostachya* (Clark, 1971). The leaves of *P. decora* proved highly toxic to horses at 440–1000 mg. per kg. of body-weight, being lethal within 24 hours. Luckily the plant is unpalatable. The toxin has an acute necrotizing effect on the intestinal mucosa and gives rise to haemorrhage in the intestines, kidney, and spleen (Hill, 1970). A labrador puppy died after eating leaves from a choke-cherry (*Prunus virginiana*) overhanging its run. The stomach was full of leaves and smelt of bitter almonds; the tree contains a cyanogenetic glycoside (Stauffer, 1970).

Gregorović and others (1970) state that the haematuria in cattle caused by bracken (*Pteridium aquilinum*) may be controlled by applying fertilizers to the pastures, and by feeding hay for 3 weeks out of every 6. Both antihaemopoietic and carcinogenic factors in bracken are subject to seasonal and regional variation (Schacham, Philp, and Gowdey, 1970). Pamukcu and others (1970) describe a method for concentrating the carcinogenic factor by solvent fractionation. The condition known as 'bright blindness' in sheep has been produced experimentally by feeding with dry bracken (Barnett and Watson, 1970). Jones, Seawright, and Little (1970) and Seawright, Groenendyk, and Silva (1970) have described an outbreak of oxalate poisoning in cattle due to the tropical grass *Setaria sphacelata*, which was found to contain 6–9 per cent of oxalate. Hunger and high-feed requirement were probably contributory factors. It is suggested that three different syndromes may follow the ingestion of oxalate by ruminants. First, an acute syndrome due to hypocalcaemia; secondly, a less acute syndrome in which damage to vascular tissues in alimentary tract and lungs caused by oxalate ions is followed by microbial invasion; and, thirdly, a chronic syndrome caused by progressive deposition of calcium oxalate crystals in the kidneys (James, Seawright, and Steele, 1971).

Solanum malacoxylon, which gives rise to the form of bovine arteriosclerosis known as 'enterque seco' in South America, has been shown to produce gross evidence of calcification of the aorta, cardiac muscle, and intercostal muscles in guinea-pigs (Camberos and others, 1970). *S. sodomaeum*, which grows in areas in Hawaii where bovine arteriosclerosis is endemic, has been found to be highly toxic to chicks and quail (Ross and Furumoto, 1970). The embryo mortality observed when quail are dosed with *Sterculi foetida* oil is due to the increased ratio of saturated fatty acids and not to the cyclopropenoid compounds in the oil (Donaldson and Fites, 1970). Cattle clinically affected by the ingestion of *Swainsona galeyifolia* were found to have up to 50 per cent of vacuolated lymphocytes, a finding which may be of considerable diagnostic value in cases of *Swainsona* poisoning (Huxtable and Gibson, 1970). Meyer (1970) has noted lactation in rams grazing subterranean clover (*Trifolium subterraneum*), although their fertility was not impaired. Cyclopamine from *Veratrum californicum* produced cyclopian deformities in the offspring of rabbits if given between the sixth and ninth days of pregnancy (Keeler, 1970). Horváth and Modor (1970) record heavy losses in pigs grazing *Xanthium italicum*; 15 g. per kg. of the plant, or 1·5 g. per kg. of the seed, produced a 100 per cent mortality.

REFERENCES

ABELSON, P. H. (1970), *Science, N.Y.*, **169**, 237.
BÄCKSTRÖM, J. (1969), *Acta pharmac. tox.*, **27**, Suppl. 3, 103.
BAIRD, J. D., HUTCHINS, D. R., and LEPHERD, E. E. (1970), *Aust. vet. J.*, **46**, 496.
BANERJEE, N. C., MILLER, G. E., and STOWE, C. M. (1969), *Indian vet. J.*, **46**, 1055.
BARNETT, K. C., and WATSON, W. A. (1970), *Res. vet. Sci.*, **11**, 289.
BASSON, P. A., ADELAAR, T. F., NAUDE, T. W., and MINNE, J. A. (1970), *Jl S. Afr. vet. med. Ass.*, **41**, 117.
BECKETT, S. D., and SHIELDS, R. P. (1971), *J. Am. vet. med. Ass.*, **158**, 472.
BEDFORD, P., and CLARKE, E. G. C. (1971a), *Vet. Rec.*, **88**, 599.
— — — — (1971b), *Ibid.*, in the press.
BERG, P., NUNAMAKER, D., AMAND, W., HARVEY, C., and KLIDE, A. (1971), *J. Am. vet. med. Ass.*, **158**, 468.
BJERK, J. E., and SUNDBY, R. (1970), *Norsk. VetTidsskr.*, **5**, 241.
BORG, K., ERNE, K., HANKO, E., and WANNTORP, H. (1970), *Envir. Pollution*, **1**, 91.
BROCKIS, D., JONES, R. J., PARKER, R. M., and GILL, A. R. (1970), *Vet. Rec.*, **87**, 638.
BRODIE, D. A., TATE, C. L., and HOOKE, K. F. (1970), *Science, N.Y.*, **170**, 183.
BUCK, W. B. (1970), *J. Am. vet. med. Ass.*, **156**, 1468.
CABADAJ, R., and GDOVIN, T. (1970), *Vet. Med., Praha*, **15**, 21.
CAMBEROS, H. R., DAVIS, G. K., DJAFAR, M. I., and SIMPSON, C. F. (1970), *Am. J. vet. Res.*, **31**, 685.
CAMP, B. J. (1970), *Ibid.*, **31**, 755.
CARAVAGGI, C., CLARK, F. L., and JACKSON, A. R. B. (1970), *Res. vet. Sci.*, **11**, 501.
CHARLTON, K. M., and PIERCE, K. R. (1969), *Tex. Rep. Biol. Med.*, **27**, 389.
CHOW, T. J., and EARL, J. L. (1970), *Science, N.Y.*, **169**, 577.
CHRISTIAN, R. G., and TRYPHONAS, L. (1971), *Am. J. vet. Res.*, **32**, 203.
CLARK, I. A. (1971), *Aust. vet. J.*, **47**, 123.
CLARKE, M. L., CLARKE, E. G. C., and KING, T. (1971), *Vet. Rec.*, **88**, 199.
COX, J. L. (1970), *Science, N.Y.*, **170**, 71.
CRISTEA, I., DULFU, R., MARIAN, P., and DULFU, V. (1970), *Recl. Méd. Vét.*, **146**, 783.

Dobos Kovács, M. (1970), *Magy. Allatorv. Lap.*, **25**, 472.
Dollahite, J. W., and Holt, E. C. (1969), *SWest. Vet.*, **23**, 23.
Donaldson, W. E., and Fites, B. L. (1970), *J. Nutr.*, **100**, 605.
Durham, P. J. K., and Sharman, J. R. (1970), *N.Z. vet. J.*, **18**, 55.
Fair, A. E., Tustin, R. C., and Adelaar, T. F. (1970), *Jl S. Afr. vet. med. Ass.*, **41**, 231.
Fountain, J. E. (1970), *Vet. Med., small Anim. Clin.*, **65**, 718.
Fox, M. R. S., and Fry, B. E. (1970), *Science, N.Y.*, **169**, 989.
Gabbedy, B. J. (1970), *Aust. vet. J.*, **46**, 223.
Giddens, W. E., Whitehair, C. K., and Sleight, S. D. (1970), *Am. J. vet. Res.*, **31**, 1779.
Gregorović, V., Jazbec, I., Šenk, L., and Skušek, I. (1970), *Zborn. bioteh. Fak. Univ. Ljubljana*, **7**, 5.
Halverson, A. W., Tsay, D.-T., Triebwasser, K. C., and Whitehead, E. I. (1970), *Toxicol. appl. Pharmac.*, **17**, 151.
Hanko, E., Erne, K., Wanntorp, H., and Borg, K. (1970), *Acta vet. scand.*, **11**, 268.
Harrison, D. L., Mol, J. C. M., and Healy, W. B. (1970), *N.Z. Jl agric. Res.*, **13**, 664.
Hill, M. W. M. (1970), *Aust. vet. J.*, **46**, 287.
Horváth, Z., and Modor, V. (1970), *Magy. Allatorv. Lap.*, **25**, 349.
Houser, W. D., and Frank, N. (1970), *J. Am. vet. med. Ass.*, **157**, 1919.
Huxtable, C. R., and Gibson, A. (1970), *Aust. vet. J.*, **46**, 446.
Ivins, L. N., and Allcroft, R. (1970), *Br. vet. J.*, **126**, 505.
Jackson, G. (1969), *Ibid.*, **125**, i.
Jago, M. V. (1970), *Aust. J. exp. Biol. med. Sci.*, **48**, 93.
James, L. F. (1970), *J. Am. vet. med. Ass.*, **156**, 1310.
— — Butcher, J. E., and Van Kampen, K. R. (1970), *J. Range Mgmt*, **23**, 123.
— — and Johnson, A. E. (1970), *J. Am. vet. med. Ass.*, **157**, 437.
— — and Van Kampen, K. R. (1971), *Ibid.* **158**, 614.
— — — — and Johnson, A. E. (1970), *Am. J. vet. Res.*, **31**, 663.
James, M. P., Seawright, A. A., and Steele, D. P. (1971), *Aust. vet. J.*, **47**, 9.
Jara, Z. (1970), *Medcyna. wet.*, **26**, 131.
Jones, R. J., Seawright, A. A., and Little, D. A. (1970), *J. Aust. Inst. agric. Sci.*, **36**, 41.
Keeler, R. F. (1970), *Teratology*, **3**, 169.
Kelsey, F. H. (1971), *Vet. Rec.*, **88**, 136.
Kitto, H. W. (1970), *Ibid.*, **87**, 73.
Kloke, A., and Leh, H.-O. (1969), *Proceedings of 1st European Congress on the Influence of Air Pollution on Plants and Animals, Wageningen, 1968*, p. 259. Berlin: Bundesanstalt für Land- und Fortswirtschaft.
Kutches, A. J., Church, D. C., and Duryee, F. L. (1970), *J. agric. Fd Chem.*, **18**, 430.
Kydd, A. M., Boswood, B., and Watts, A. E. (1970), *Vet. Rec.*, **87**, 518.
Labadie, M., Nicolas, A., Breton, J.-C., and Pestre-Alexandre, M. (1970), *Revue Méd. vét.*, **121**, 885.
Lane, P. J. (1970), *Vet. Rec.*, **87**, 812.
Lanigan, G. W. (1970), *Aust. J. agric. Res.*, **21**, 633.
— — and Smith, L. W. (1970), *Ibid.*, **21**, 493.
— — and Whittem, J. H. (1970), *Aust. vet. J.*, **46**, 17.
Larson, K. A., and Young, S. (1970), *J. Am. vet. med. Ass.*, **156**, 626.
Liska, B. J., and Stadelman, W. J. (1969), *Residue Rev.*, **29**, 51.
Lüke, F., and Wiemann, H. (1970), *Berl. Münch. tierärztl. Wschr.*, **83**, 253.
McClure, T. J., and Farrow, B. R. H. (1971), *Aust. vet. J.*, **47**, 100.
de Malmanche, I. (1970), *N.Z. vet. J.*, **18**, 96.
Meek, D. G., and Keatts, W. H. (1971), *J. Am. vet. med. Ass.*, **158**, 491.
Menges, R. W., Kintner, L. D., Selby, L. A., Stewart, R. W., and Marienfeld, C. J. (1970), *Vet. Med., small Anim. Clin.*, **65**, 565.
Meyer, E. P. (1970), *Aust. vet. J.*, **46**, 305.
Milhaud, G., and Riet Alvariza, F. (1970), *Recl. Méd. vét.*, **146**, 345.
Mugera, G. M. (1970), *Bull. épizoot. Dis. Afr.*, **18**, 41.
Mustaffa-Babjee, A., Lee Chin Hua, and Nazarddin, M. S. (1970), *Malay. Agric. J.*, **47**, 309.
von Oettingen, W. F. (1958), *Poisoning*. Philadelphia: Saunders.

OLSEN, P. (1969), *Acta vet. scand.*, **10**, 288.
ÖSTLUND, K. (1969), *Acta pharmac. tox.*, **27**, Suppl. 1, p. 132.
PAMUKCU, A. M., PRICE, J. M., and BRYAN, G. T. (1970), *Cancer Res.*, **30**, 902.
PETERSON, P. J., and BUTLER, G. W. (1971), *Aust. J. biol. Sci.*, **24**, 175.
PETTERSON, D. S., and PARR, W. H. (1970), *Res. vet. Sci.*, **11**, 282.
PINSENT, P. J. N., and LANE, J. G. (1970), *Vet. Rec.*, **87**, 247.
PIPER, R. C., MILLER, V. L., and DICKINSON, E. O. (1971), *Am. J. vet. Res.*, **32**, 263.
PLATONOW, N. S., and FUNNELL, H. S. (1970), *Vet. Rec.*, **87**, 786.
PRESTT, I., JEFFERIES, D. J., and MOORE, N. W. (1970), *Envir. Pollution*, **1**, 3.
ROBERTS, H. B., and HEALY, P. J. (1971), *Aust. vet. J.*, **47**, 123.
ROBISON, W. H. (1970), *J. Wildl. Mgmt*, **34**, 647.
ROSCA, V., and PAVEL, A. (1969), *Revtă Med. vet. Zootech.*, **19**, 81.
ROSS, D. B. (1970), *Res. vet. Sci.*, **11**, 295.
ROSS, E., and FURUMOTO, H. H. (1970), *Poult. Sci.*, **49**, 13.
ROWE, L. D., OHLENBUSCH, P. D., and DOLLAHITE, J. W. (1970), *SWest Vet.*, **23**, 219.
RÜSSEL, H. A. (1970), *Bull. envir. Contam. Toxic.*, **5**, 115.
RYBOLT, D. (1970), *Iowa St. Univ. Vet.*, **32**, 4.
SCHACHAM, P., PHILP, R. B., and GOWDEY, C. W. (1970), *Am. J. vet. Res.*, **31**, 191.
SEAWRIGHT, A. A., GROENENDYK, S., and SILVA, K. I. N. G. (1970), *Aust. vet. J.*, **46**, 293.
SELYE, H. (1970), *Science, N.Y.*, **169**, 775.
SHARMA, D. D., CHANDER, S., and NEGI, S. S. (1969), *J. Res., Ludhiana*, **6**, 388.
SINCLAIR, D. (1970), *Vet. Rec.*, **87**, 764.
SMALLEY, H. E., and RADELEFF, R. D. (1970), *Toxic. appl. Pharmac.*, **17**, 305.
STAUFFER, V. D. (1970), *J. Am. vet. med. Ass.*, **157**, 1324.
STOPFORTH, A. (1970), *Vet. Rec.*, **87**, 788.
STUCKEY, G. M. (1971), personal communication.
TAIT, R. M., KRISHNAMURTI, C. R., GILCHRIST, E. W., and MACDONALD, K. (1971), *Can. vet. J.*, **12**, 73.
TESINK, J. (1969), *Proceedings of 1st European Congress on the Influence of Air Pollution on Plants and Animals, Wageningen, 1968*, p. 281. Berlin: Bundesanstalt für Land- und Fortswirtschaft.
TUTT, J. B. (1970), *Vet. Rec.*, **87**, 107.
VAN KAMPEN, K. R., JAMES, L. F., and JOHNSON, A. E. (1970), *J. Am. vet. med. Ass.*, **156**, 328.
— — — — RASMUSSEN, J., HUFFAKER, R. H., and FAWCETT, M.O. (1969), *Ibid.*, **154**, 623.
— — SHUPE, J. L., JOHNSON, A. E., JAMES, L. F., SMART, R. A., and RASSMUSSEN, J. E. (1970), *Ibid.*, **156**, 1032.
VAN WARMELO, K. T., MARASAS, W. F., ADELAAR, T. F., KELLERMAN, T. S., VAN RENSBURG, I. B. J., and MINNE, J. A. (1970), *Jl S. Afr. vet. med. Ass.*, **41**, 235.
VERWEY, J. H. P. (1969), *Proceedings of 1st European Congress on the Influence of Air Pollution on Plants and Animals, Wageningen, 1968*, p. 269. Berlin: Bundesanstalt für Land- und Fortswirtschaft.
VOS, J. G., and KOEMAN, J. H. (1970), *Toxic. appl. Pharmac.*, **17**, 656.
WHITE, R. C., and VONESCH, R. J. K. (1970), *Vet. Rec.*, **87**, 731.
WILLIAMS, M. C., NORRIS, F. A., and VAN KAMPEN, K. R. (1970), *Am. J. vet. Res.*, **31**, 259.
WILSON, B. J., YANG, D. T. C., and BOYD, M. R. (1970), *Nature, Lond.*, **227**, 521.
WOMACK, H. D. H. (1971), *Vet. Rec.*, **88**, 200.
WRAY, C., and MATHIESON, A. O. (1970), *Ibid.*, **87**, 797.
YOUNG, S., BROWN, W. W., and KLINGER, B. (1970), *Am. J. vet. Res.*, **31**, 1393.
ZOOK, B. C., SAYER, R. M., and GARNER, F. M. (1971), *J. Am. vet. med. Ass.*, **157**, 691.

LEGAL DECISIONS AND LEGISLATION

A. R. W. Porter, M.A., Barrister-at-Law

LEGAL DECISIONS AND LEGISLATION

A. R. W. Porter, M.A., Barrister-at-Law

LEGISLATION

The Animals Act, 1971.—This Act, which does not apply in Scotland or Northern Ireland, gives broad effect to the recommendations of the Law Commission's report on Civil Liability for Animals. It replaces by statutory provisions the common law rules relating to liability for cattle trespass and provides for the detention and sale of trespassing livestock under stated circumstances. The old common law rules relating to damage caused by dangerous animals are also replaced. Fresh provision is made for liability caused by dogs to cattle or poultry, and for the protection of livestock against dogs. The former common law rule (which was much criticized), excluding or restricting a person's duty to take care to avoid damage being caused by animals straying on the highway, is abrogated. The Act came into force on 1 Oct., 1971.

The Brucellosis (*Eradication Areas*) (*England and Wales*) *Order*, 1971, *and the Brucellosis* (*Eradication Areas*) (*Scotland*) *Order*, 1971.—These Orders, which came into operation on 1 April, 1971, establish areas in which a start is being made on the eradication of brucellosis from Great Britain. Such areas are delineated in North-west England, in Scotland, and in Wales, and certain islands including the Shetlands, the Uists, and the Isle of Wight are also named as eradication areas. The Orders prohibit the vaccination of cattle against brucellosis in any eradication area, unless the vaccination is carried out by an officer of the Minister of Agriculture, Fisheries, and Food, or a person acting on the Minister's behalf *or* the vaccination is carried out under licence and in strict accordance with the terms and conditions thereof.

The Diseases of Animals (*Approved Disinfectants*) *Order*, 1970, sets out in the Schedule lists of disinfectants approved by the Minister and the Secretary of State in relation to orders under the Diseases of Animals Act, 1950, dealing with foot-and-mouth disease, fowl pest, and tuberculosis and other orders under that Act which require the use of an approved disinfectant. The rate at which an approved disinfectant is to be diluted with water in general circumstances is also specified. The Order came into force on 17 Sept., 1970.

The Misuse of Drugs Act, 1971, will, when fully operative, replace the Dangerous Drugs Acts of 1965 and 1967 and the Drugs (Prevention of Misuse) Act, 1964, with new and more extensive provisions for controlling drugs. The Act provides for the establishment, functions, and procedure of a new advisory body to be known as the 'Advisory Council on the Misuse of Drugs'. The Council has the duty of keeping under review the situation in the United Kingdom with respect to drugs which are being or appear likely to be misused in such a way as to constitute a social problem, and to advise the appropriate Ministers on the action which should therefore be taken. The Act also provides for the classification of drugs according to their relative harmfulness, and the control of their import, export, production, sale, supply, and use.

Section 13 of the Act provides that if any doctor, dentist, or veterinarian has been prescribing, administering, or supplying controlled drugs 'in an irresponsible manner' the Secretary of State may give a direction prohibiting the offender from prescribing, administering, or supplying such drugs as may be prescribed in the direction. The term 'in an irresponsible manner' is not defined, and would seem more apt (in the context of the intention of the Act) in relation to the practice of human than veterinary medicine. However, machinery is provided by Sections 14 and 15 of the Act whereby consideration can be given to whether the veterinary surgeon, for instance, can be said to have been prescribing, etc., in an irresponsible manner. The Secretary of State is empowered:—

1. Either to refer the matter for advice under Section 14 (1) to a tribunal consisting of a legally qualified chairman and four members of the veterinary profession;

2. Or in cases where urgent action is necessary, to take advice under Section 15 (1) from a panel consisting of a chairman and two other members of the veterinary profession with a view to making an interim order before the matter is referred to the tribunal mentioned above.

In either case the tribunal or panel will advise the Secretary of State as to whether there has been any prescription, administration, or supply of controlled drugs in an irresponsible manner and whether the evidence would justify the making of an appropriate direction against the offender. The Act will come into operation on such day as may be appointed and different operative days may be appointed for different parts.

The Slaughter of Poultry (*Humane Conditions*) *Regulations*, 1971, came into operation on 1 Aug., 1971. They relate to turkeys and domestic fowls. The main provisions are that poultry awaiting slaughter must not be subjected to unnecessary pain or distress, must be slaughtered as soon as practicable, and must be provided with adequate ventilation and with protection from sun and adverse weather. Maximum periods are prescribed beyond which birds may not be suspended head downwards before slaughter or stunning with an instrument of an approved kind. Provision is also made for minimum periods which must elapse before birds are immersed in a scalding tank or plucked after slaughter by cutting the neck.

The Therapeutic Substances (*Supply of Antibiotics and Chemotherapeutic Substances for Agricultural Purposes*) *Regulations*, 1971, and *The Therapeutic Substances* (*Control of Sale and Supply*) (*No.* 2) *Regulations*, 1971.—These two sets of Regulations, which came into operation partly in March, 1971, and partly on 1 Sept., 1971, implement certain of the recommendations of the Swann Committee which reported on the use of antibiotics in animal husbandry and veterinary medicine. The Swann Committee recommended, and the Government accepted, that in agriculture there should be two groups of antibiotics: (1) Therapeutic antibiotics, for use on veterinary advice for the treatment of particular disease conditions; (2) Feed antibiotics, for use at low levels in animal feedingstuffs. Included in group (1) by virtue of the Regulations are penicillin, chlortetracycline, oxytetracycline, tylosin, nitrofurazone, furazolidone, introfurantoin, and furaltadone. These antibiotics may only be sold or supplied on the prescription or written direction of a veterinarian. The sulphonamides are also included in group (1) except that sulphaquinoxaline and sulphanitran continue to be available as coccidiostats without prescription. It is not, however, possible to use sulphaquinoxaline at more than 75 p.p.m. except on prescription or on the written direction of a veterinarian. Sulphanilamide wound powder also continues to be available without prescription, provided the level of sulphanilamide does not exceed 5 per cent.

In group (2), subject to some restrictions on mixture rates, flavomycin and zinc bacitracin are available for pigs and poultry, and virginiamycin for poultry without a prescription or written direction.

Where a written direction is required from and is given by a veterinarian in terms of the Regulations he must give it, sign it, and date it personally, specify the quantity of the substance with which a stated quantity of animal feedingstuff or diluent is to be mixed, authorize the quantity of feedingstuff or diluent which may be sold or supplied after mixing to the client named in the direction, and state that the product is for administration to animals under the veterinarian's own care.

The Veterinary Surgery (*Exemption*) *Order*, 1970, permits lay persons, who meet certain requirements, to take blood from cattle for the purpose of the diagnosis of brucellosis. The requirement in relation to a person undergoing training in this technique is that he shall take blood only under the direct personal supervision of a registered veterinarian. In relation to a fully trained person it is required that he shall hold a certificate issued by or on behalf of the Minister of Agriculture, Fisheries, and Food, the Secretary of State for Scotland, and the Minister of Agriculture for Northern Ireland, certifying his proficiency in taking blood from cattle, and that he shall do so only while acting under the general direction of a registered veterinarian. Such certification follows a period of formal training and practical experience. The Order came into operation on 17 Sept., 1970.

The Weights and Measures (*Equivalents for dealing with Drugs*) *Regulations*, 1970.—These Regulations, which came into force on 1 Jan., 1971, re-enact with amendments the 1969 Regulations of the same name. Those Regulations prescribed, for the purpose of any dealings with drugs, equivalents between imperial and metric units of measurement and required, as from specified dates, that orders or prescriptions for the supply of drugs expressed in imperial units should be carried out in terms of the metric equivalent prescribed by the Regulations. The principal changes made by the new Regulations are:—

1. The provision of metric equivalents for dealings with larger quantities of ingredients of veterinary drugs than were provided for in the earlier Regulations.
2. A variation of the metric equivalents for dose quantities of prescriptions for liquid paraffin, fixed oils, and certain mixtures.
3. The exclusion from the ambit of the Regulations of dealings in drugs included in medicated animal feedingstuffs or medicated feed supplements.

Legal Decisions

Three cases of interest to veterinary surgeons have taken place during the past twelve months, two of them being reported in the Law Reports, and the other merely being noted in the press.

The first case was that of *Faridian* v. *General Medical Council* (1971), 1 *All E.R.* 144. Dr. Faridian was a registered medical practitioner who held shares in a company which managed a clinic. His shareholding was such that he had a controlling interest in the company. It was alleged that the company had advertised its services by sending letters to doctors in West Germany offering financial inducements to them to refer or introduce patients to the clinic, by sending £20 to a medical practitioner (who returned the money) for introducing a patient to the clinic, and by providing material for an article on the clinic in a newspaper. It was further alleged that the matron of the clinic had advertised its services on television.

Dr. Faridian was charged before the Disciplinary Committee of the General Medical Council with infamous conduct in a professional respect in that he had had controlling interest in the company owning the clinic, and that that company had advertised services connected with the practice of medicine. The General Medical Council found the allegations set out in the last paragraph to be proved, and on that basis found Dr. Faridian guilty of infamous conduct in a professional respect, and directed the Registrar to erase his name from the register. Dr. Faridian appealed to the Judicial Committee of the Privy Council, the question for decision being broadly whether his failure to exercise his power to control the activities of the company was, in the light of the proved facts, capable of amounting to infamous conduct in a professional respect.

The ruling of the Judicial Committee was that since there was no proof that Dr. Faridian had prior knowledge of what was done, or reason to suspect that it would be done, the fact that he had a controlling interest as a shareholder in a company which did these things was insufficient to render him guilty of infamous conduct. In delivering the Committee's judgment, Lord Dilhorne said:—

> In their Lordships' view it cannot be said that the appellant acted disgracefully or dishonourably in failing to exercise his power by virtue of his shareholding to control Langham Street Clinic Ltd. If there had been any evidence that he knew that the four acts complained of would be perpetrated by those engaged in running the clinic or had any reason to suspect that they might be, the position would be different.
>
> It may be said that a person so closely associated as the appellant was with the clinic at its inception, must do all in his power to prevent misconduct such as occurred in this case, and that, if he does not do so, he must have connived at or acquiesced in what was done and so is guilty of infamous conduct. But in this inquiry the appellant was not charged with acquiescing or conniving at what was done and there was no investigation as to what steps, if any, were taken by him to prevent malpractices. His failure to exercise the power he had when it was not shown that he had any prior knowledge of what was done or reason to suspect that it would be done is not, in their Lordships' opinion, capable of being held to be infamous conduct on his part.
>
> Their Lordships have therefore humbly advised Her Majesty that the appeal should be allowed.

The case has obvious relevance to veterinary ethics also, although a company may not in law itself practise veterinary surgery as such.

The second case is that of *Ashington Piggeries Ltd.* v. *Christopher Hill Ltd.* (1971), 1 *All E.R.* 847, which was heard in the House of Lords on appeal together with the case of *Christopher Hill Ltd.* v. *Norsildmel* in which the respondents claimed an indemnity from the suppliers of the herring meal which featured so prominently in this case. The facts were briefly as follows.

In 1960 the appellants asked the respondents, who were well-known animal feedingstuff compounders, if they would compound for them a mink food, called 'King Size', in accordance with a formula prepared by a Mr. Udall who controlled the appellant company. Mr. Udall was a leading mink farmer and an expert in mink nutrition. One of the ingredients included in the formula was herring meal. The respondents had a great deal of experience in compounding animal foods, but had never previously prepared food for mink. The respondents were expected to supply all the ingredients to the best quality available. Agreement was reached, the food was compounded, the mink ate it and all appeared to be well. However, in July, 1961, the first case was noticed of a new and hitherto unknown disease afflicting mink. A male kit was found with a grossly enlarged abdomen and died within a few days. Other cases followed, and it was realized that all the mink involved had been eating 'King Size'. The losses of mink were considerable.

Investigations revealed that the harm was being caused by the Norwegian herring meal which was the herring meal the respondents had recently started using in the production of 'King Size'. This herring meal was found to include dimethylnitrosamine (DMNA) which in certain quantities appeared to be toxic to mink. The presence of DMNA in the meal was unknown to the respondents and to their suppliers. It was produced by a chemical reaction caused by the use of sodium nitrate as a preservative—but this was a completely new discovery. There was no evidence as to the lethal dosage for other animals, but it was discovered that all animals were sensitive to DMNA, with sensitivity varying from species to species. Prior to 1960, it should be added, the use of herring meal as a mink food was unknown in the United Kingdom but it had been used in other countries including Norway.

Their Lordships held that the respondents were liable to the appellants, even although the appellants had provided the formula, and in spite of the fact that in the existing state of scientific and commercial knowledge no deliberate exercise of human skill or judgment could have prevented the meal from having its toxic and lethal effect on mink. The reasons for their Lordships' finding for the appellants were:—

1. Although the appellants relied on their own skill and judgment in making up the formula, they relied upon the skill and judgment of the respondents to see that the ingredients were of a quality suitable for compounding animal feeding stuffs.

2. The respondents would not have been liable if it could have been shown that the herring meal containing DMNA was toxic only to mink owing to some factor peculiar to mink, since the respondents' expertise was in the field of animal feed compounding generally and not in mink feedstuffs in particular. There was, however, evidence that all animals were sensitive to DMNA to some degree or another.

3. The respondents were in breach of section 14(1) of the Sale of Goods Act, 1893, which provides that:—

'Where the buyer, expressly or by implication, makes known to the seller the particular purpose for which the goods are required, so as to show that the buyer relies on the seller's skill or judgment, and the goods are of a description which it is in the course of the seller's business to supply . . . there is an implied condition that the goods shall be reasonably fit for such purpose. . . .'

4. The respondents (by a majority view) were also in breach of section 14(2) of the same Act which, so far as is material, provides that:—

'Where goods are bought by description from a seller who deals in goods of that description (whether he be the manufacturer or not) there is an implied condition that the goods shall be of merchantable quality. . . .'

The appellants were therefore able to recover damages from the respondents although they in turn were able to recover from the third party.

The third case which was heard in the Court of Appeal was not published in the Law Reports and appeared only in the press. Nevertheless, it is worth noting as being one of the first cases brought under the Trade Descriptions Act, 1968, in relation to an animal. Most people are aware that prosecutions may be brought under this Act in relation to a false trade description, but it is commonly believed that the Act applies only to shopkeepers, merchants selling other goods, travel agencies advertising holidays abroad, and the like. In fact, section 2 of the Act provides that, among the matters which can be the subject of a trade description, are, for example, fitness for purpose, strength, performance, behaviour or accuracy, and any other physical characteristics not covered by those terms. In relation to an animal it is specifically stated that a trade description can include any indication, direct or indirect, of the sex, breed or cross, fertility or soundness of the animal, and in relation to any semen, the identity and characteristics of the animal from which it was taken and the measure of dilution.

The animal concerned in the case in question was a puppy which was sold as a pedigree Sheltie, when in fact it was not. The dealers who had sold the dog sought to establish that they had taken 'all reasonable precautions and exercised all due diligence' to avoid giving a false description of the puppy. Had they been successful in establishing this, the dealers would have had a good defence by virtue of section 24(1)(b) of the Act. One of the facts which the dealers relied on to show that they had taken all reasonable precautions was that the puppy had been seen by a veterinary surgeon. It was made abundantly clear, however, that the veterinary surgeon had been asked only to inoculate the puppy and to examine its health state. There had been no request to the veterinarian to check the puppy's pedigree which would in any event have been exceedingly difficult to do from a visual examination. The fact that the veterinary surgeon did not say that the puppy was *not* a Sheltie but accepted this identification for the purpose of completing the inoculation certificate could not be relied upon as providing a defence for the dealers.

ANIMAL HUSBANDRY

T. K. Ewer, B.V.Sc., Ph.D., H.D.A., M.R.C.V.S.
Roger Ewbank, B.V.Sc., M.R.C.V.S.

ANIMAL HUSBANDRY

T. K. Ewer, B.V.Sc., Ph.D., H.D.A., M.R.C.V.S.

Grass Conservation

The importance of grassland in the animal production of this country is self-evident. Just how great a part it plays in the dairying, beef, and sheep industries varies according to location but its continuing importance is not in doubt. Grass, as Woodford (1971) has pointed out, occupies 73 per cent of the surface of mainland Britain and 50 per cent of the enclosed agricultural land of England and Wales. The factor that causes the biggest variation in the area down to grass is the price of cereals, itself related in the past to Government policy of price support for cereal production. The profit to be made from cereals now is not as high as it was some years ago and there are considerable problems arising from continuous cereal production in the east of the country in terms of soil structure. The combined effect is to turn many farmers' minds towards the use of the grass ley. High prices of imported cereals and oil meals are encouraging a greater dependence upon grassland for animal production. We must remember that land is being taken for forestry, urban development, and amenities of the order of 120,000 acres a year. On the other hand, it is possible by the clearing of heather and the drainage of some upland soils to increase grassland productivity as some offset to the loss of grassland.

The present division of grassland in the United Kingdom is thought to be: (1) rough grazing, 18 million acres; (2) temporary grassland, 12 million acres, consisting of 9 million short-rotation grassland and 3 million over 20 years old; (3) permanent grassland, 6 million acres.

The importance of hill pastures is clear enough. This is where two-thirds of all our sheep are to be found. Its productivity is low, often far too low. The Hill Farming Research Organisation (1969–70) has been able to show the degree of improvement in terms of animal output which many upland and hill grazing areas can be made to produce. For many years past there is no doubt that cows and sheep are kept on much of the hill country of Britain only because of the generous Government subsidies. There will be more co-ordinated planning in attempts to combine recreational and forestry use of the rough hill land, along with new methods of management to raise the productivity of the permanent pasture (or heather) in these areas. It is the remainder of our grassland, whether it is classified as temporary or permanent, that provides the overwhelmingly large part of the nutritional needs of dairy herds, the grassland beef and lamb that contribute 60 per cent of home-produced meat. All these animals are wholly dependent upon the value of spring and summer grazing and a sufficiency of high-quality conserved grass for the late autumn and winter feeding.

The problem in our uncertain climate is how the excess grass of the summer can be most appropriately conserved. In spite of the great efforts made by the Government advisory service, private industrial interests, and the many publications to show the value of silage as the most certain and economical way to conserve summer pastures, the proportion of grass put down to silage throughout the country only slowly increases. It would appear that hay still represents about 80 per cent of all fodder conserved. It was as interesting as it was unexpected to read (Copeman, 1971) that in Aberdeenshire there is now as much silage conserved as hay. Maybe this is a sign of things to come.

Formic Acid as Silage Additive

An interesting development in silage-making over the past two or three years has been the very rapid increase in popularity of formic acid as an additive. Henderson and MacDonald (1971) point out that formic acid used in this way is not new since it was first advocated by Dirks as early as 1926. In many European countries either formic acid alone or mixed with hydrochloric acid has been quite widely used and a comparison made with the mixture of mineral acids popular for many years in Scandinavian countries and known as the A.I.V. process. Two events have made the use of formic acid suddenly of great interest to farmers in this country; the first was the fact that B.P. Chemicals Group began marketing formic acid in this country in 1968 under the trade name 'Add-F' with appropriate advertising; the second was the availability of plastic containers for attaching directly to the forage harvester, thus making the actual process of adding the acid to the freshly cut grass relatively easy. 'Add-F' is in fact an 85 per cent formic acid solution which is recommended to be added to silage at the rate of 0·5 gal. per ton of fresh grass equivalent, to a concentration of 0·265 per cent.

The reasons for using this or any other additive to silage is to reduce the oxidation and loss of nutrients that occurs during the fermentation of the cut grass as soon as it is ensiled. The process continues until the organic acids, mainly lactic and acetic acids, lower the *p*H and virtually stop bacterial action. The longer this continues, the greater the likelihood of clostridial build-up and the production of butyric acid. Early in the season when the easily fermentable sugars are highest in the grass, the fermentation process is a very rapid one and there is no need to add anything. It is during the later parts of the spring and summer and in the autumn that the fermentation is slower and the adding of formic acid reduces the losses from oxidation. This is particularly marked if grass is not wilted before ensiling or if silage-making is undertaken in wet weather.

There are a number of laboratory and field experiments being published endeavouring to assess the usefulness of formic acid as an additive. Its cost at the present time is approximately 30p per ton of fresh grass. This is not expensive since if milk yields during the winter months were raised by more than 10 gal. per cow or if 1 cwt. of concentrates per cow could be saved then the use of an additive is justified. One of the most complete series of trials over the past 4 years has been conducted at the Hannah Dairy Research Institute, near Ayr (Watson, 1971). Here about 1500 tons of silage have been treated with formic acid and two feeding experiments have been conducted.

Experiment 1.—Two silages were made without the acid and two with the acid. All the herbage for the four experimental silages was cut from an old Timothy/perennial ryegrass ley. The silages were made in vacuum silos filled over a period of 2 days, 25 tons of grass in each and the air being evacuated immediately after filling. All the grass was cut directly with a forage harvester and alternate loads were either treated or not treated. The silages were made in June and in September with good weather for the first and dull, damp weather for the second lot of silage. When grasses were cut there was no difference in the grass dry-matter contents but there were consistent differences between the silages when they were fed. These can be seen in *Table I*.

The *p*H values and the lactic and butyric acid contents of the silages show that as a result of the acid there has been better fermentation in the grass with

Table I.—DETAILS OF FOUR SILAGES MADE EITHER WITH OR WITHOUT FORMIC ACID

DATE CUT (1968)	ADDITIVE	DRY MATTER (per cent)	*p*H	LACTIC ACID CONTENT (per cent)	BUTYRIC ACID CONTENT (per cent)	MAXIMUM TEMP. IN SILO (°F.)
4–5 June	Formic acid	22·0	3·8	2·45	0·04	64
	None	21·1	4·2	0·78	0·34	90
10–11 Sept.	Formic acid	20·1	3·7	3·30	0·05	62
	None	19·1	4·5	1·63	0·29	80

the acid added. Digestibilities of the acid silages were measured and were found to be slightly higher than those of the untreated silages.

During the winter the silages were fed to Ayrshire cows for a 16-week period with three feeds a day at amounts to leave no residues. In addition to the silage, moist barley was fed at the rate of 3·9 lb. per gallon of milk plus 1 lb. of groundnut cake to each cow daily. *Table II* shows that the intakes of silage dry matter were significantly better for the treated silage than for the untreated silage.

Table II.—SILAGE INTAKE, AVERAGE DAILY MILK YIELD, AND MILK COMPOSITION

TYPE OF SILAGE	INTAKE OF SILAGE DRY MATTER (lb. per cow per day)	MILK YIELD (lb. per cow per day)	MILK COMPOSITION (per cent)		
			Total Solids	Solids-not-fat	Crude Protein
June cut: +formic acid	18·8	36·3	13·08	8·60	3·10
June cut: no acid	16·8	33·8	12·92	8·50	3·00
Sept. cut: +formic acid	17·0	35·4	12·90	8·60	3·14
Sept. cut: no acid	15·3	34·1	12·83	8·50	3·04

It was suggested that the higher intakes were due to the better palatability, itself due to the higher lactic and lower butyric acid content of the treated silage. It was found that the mean daily milk yields of the cows eating the formic acid silages were significantly higher than with the untreated silages. This increase was 2·5 lb. per day with the June silage and 1·3 lb. per day with the September silage. There was virtually no effect of the treatment on the fat content of the milk but the percentages of the solids-not-fat and crude protein were significantly higher with the acid-treated silage. The additional cost of the formic acid and the extra silage eaten was about 2p per cow per day, but the returns in extra milk sales from the June and September silages were 5p and 2½p per cow per day respectively.

Experiment 2.—During the winter 1969–70 another experiment was conducted at the Hannah Institute to see if wilting could replace formic acid as an effective silage treatment. It was found that the formic acid silage was a good deal better than untreated silage, while the wilted silage, although rather more palatable than the untreated silage, was still not eaten in as large an amount as the formic acid-treated silage.

The testing of a new technique such as this is peculiarly appropriate for the experimental husbandry farms. They have indeed been testing this silage additive at three of the farms (Williams, 1971): at Greathouse and Drayton in 1967 and 1968, at both these farms, and at the Liscombe Experimental Husbandry Farm in the south-west in 1969. The method of testing was to cut all grass areas with a cutterbar mower to wilt the silage and then collect with a flail harvester, except at Drayton where a double-chop harvester was used. The period of wilting was 24 hours and the formic acid was applied to half the silage which varied in amount from 14 to 140 ton lots, at the rate of ½ gal. per ton of herbage in 1967 and 1968 and ¾ gal. per ton in 1969. Silages were all put into roofed bunker silos with concrete or wooden walls and care was taken to seal the silos as efficiently as possible after consolidation by using plastic sheets weighed down with straw bales. In other words, the controlled silages were of very high quality and likely to be very much better than the sort of silage that might be made by a farmer who, for whatever reason, does not wilt and conserve grass when it may be more mature than is desirable. Under such conditions it is likely that the addition of formic acid at the appropriate level will have a more pronounced effect than when it is used with wilted silage. The silages from these E.H.F. trials were fed in the main to fattening cattle, although at Greathouse Friesian dairy cows were fed both silages. In the latter case it was found that the formic acid-treated silage gave some 2 lb. (1 kg.) of milk extra per day over the winter period. They also maintained their weights more consistently on the treated silage than on the untreated, wilted silage. The most consistent feature of these trials was the higher digestibility of the silages treated with formic acid. The maximum improvement was found at Greathouse Experimental Husbandry Farm in 1967 where the treated, wilted silage contained about 9 per cent more digestible dry matter than the control. Nevertheless, the energy value of this improvement could have been supplied by less than 25 lb. (11·1 kg.) of barley, whereas the cost of applying a half to three-quarters of a gallon of formic acid per ton of silage was between 30–45p. Under these conditions of making excellent quality-controlled silage the direct financial benefit of an additive was nil.

The results from another series of experiments, on a small scale but under fully controlled conditions, have recently been published by Edinburgh workers (Henderson and MacDonald, 1971). They used grasses that were low in dry matter (11·8–17·3 per cent) and low in water-soluble sugars and high in nitrogen as a result of heavy fertilizer application. Formic acid was applied at the recommended rate of 0·22 per cent and at higher rates of 0·34 and 0·51 per cent. Very careful monitoring of chemical changes, effluent losses, and digestibility trials on the silages was undertaken. The conclusions arrived at were that the *p*H of treated silage was lower but effluent losses were higher. There was no improvement in the feeding value as a result of treatment, but the control silages were of high quality.

Perhaps the most active group studying quality and nutritional value of silages are workers at Hurley. Raymond (1971a) has pointed out that they have measured the voluntary intakes of about 90 different silages over recent years in feeding experiments. These were also analysed in the laboratory and calculations made of the possible relationships between their chemical compositions and the measured intakes. No single factor was found which seemed to account for the low intake of many silages. This reluctance of cattle and sheep to consume silages with relish was found over a wide range of silages, from those of low *p*H where the high acidity might be the main factor to those of high *p*H where there has been some breakdown in protein. It is difficult to decide what is likely to be an optimum *p*H for high intake. In so far as the addition of formic acid tends to lower the *p*H, this is not likely to result in greater palatability, although of course it will reduce protein breakdown, probably making the silages more attractive to animals.

Sterilization of Grass

The results with formic acid suggested to the Hurley workers that a stage further in the process of grass preservation might be the use of substances whose purpose would be virtually to prevent altogether the fermentation of freshly cut grass. The use of sodium metabisulphate some years ago had not proved effective, partly because it was difficult to mix evenly with the grass and also because there was difficulty in sealing the silo to exclude air. During 1970, Wilkins at Hurley has made some small quantities of 'silage' using formaldehyde and formaldehyde–formic acid mixtures. The preliminary results were very encouraging with losses being virtually eliminated and the animals readily eating the preserved grass during the winter. Larger field-scale trials will be made during 1971.

Another approach to the sterilizing of grass for preservation is the use of antibiotics. This is being studied by Edinburgh workers. The difficulty with such methods is the fact that when the 'silo' is opened for feeding-out the rate of moulding of the sterilized grass is likely to be at a high rate. In co-operation with the National Institute for Agricultural Engineering at Silsoe some novel types of storage and feeding-out equipment are being investigated.

Hay Additives

There have been a number of substances put on the market over the past few years designed to prevent moulding of hay in storage. These ('Hayguard' and 'Haysaver') have contained proprionic acid and formic acid and mixtures of both. Over the past three seasons a considerable number of trials of both commercial additives and various mixtures of acetic, formic, and proprionic acids have been tried (Badger, 1970). They have been conducted at five of the experimental husbandry farms. In the great majority of cases there has been no beneficial effect as a result of putting these substances into hay bales. The cost is not inconsiderable, adding around £3 per ton, but the effect has been either very small or negligible. There is difficulty in applying proprionic acid evenly. This is the most hopeful substance, but at present there does not seem to be a useful purpose in these substances being added to hay.

The Production of Dried Grass

Reference in previous VETERINARY ANNUALS (1969, 1970) to the increasing number of trials at research institutes and universities, concerned with how dried grass can be used, emphasizes how interest has mounted in the use of this material. As Raymond (1971b) points out, grass-drying is not new, but it is a fact that most of the large number of drying plants which operated at the end of the last war and in the early '50s were closed down when feedstuffs were derationed in 1952. Until the past two or three years only about 50 operators were left to produce a high-grade meal for use in poultry and pig rations. The marked upward swing in the price of cereals, which occurred towards the end of 1970 and which bids fair to become a permanent feature of livestock feeding if Britain joins the European Economic Community, has added point to a careful consideration of feeding value and costs if dried grass is to become incorporated in a regular fashion in the feeding of ruminants. Other factors are involved; the availability of more efficient machinery, better varieties of grasses and other crops to be dried, and the need for more break-crops in arable rotations. The latter need is, of course, felt most widely in the eastern counties where facilities for stock-keeping are often non-existent now. If grass or lucerne is to be widely used as a break-crop to maintain soil structure, the opportunity seems ready made for a large increase in dried crop production.

There are two types of driers being used in Great Britain now; *fixed driers* which produce most of the material and are likely to continue to do so, and *mobile or semi-mobile* machines designed for use on small or medium-sized farms.

1. *Fixed Driers.*—There are two main types: (*a*) low temperature operating at about 250° F.; or (*b*) high-temperature driers operating at 1300° F.

a. Low-temperature driers with the grass drying slowly, passage taking up to 30 minutes. The grass is loaded on to a moving belt which passes slowly through the drying chamber. The recent development by Alvan Blanch is illustrated in *Fig.* 24. The speed of the belt and the thickness of the bed of

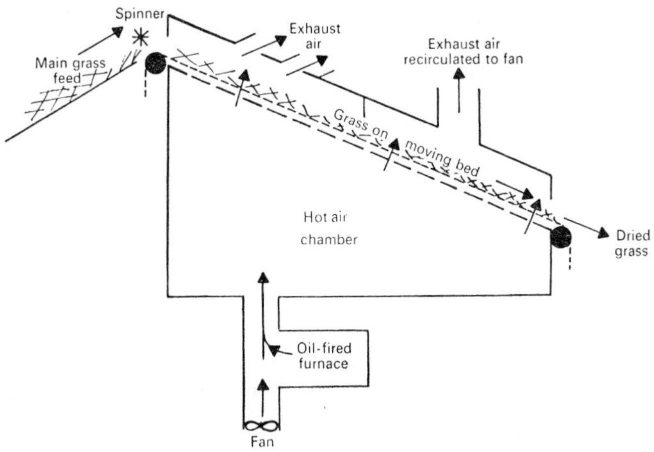

Fig. 24.—Diagram of Alvan Blanch low-temperature grass drier.

cut grass are adjusted so that the grass leaving the machine is dried to 10–12 per cent residual moisture. It is suitable for drying fairly long grass, allowing the product either to be baled or packaged directly into cobs, or after hammer-milling into pellets. It has the advantage of being able to be used for drying grain. The rate of output of the different sizes ranges from 5 to 15 cwt. per hour.

b. High-temperature driers operate with an inlet air temperature between 800° F. and 1500° F. The grass is carried in the air-stream which cools as the grass dries towards the outlet end so that the dried grass is not subject to extremely high temperatures. Usually the finely chopped crop with the average of ¾ in. length is dropped into the hot air-stream as it enters the drying drum (*Fig.* 25). The drum containing a complicated series of baffles is rotated

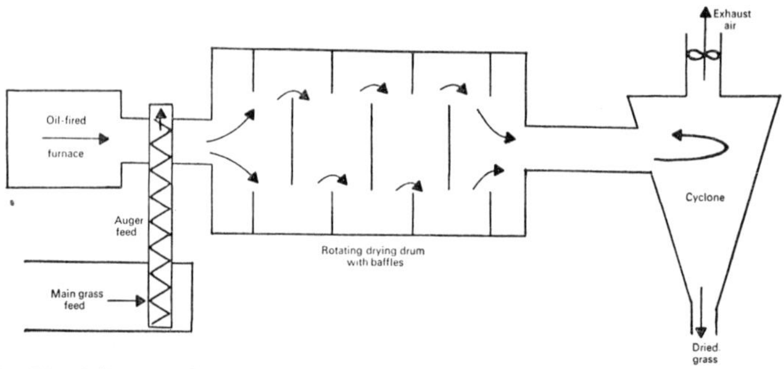

Fig. 25.—Diagram of single-pass high-temperature driven drier (pneumatic drier.)

along the axis of the air stream. A piece of stem which loses its moisture more slowly than the leaf is carried through the drum more slowly so that it also is dry when it reaches the cyclone whose effect is to separate the dried material from the air-stream from which it drops to the milling and packaging equipment. Smaller-sized driers work at between ½–1 ton per hour using light fuel oil while the larger driers do 10 tons per hour and use high-viscosity oil.

2. *Mobile Driers.*—These again may operate at low temperature or at high temperature. In the former category there is a promising new type called the 'Avon Hay Flaker', developed by a Berkshire farmer, and this is now being evaluated at the Broxworth Experimental Husbandry Farm and the Shell Farm at Ilmer. Its capacity is approximately 10–15 cwt. per hour. There are only Continental makes of high-temperature mobile driers now available and these are expensive and have rated outputs of about 10 cwt. per hour. Such an output is considerably more than would be needed by any but the largest livestock enterprise so that co-operative use of mobile driers, as is being undertaken by companies owning the larger fixed type of drier, will probably be the pattern of development.

Costs.—The costs involved in setting up new green crop-drying enterprises is being examined very closely by a number of people. At the present time it would appear that the cost before grant of the operation of a drier with an output of 1 ton per hour is about £50,000, although a drier with three times this output is likely to cost about £100,000.

The whole question of the use of dried grass was considered by a residential course conducted in November, 1969, at the Grassland Research Institute, Hurley. An account of some of the more important points covered has been published (Anon., 1970). The reports presented at this Conference by Advisory Officers indicated that farmers who had been trying dried grass or dried lucerne cobs with dairy cows were very satisfied with the results. These had been fed at levels as low as 4 lb. per cow per day or up to 20 lb. of dried grass per cow per day. Where the larger amounts were fed, the remainder of the ration had been made up with barley straw and balancer to give a total of 3 and occasionally 4 gal. as well as maintenance requirements. For production above this a dairy concentrate mixture fed in the parlour at the usual rate was used.

An account was given by the manager of a new crop-drying enterprise in Essex of the first year of operation of a large drier. It was found that the total cost of drying was £15·30 per ton with a season's output of 3000 tons which required 3000 hours of drying. At the present time artificially dried fodder is sold on a protein-content basis so that lucerne is the most profitable crop to dry. It has been pointed out that a useful development would be the specification of digestibility or of D value,* as well as a statement of crude protein levels.

Assuming the availability of adequate supplies of dried grass in various specified forms and quality, the question a farmer has to answer is, When does it pay him to include this ingredient in a ration? An important and most interesting contribution to this subject is a paper by Crabtree (1970). He examines the economics of the inclusion of dried grass in rations for dairy cows. He has applied the powerful technique of linear programming, using the computer, explaining clearly how it is done. This simply means that a number of nutritional conditions (or 'constraints', as they are called) are specified which together with an array of foodstuff prices and a matrix describing the contributions of the foodstuff towards meeting the constraints are subjected to an iterative procedure whose purpose is to find the minimum cost ration which satisfies the specified conditions. In other words, it discovers the price at which any particular feedingstuff does become an economically viable component of a ration. He uses the increasingly widely accepted feeding standards of metabolizable energy (ME)† and digestible crude protein (DCP) in computing the constraints of his ration. The ration itself is as shown in *Table III*.

Table III.—Composition of Least-cost Ration

Feed	*kg. DM per day*
Dairy cubes	4·50
Barley	3·02
Hay	0·00
Straw	1·68
Silage	5·00
Cost £0·27	

This is based upon the price and composition of the available feeds as shown in *Table IV*. The problem then becomes one of discovering the price at which various qualities of dried grass at the current market prices would just be included in a ration. He took a number of dried grasses in long form

* D value is the percentage digestibility of the organic matter in the dry matter of the feedingstuff.

† Metabolizable energy (ME): that part of the energy in the ration that is absorbed and available to the animal.

which ranged in their energy concentration from 2·2 to 2·8 Mcal.* per kg. with digestible crude protein contents ranging from 9 to 15 per cent. The result of his computing is a table which shows in relation to different qualities of dried grass what price can be paid for the various qualities to be profitable in the dairy cow ration.

Table IV.—PRICE AND COMPOSITION OF AVAILABLE FOODS

	DAIRY CUBES	BARLEY	HAY	STRAW	SILAGE
Price (£3 ton DW)	38·4	29·1	17·5	6·4	—
MD (Mcal./kg. DW)	3·23	2·89	2·00	1·45	2·20
DCP (per cent)	15·0	5·8	4·5	0·93	8·0

It is very obvious that the price of various other ingredients of the ration will have an important effect upon the decision of when it pays to include dried grass. It was interesting to see that when this account was being written in September, 1970, a large increase in the price of cereals and roughage feeds occurred. The author therefore examined the effect of a 10–20 per cent higher price for both barley and dairy cubes. Since both are included for their energy content, it meant that the inclusion price for the dried grass becomes increasingly dependent upon its energy value as the price of concentrate increases. The forward contract price for dried grass produced in 1970 was between £26 and £27 per ton at 15 per cent crude protein, with an increase with increasing crude protein content of about £1 per ton per percentage unit. On this basis and assuming the persistence of a 10 per cent increase in the barley and dairy cube prices from the earlier part of 1970, then the dried grass market price is the same as the inclusion price. Put in another way it could be said that when the marginal costs for digestible crude protein of dried grass was 57p per kg. and the price of metabolizable energy of grass was 9·6p per Mcal. then it paid to include dried grass in the rations of lactating dairy cows.

THE FUTURE OF ANIMALS AS SOURCES OF HUMAN FOOD

In a world where the majority of people are inadequately nourished if not positively hungry, there is bound to be a continuing discussion about the place of farm and wild animals as part of the human diet. It is widely accepted that where the main deficiency is one of energy, the various food crops are more important users of the cultivable land than the utilization of pastures or fodder crops for animals. It is a fact, however, that the greatest dietary deficiency is one of high-class protein. This animals can so far most conveniently and efficiently provide.

A recent symposium organized by the Nutrition Society has sought to consider the problems of various types of animal production in the widest context of providing human food over the next two decades. The first paper (Holmes, 1970) was a useful summary of the world situation and the problem of how animals can make their best contribution to human diets, at the same

* Mcal.: megacalorie=1 million calories or 1000 kilocalories.

time recognizing that social status and custom are probably more powerful factors in determining how much and what sort of meat is eaten. Based upon the latest figures published by the Food and Agriculture Organization of the United Nations (1969), he summarizes the average diets for certain Asian, West Indian, and African countries compared with that of the United Kingdom (*Table V*).

Table V.—AVERAGE NATIONAL DIETS

COUNTRY	DATE OF ESTIMATE	ENERGY PER DAY (kcal.)	TOTAL PROTEIN PER DAY (g.)	PROTEIN CALORIES (per cent of total calories)	ANIMAL PROTEIN PER DAY (g.)	ANIMAL PROTEIN (per cent)
United Kingdom	1967–8	3150	87·5	11·4	53·8	61·5
Ceylon	1967	2170	48·0	9·1	8·3	17·3
Jamaica	1966	2260	52·6	9·5	18·7	35·6
Pakistan	1966	2230	51·5	9·5	11·2	21·8
Uganda	1961–3	2070	50·1	9·9	10·2	20·3

It will be seen that the average calorie and protein intake of those living in the United Kingdom agrees with the desirable levels in which 11 per cent of the energy is derived from protein and 62 per cent of the protein is of animal origin. In the developing countries, of which those in the table are illustrations, the calorie intakes are low, the protein provides about 9 per cent of the calories and the animal protein supplies from 17 to 36 per cent of the total protein. It has been pointed out (Clark, 1970) that such diets in tropical countries may be less deficient than they at first appear since the adult energy requirements are of the order of 2500 kcal. per day. It also appears likely that an adult really only needs 6 per cent of the calories in the form of protein, and that mixed vegetable proteins can equal animal proteins. A way in which average can mislead is illustrated by a recent U.N.E.S.C.O. report which points out: 'If the stable foods of a country are relatively poor sources of protein, such as maize or rice, or very poor sources, such as cassava, sago or plantains, young children are unlikely to obtain the quantity and quality of protein they need.' We know that the time of danger and the reason for the high incidence of kwashiorkor in so many countries is the fact that during infancy and particularly when the child is weaned there is not enough good-quality protein available amongst poor families where staple foods are very low in protein.

An indication of the way in which different types of farm animals convert food both in terms of energy or protein expressed as a percentage, and the amount of food from both animals and crops which can be obtained per unit area, are indicated in *Table VI.*

The pig is the most efficient converter of energy although only slightly ahead of dairy cows with beef, but, in terms of protein, poultry are ahead of the pig. This result follows from the greater reproductive capacity of pigs and poultry.

It is not at all surprising that the production of crops is a better way than animal production in terms of food production per unit area. This knowledge has always formed the basis of advice to developing countries that they should concentrate upon using crops for food in the first instance. In spite of great efforts during recent years to industrialize the photosynthetic capacity of plants, no great success has so far been achieved. It is very difficult to get people to change their food habits, a fact recognized by Pirie (1969), who has worked devotedly to develop home- or village-scale plant protein extraction processes.

Table VI.—FEED EFFICIENCY IN WHOLE FARM SITUATIONS: ANNUAL YIELDS FROM ANIMALS AND FROM CROPS

	ME (per cent)	PROTEIN (per cent)	ENERGY (Mcal. per ha.)*	PROTEIN (kg. per ha.)
Dairy herd	21	23	2,500	115
Dairy+beef herd	20	20	2,400	102
Beef herd	7	6	750	27
Sheep flock	3	3	500	23
Pig herd	23	12	1,900	50
Broiler flock	13	20	1,100	92
Egg flock	15	18	1,150	88
Wheat	—	—	14,000	350
Peas	—	—	3,000	280
Cabbage	—	—	8,000	1100
Potatoes	—	—	24,000	420

* ha. = hectare, 2·5 acres. (*From Holmes*, 1970.)

The industrial extraction and treatment of soya-bean protein, whose yield of 2000 kg. beans per ha. from which is extracted 600–800 kg. edible protein, is proceeding. The spun and 'textured' material is competitive in price with the cheaper meat cuts in the U.S.A. Less-processed soya protein is cheaper, as can be seen from the following relative costs (Braude and others, 1970):—

Spun soya protein fibre	100
Protein isolate	37
Protein concentrate	18
Grits	9
Flour	7

The cheaper derivatives are much used in sausages and pies.

The fact remains that ruminants harvest forage from unploughable land which makes up a high proportion of many countries. They also help to maintain the fertility of cultivable land by grazing sown pastures and eating the by-products of arable farming, straw, haulms, sugar-beet tops; as well as industrial residues such as brewers' grains, molasses, or surplus grain.

The following paper (Blaxter, 1970) was concerned with the part played by ruminants and began by presenting evidence that suggests that increases in wealth are associated with an increased demand for milk and meat, and that the wealth associated with a considerable degree of industrialization is also associated with an enhanced demand for meat. When meat consumption increases, cereal consumption falls. This pattern is well illustrated by changes over the past 20 years in the U.S.A. The mean consumption of meat from ruminant animals increased by 40 per cent, the consumption of non-ruminant meat increased by 26 per cent, while the consumption of milk fell by 12 per cent. Flour and cereal consumption fell by 18 per cent.

Beef accounts for 66 per cent of this increased consumption, while lamb and mutton declined by 24 per cent. The increase in non-ruminant meat was accounted for by 109 per cent increase in poultry meat consumption, but 3 per cent less pork and bacon is being consumed now.

The picture is somewhat similar in the United Kingdom today. The influence of income is clearly seen if the weekly consumption of two social classes, A1 and D2, is compared (M.A.F.F.: National Food Survey Committee, 1969). This reveals that well-to-do people increase their consumption of beef and pork and discriminate against other meat. They hardly increase their consumption of milk and mutton at all. A somewhat similar survey amongst professional people, skilled workers, and rural workers in France (Claudian and Serville, 1968) shows that the French people, if their financial state improved, wish to increase their meat consumption more than that of any other food. It indicated a greater proportional consumption of beef by professional people than by manual workers and a general wish to increase its consumption to that of other meats. This was stronger in the lower socio-economic groups.

If those peoples of the world currently aspiring to Western standards of living could instantaneously achieve them, then our current world production of milk needs to increase by 50 per cent and the production of ruminant meat needs to double. Milk production can be expected to increase until in societies aspiring to Western standards it averages 600 g. per person per day. Meat production will increase to provide 200 g. per person per day.

We have to remember that world population is far from static and since Western standards of living appear to be highly infectious, it is probable that by A.D. 2000 we need to cater for a potential demand equivalent to a doubling of current world milk production and a quadrupling of current world meat production.

An important point made by this contributor was that recent experimentation shows that the intensive utilization of grassland in northern temperate regions can result in an output of beef per hectare which is two and a half times that achieved by cropping policy with coarse grains and cereals. This enables one to calculate that per unit area of land beef production, which, from an energy point of view, is the least efficient of agricultural production processes, results in as much muscle protein when cropping is designed to provide feed specifically for ruminants as does a pig production system in which the cropping is with cereal grains and pulses which could be used after refining by man. Similarly, milk protein per unit area is very much greater than the production of either pig meat or beef.

Planted crops account for a world acreage only half that occupied by natural grassland and only a third that of the world's natural forests. Grasslands and part of the forest country can only be converted into food for man by grazing herbivores, the most important of which are the ruminants. The idea that animals generally are competitors for human food is inaccurate. Ruminants are commensals of man.

The role of poultry was covered by Bolton (1970), who traces the extraordinary changes in numbers and methods of husbandry that have occurred in the United Kingdom over the past few years. He admits that the long-term survival of poultry as farm animals may be determined by whether or not a replacement for the energy-supplying part of the diet can be found. It is to be remembered that poultry food is made up of approximately 75 per cent cereals, 15 per cent of vegetable protein, and 7·5 per cent of animal protein. The suggestion is made that since the world is becoming deluged with paper, and paper is largely cellulose, a polymer of glucose, it should become feasible to hydrolyse used paper into glucose and use the latter as human and poultry food.

An interesting account is given of the potentialities of ducks as the providers of eggs. It is pointed out that while *Salmonella* can be excreted in the duck egg, modern intensive housing has greatly reduced the chances of the duck becoming infected. The chances are no greater than with the fowl. It appears that the laying hen has reached a plateau of egg production at about 270 eggs per bird per year; but Khaki Campbell ducks can lay 300 eggs per bird per year. Breeding research should rapidly produce strains of ducks that could outlay strains of fowls.

Other competitors of the fowl, as producers of meat and eggs respectively, are the guinea-fowl and the Japanese quail. Guinea-fowls have a much more acceptable taste, being akin to the pheasant or grouse, than the modern, almost tasteless, broiler. Again, more research upon breeding and nutrition might well lift the guinea-fowl out of the luxury food category. The Japanese quail become sexually mature at 5 weeks, require much less space than a hen, and produce twice the annual egg mass than the modern hybrid hen per unit of body-weight. The drawback, of course, is that quail eggs weigh only 9 g. but this is equal to about 7 per cent of the adult body-weight; the eggs layed by a modern light-weight strain of fowl represent about 3·5 per cent. This means that the cost of rearing the birds is less and the efficiency of conversion of food to eggs is higher.

There has recently been much greater efficiency in the utilization of waste from poultry production. Offal from poultry-dressing stations, incubator refuse, and dead birds are being processed into a protein-rich animal food. Now the manure from the large caged units is being dried and has been shown to provide a valuable food for ruminants. It contains all the cellulose of the original food and up to half the crude protein, mainly as urates.

The advantages of poultry over other farm animals in developing countries is steadily being exploited. There is no disadvantage from religious objection to the consumption of fowls and eggs. The latter are produced ready wrapped and have a better shelf life than meat or milk. The live animal can be carried home; its rate of reproduction is rapid, for one breeding hen can produce a hundred daughters a year, thus permitting the rapid spread of improved strains. Housing in tropical countries can be very simple. An illustration of what can be achieved in a very short period is that of Chad. Between 1961 and 1968 the production of eggs was increased to the extent that the average consumption rose from 5 eggs per head per year to 10 eggs per head per year. It was done by a combination of better strains of fowl and better husbandry.

The remarkable potentialities of the pig were clearly and persuasively set out by Braude and others (1970). To provide a basis on which to discuss possible ways of improvement, the pig population in the United Kingdom and in the world is summarized in *Table VII*.

The place that pig products play in our annual consumption of meat is set out in *Table VIII*.

This indicates the continued growth of consumption of pig products compared with a decline in the consumption of beef and mutton and lamb. Braude says that he expects the total of pork and bacon consumption to

Table VII.—PIG POPULATION (MILLIONS) IN THE UNITED KINGDOM AND IN THE WORLD

YEAR	U.K.	WORLD	U.K. AS PER CENT OF THE WORLD	INCREASE PER YEAR	
				U.K.	World
1934–8	4·6	249	1·85		
1958	6·5	455	1·43	2·1	4·1
1968	7·8	605	1·29	2·0	3·3
1978	9·2	786	1·17	1·8	3·0
1988	10·7	982	1·09	1·6	2·5

Table VIII.—PER CAPITA ANNUAL CONSUMPTION (kg.) OF MEAT IN THE UNITED KINGDOM

	1934–8	1958	1964	1968	INCREASE OR DECLINE IN 30 YEARS
Pork	4·8	8·7	10·3	10·6	+5·8
Bacon and ham	12·8	11·5	11·5	11·5	−1·3
Total pork, bacon and ham	17·6	20·2	21·8	22·1	+4·5
Beef	25·0	23·5	21·5	20·4	−4·6
Mutton and lamb	11·5	10·3	10·7	10·5	−1·0
Poultry	2·3	4·3	7·2	9·1	+6·8
Offal and canned meat	5·4	8·9	9·5	8·2	+2·8
Total meat	61·8	67·2	70·7	70·3	+8·5

increase at least a further 10 per cent in the next decade and probably a similar increase in the subsequent decade. Recent figures that I saw presented at a whole-day meeting at the Meat Research Institute early 1971 and so far unpublished indicate that pork and bacon consumption are certainly continuing to maintain their position as the most popular meats in this country. This, of course, is due to pig meat's competitive price.

This will only be maintained if efficiency of food conversion and production can be further improved. There is a big range in the annual production from each sow in this country at the present time, due to a combination of genetic factors, husbandry, and disease control inadequacies. This is summarized in *Table IX*, along with Braude's suggestion for the performance of the future pig.

It is possible, he claims, that there will be a fivefold increase over the present average in the amount of lean meat produced daily by the offspring of a sow. This would mean that the annual production by the offspring of one sow could be 2730 kg. liveweight, of which 1354 kg. would be lean meat, or 303 kg. of very high-quality protein. If a baconer is produced capable of not storing excessive amounts of fat at higher weights, the optimum slaughter weight may reach 105 kg. by the end of the second decade. If this is so, then the above values could be increased to 1563 kg. of lean meat or 350 kg. of protein.

Table IX.—PAST, PRESENT, AND FUTURE ANNUAL PRODUCTION PER SOW

		PRESENT PIG			FUTURE PIG		
	Wild Pig	Average	Good	Excellent	Without Artificial Rearing	First Decade	Second Decade
No. of pigs	4	14	18	22	24	28	30
Weight at 8 weeks (kg.)	7	16	18	20	23	32	32
Daily gain (g.) from 8 weeks to slaughter at 91 kg.	(225)	550	650	730	860	860	1000
Days to reach 91 kg.	(429)	192	168	153	135	125	115
Killing out (per cent)	—	72	75	78	80	80	80
Lean in carcass (per cent)	—	50	54	58	62	62	62
Total lean meat (kg.) per sow per year	—	459	663	906	1083	1264	1354

Braude's confidence in the great improvement in the efficiency of food utilization, as well as the improvement in daily weight-gain, is based upon the evidence emerging from the published papers from the National Institute for Research in Dairying during the past 30 years of his work there. These are summarized in a striking figure (*Fig.* 26).

It should be possible to reduce the amount of feed required to produce 1 kg. of live-weight, dead-weight, or lean meat to 2·28, 2·85, or 4·60 kg. respectively, which certainly is a very high efficiency of conversion.

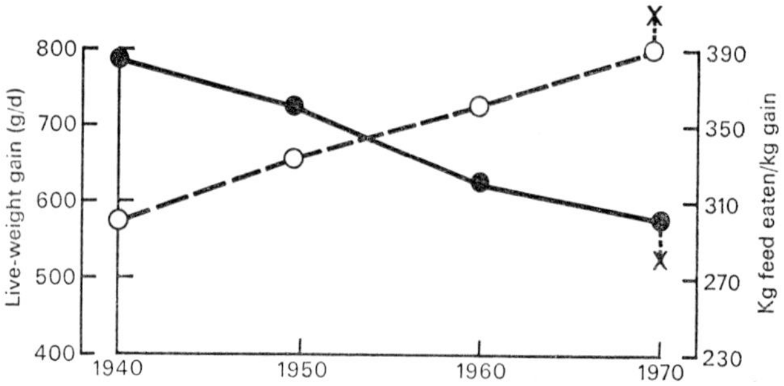

Fig. 26.—Improvement in live-weight gain (grammes per day) and feed conversion efficiency of Large White pigs at the National Institute for Research in Dairying during 1940 to 1970. ○ - - - ○, daily live-weight gain; ●——●, feed-conversion efficiency. Values for 1940 from Braude and Foot (1942); for 1950 from Braude, Mitchell, and Robinson (1950); for 1960 from Barber, Braude, and Mitchell (1960); for 1970 from Braude and others (1970). ×, Average for the best 6 pigs in an experiment now in progress.

He sees the situation in these terms. Either by maintaining the present standards and accepting the projected increase in human population and its pork consumption, then at the end of the second decade from now about 55 per cent more sows and feed would be needed. Or, if the specified targets are attained by the end of the 1980's, 28 per cent fewer sows and 10 per cent less feed will be required. On that basis also it is possible to reduce the cost of production very considerably and even if the price of feed is very substantially increased the improved efficiency standards would more than cover the increased production costs. It seems too unlikely to state, but he says that the retail price of pork and pork products could eventually be lower than it is at present without sacrificing the legitimate interests of producers.

There are, of course, some very serious difficulties. Braude recognizes that his targets can only be attained if artificial rearing of pigs from birth or soon afterwards becomes possible. That means that several major problems will have to be solved before artificial rearing can be satisfactorily applied under practical conditions of pig-keeping. Immunological and disease problems of baby pigs and difficulties over reproduction in the early weaned sow are the present major stumbling blocks. There is much active research being done and he believes that this will be successful.

On the improvement of the genetics of the pig, he is not a believer in the virtues of hybrids. He quotes the evidence from Sweden where no benefit from cross-breeding in terms of the numbers of pigs born and reared and their weights at 3 weeks of age has been observed. On the other hand, he admits that there is evidence pointing to benefits from cross-breeding under poor conditions of production, but these will have to be removed if the future targets are to be attained. The advantages and the practical ways of eliminating losses from enzootic pneumonia are already understood. Enteric disease will certainly have to be brought under control. He says: 'Genetic improvement must go hand-in-hand with improvement in health. It just does not make sense to establish genetically superior herds which harbour infectious diseases, and thus may be responsible for their transfer to herds which purchase stock from them.'

Finally, there was an interesting contribution from Kay (1970) dealing with meat production from wild herbivores. Over recent years there have been many publications advancing proposals and examining the evidence for the utilization of various types of wild herbivore, many of which are to be found in Africa. The overriding reason for giving attention to wild animals in difficult habitats is precisely that they live in environments which are unsuitable for domesticated animals. It is a fact that about 30 per cent of the land surface of the world is too arid for intensive development, while there are other large areas which are mountainous or only have tundra or taiga vegetation. It has been estimated that the East African acacia savannah and bushland is able to carry roughly a five times greater biomass of wild ungulates than of domestic animals.

From the most distant times up to the present day, clumsy attempts to introduce domestic species of plants or animals into marginally arid regions have led to catastrophic collapse of the ecosystem and the appearance of dust bowls and desert. The adaptation of certain species such as the camel and the eland to the great stretches of hot, dry country that are to be found in Africa has been fairly well documented. In addition there are some other advantages. Endemic disease often rules out the introduction of exotic domestic species. Trypanosomiasis and swine fever are the scourge of cattle and pigs over large tracts of Africa, though the diseases scarcely affect native ungulates.

There is little evidence to indicate whether they have as great a digestive efficiency as cattle and sheep. A recent useful study by Skinner (1970), from South Africa, claims that game are not as efficient. What is not in doubt is that their choice of food is better and their capacity to manage on much less water is very evident. In their favour is the killing-out percentage being if anything better than ruminants. African ungulates are characteristically very lean, with carcasses rarely containing more than 2·5 per cent of fat. Recent studies on the springbok (von la Chevallerie, 1970) have shown that not only are the hindquarters relatively heavy but the longissimus dorsi muscle is very well developed in comparison with sheep of the same weight. Unfortunately the eating quality of venison is frequently adversely affected by spoilage with blood and ingesta at slaughter.

There are two management systems that can be considered as applying to wild animals: hunting and game cropping. Hunting is a popular tourist activity in many African countries and indeed is undertaken in many parts of the world. Kangaroos in Australia provided about 2000 tons of meat for export in 1960–1. In 1966 Ghana produced nearly 28,000 tons of meat from wild game; and in 1968 New Zealand, as a by-product of a drive to control red deer, exported about 3000 tons of venison. This, none the less, is a poor way to exploit a population of wild herbivores.

Game Cropping

This is the traditional method of dealing with reindeer and is still practised in northern countries. A stable animal/environment relationship can be fairly readily established. In Africa, if this is to be achieved, it is necessary to have a mixture of browsers such as giraffe and elephant, grazers such as buffalo and kob, and rooters such as warthog and bushpig. Some workers have calculated that the sustained yield, based on a 10 per cent annual cull of the nine most abundant large ungulates found in the Serengeti National Park, amounts to 12,675 tons live-weight a year (4·17 kg. per ha.). It almost certainly exceeds the yield from cattle pastured on such country.

In terms of advancing towards game farming and thus to domestication of ungulates, it would appear that in Africa in the dry tropical regions the most likely species is the eland. It is very well adapted to the country. It is docile and the quality of its carcass is excellent. Incidentally, a herd of eland has been maintained for 72 years in the southern Ukraine. The young eland gain about 0·8 kg. per day when fattened and lactating cows produce 100–600 kg. of milk rich in protein and fat at each lactation. I myself have seen giraffe and eland being farmed on a modest scale along with Boran cattle on a ranch in Kenya. The giraffe were mainly for their browsing habits, to keep the thorn tree cover high, possibly reducing the tsetse-fly concentration. On 50 square miles of a game ranch in Rhodesia studied by Dasmann (1963) the production of game meat has equalled the production of beef and has been more profitable owing to the lower cost chargeable to the game animals.

Nevertheless, there are great difficulties associated with the utilization of wild ungulates until they are fully domesticated. The problem of slaughter is clearly of great importance. At the present time there is a loss of hides and carcass meat as well as other offal which has been estimated to amount to 10 per cent of the carcass weight. Transport and marketing problems have hardly been tackled. Finally, there is the fact that such wild ungulates may act as a reservoir of disease which, though not deleterious to themselves, makes them unsuited to being mixed with susceptible domestic animals.

Kay concludes with a short discussion of the future possibilities of farming red deer in the remoter parts of the United Kingdom. The Nature Conservancy (1967) is making a thorough study of wild deer and some laboratory research is in progress. A meeting was held in 1969 by the Highland and Islands Development Board and the Rowett Research Institute to consider the whole question of the husbandry of red deer for meat production. The proceedings of this meeting have been published (Bannerman and Blaxter, 1969). It appears that there are about 180,000 red deer in Scotland, remarkably free from disease. At present one-sixth are killed each year yielding 1500 tons of meat (about 0·7 kg. per ha.) which is mainly exported to West Germany. So far little husbandry is practised, few of the estates are fenced, although some provide the deer with supplementary food in winter. It is this period that limits the deer to their present number and causes the death of about a third of the calves.

Breeding Policies for Beef in the United Kingdom

During the past year there has been general interest in the moves by groups of producers to import into Great Britain some Continental beef breeds. These have been the Simmental, the Limousin mainly from France, and a few of the Meuse-Rhine-Yssel (MRY), a breed from the Netherlands. These moves have focused attention upon the desirability of having a clearer understanding of what qualities the various beef breeds can contribute. Two recent publications are concerned with this subject. Mason (1971) has for the first time brought together a large body of work from many countries where performance testing of various European beef breeds has been undertaken. The Meat and Livestock Commission (1971) has just published the report of a Scientific Study Group charged with the task of advising upon beef improvement in the United Kingdom.

Apart from the Friesian, the commonest European breed in Britain today is the Charolais. There have been 111 bulls and 743 females imported since the first permits were issued in 1961. In 1970, 34 bulls and 224 females of the Swiss Simmental breed and 13 bulls and 259 females of the German Simmental breed arrived. The Limousins and the MRYs should be released from quarantine during 1971. The latter breed are only in small numbers and presumably will be used along with other dairy and dual-purpose breeds such as the Canadian-Holstein, the Danish Red, and the Finnish Ayrshire to help with both production and size in producing cows whose male calves can be used for beef but whose heifers can enter the dairy herd. The MRY cattle are about 9 per cent heavier and 2 per cent taller than the Dutch Blackpied or Friesian.

Just how different in production characteristics are Simmental cattle coming from Switzerland, France, and Germany? There has been a large-scale Swiss experiment which involved 754 animals, aimed at comparing the three varieties. The only obvious differences between the breeds were the higher milk yield of the French Simmental (or Montbéliard) heifers and their greater height at the withers. Apparently the frequency of stillbirths and the disease incidence were the same in the three groups. As one might expect, the differences between individual bulls were greater than those between the breeds.

Mason has gathered all the information that exists to make a comparison between the main French and German beef breeds; that is, to answer the question of how does the Charolais compare with the Simmental? In Germany some direct comparisons showed no difference in the growth-rate. In Canada and the Argentine there was no difference between Charolais and Simmental crosses either in the amount of calving difficulty or in the growth-rate.

It is, of course, of the utmost interest to us to know how the other European breeds would compare with our own pure beef breeds. While the United States of America have begun a comprehensive comparative test, there are no results yet from it. In South Africa there are large populations of pure-breds and they have been compared over many years starting in 1957. *Fig.* 27 indicates the growth-rate of steers of the various breeds.

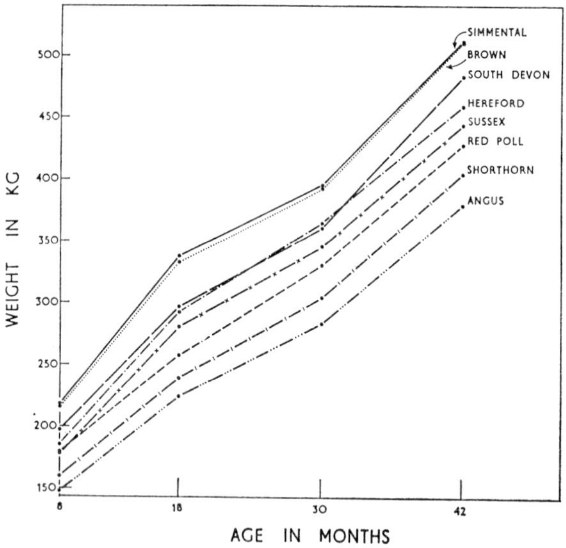

Fig. 27.—Growth-rate of steers of various breeds in the experimental farm at Omatjenne, South West Africa. (Drawn from figures in Borstlap, 1968.)

The climate and pastures in South Africa are very different from those of western Europe or North America but the British breeds appear in about the same weight order as in Britain, so there is no obvious sign of breed/environment interaction. Close examination of the figures show that the South Devon and Hereford are superior to the Simmental and the Brown cattle in terms of food conversion and daily gain.

The carcasses of 40 bulls and 40 steers of 7 breeds and 4 crosses in this South African experiment showed that the Simmental and Brown had the largest eye-muscle area, the highest percentage of lean, and the highest percentage of valuable cuts but the carcasses graded low. The Hereford had the smallest eye-muscle area, low percentage of lean, and the highest percentage of fat, leading to high carcass grade. The Sussex had a high eye-muscle area, low percentage of lean, thin subcutaneous fat, low percentage of fat, and a low carcass grade.

The M.L.C. have been conducting comparisons of the Charolais with British beef breeds in their Performance Testing Station at Warren Farm for some years now. The most recent figures show that as pure-breds the Charolais exceeds all British breeds in size and growth-rate. This is clearly shown in *Fig.* 28.

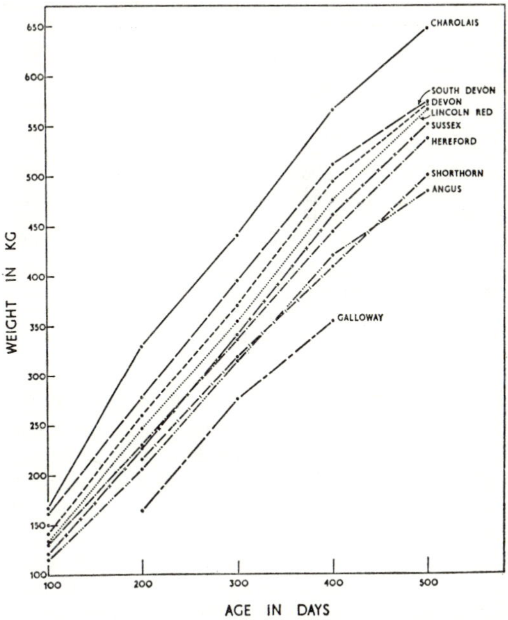

Fig. 28.—Results of recording of weights of pure-bred bulls (farm records plus performance-test records). (Drawn from M.L.C. figures supplied by Lewis, 1970.)

The effect of crossing the beef bulls with the Friesian cows has also been studied in the progeny and some of the results are shown in *Table X*. The surprise here is the Sussex breed which shows itself superior to all other breeds.

Mason summarizes his study by saying that there is a group of breeds which grow at about the same rate. These include the Charolais, Simmental, German Yellow, Romagna, Marche, and Chiana. More extensive testing may show that there are no real differences between these breeds. The breeds in the next group are a little smaller and they include the Limousin, the Acquitane Blond, the Maine-Anjou in France, the Brown Mountain cattle in the Alps, the Piedmont in Italy, the MRY in the Netherlands, and the British Friesian and South Devon. The next group, which may not be easy to separate from the preceding one, includes the Continental Friesians based on Dutch and German blood and possibly the Normandy, the Swedish Red and White; the Danish Red and the Devon and Sussex should also be included in this group. The last group includes the remaining British breeds headed by the Hereford and followed by the Shorthorn and Aberdeen Angus.

Table X.—PURE-BRED AND CROSSING PERFORMANCE OF BULLS IN BRITAIN—200-DAY WEIGHTS (kg.)

	PURE-BRED BULLS*		CROSS-BRED SUCKLED CALVES MEAN OF BOTH SEXES†	
	No.	Mean	No.	Mean
Charolais	617	330	980	217
South Devon	312	278	562	215
Devon	356	260	602	211
Lincoln Red	248	247	416	211
Hereford	2706	230	2121	191
Sussex	249	227	298	219
Welsh Black	86	227	270	191
Beef Shorthorn	143	216	549	171
Aberdeen Angus	1082	206	1621	179
Galloway	69	163	494	170

* Data from performance testing in stations and on-farm pedigree recording during 1968–70 except Beef Shorthorn and Galloway (1967–70) and Welsh Black (1966–70).

† Data from on-farm commercial recording during 1966–70.

There is a positive correlation between daily gain and weight and a negative one between daily gain and fatness. In other words, breeds with a large mature size grow most rapidly and mature most slowly, i.e., they reach their mature weight at a later age and therefore start to put on fat later. The greater amount of fat in the carcass of the smaller breeds is most conspicuous when they are compared at the same age. Rapid gainers use a smaller proportion of their food for maintenance and less fat is laid down as they grow. If the larger breeds are compared with the smaller breed at similar weight, the former have more muscle in the carcass and thus a higher muscle/bone ratio. The less desirable results of large size are greater gestation lengths, heavier calves at birth, and thus more calving difficulties and more still-births.

Mason points out that more important are the breeds which deviate in some way from the general regression on size. Here the Limousin should be specially noted since it has a higher muscle/bone ratio than would be expected from its size. This is reflected in the large eye-muscle area. There seems to be little to choose between the beefing characters of the large breeds in Group 1 but the Simmental is the breed to use, especially the French variety, in a dual-purpose breed or in the production of a suckler cow. But the breed which will produce most weight in a dairy cross is undoubtedly the Charolais.

The value of the United Kingdom pursuing a liberal policy in the importation of new genetic material is recommended by the Study Group in their report to M.L.C. on beef improvement. They also say that work on the comparisons of different breeds and crosses leading eventually to breed substitution 'is likely to be highly cost-effective and is recommended'.

Top priority is given to their recommendation that M.L.C. itself set up a herd of beef cattle and select for improved performance. They say the herd should consist of at least 200 cows. All the males would be weaned at a few days of age, reared together, and performance tested over a weight range from about 220 to 880 lb. (100–400 kg.) using a single complete diet in order to measure feed-conversion efficiency. Ultrasonic measures of fat deposition and eye-muscle area would be taken, initially for development purposes but later as selection criteria. The details of the proposed breeding programme and the progress predicted are given in an appendix. It is calculated that the annual rate of improvement of 17 lb. (7·6 kg.) or 1·7 per cent in live-weight at about 400 days should be possible. The selected bulls from this M.L.C. herd would be used in A.I. with the active co-operation of the A.I. services to promote the use of these bulls.

If bulls from the herd were used to sire 100,000 crossbred animals for slaughter each year with a similar number of the grand progeny being reared in single suckler herds, they predict that a rate of return on the capital invested of 23 per cent would be obtained. Surveying the breeds available in the country at the present time in terms of numbers which could be obtained to establish the herd, they come to the conclusion that the Hereford must be chosen. The possibility of introducing animals from other breeds should be considered at frequent intervals as more information on the performance and acceptability of breeds other than the Hereford becomes available.

Cross-breeding for Beef

The question of the suitability of breeds for particular parts of the world and the differing climatic and pasture conditions that are to be found there is highlighted by two interesting articles recently by Moran (1970a, b). He examined the performance of a $\frac{3}{4}$ Brahman and 4 pure-bred Hereford steers over a 12-month period, kept together on the high country of New England in N.S.W. where the climate is temperate with very cold nights through the winter. Brahman cattle are a combination of Indian and Pakistan zebu breeds. Many studied in the southern United States and Australia have revealed their special attributes of being able to utilize poor pastures, their ability to withstand high temperatures, resistance to tick infestation, and a greater capacity to pass on increased growth-rates following crossing with British breeds, as a manifestation of hybrid vigour, than occurs when British breeds are crossed among themselves.

This new study, carried out in two parts, was undertaken firstly to investigate live-weight gains and carcass characteristics between the Hereford and the $\frac{3}{4}$ Brahman, and secondly to examine the behavioural characteristics of the two breeds under cold winter conditions. It has shown that while the highest live-weight gains over the whole year were made by the Herefords, during the time when the nutritional level was poor the Brahmans had an advantage on average daily gain. The latter had a higher dressing percentage because of their smaller alimentary tracts and also exhibited a greater carcass muscle and smaller carcass fat content than the Herefords. The result was that the retail value index of Herefords fell to a level below that of the Brahmans in a market which discriminated against excess fat.

A series of 24-hour grazing studies made of the two breeds throughout the year showed that both breeds spent approximately the same time grazing. There were no signs of cold stress in either breed even when the dry-bulb temperature frequently fell below freezing point. Perhaps the usefulness of Brahmans and Brahman crosses for use in some of our single suckler herds on the rough hill country might be examined.

United States Experience

Animal scientists in the United States have for many years conducted fairly large-scale field experiments with various British breeds of beef cattle and their crosses, seeking suitable cattle for fattening in the large feed-lots. It was interesting to see in some recent papers describing current work, presented at a special beef cattle symposium, that their problems in terms of breeding policy for the future are similar to those of our own. A paper by Cundiff (1970), summarizing experimental results on cross-breeding of cattle for beef production, points out that the production per cow can be increased 20–25 per cent by systematic crossing of British breeds; and that about half of this advantage is dependent upon the use of cross-bred cows to take advantage of heterosis for maternal ability and reproduction. It appears that the Charolais has promise as an important sire breed because of its transmission of growth-rate. He also comments upon the advantages of Brahman crosses with British breeds where the effect of heterosis with a Hereford/Brahman cross was 15·9 per cent and in a comparison between cross-bred Brahman British calves and British straight-bred calves the former exceeded the latter by about 11 per cent in weaning weight.

In a paper discussing just what should be the selection criteria for beef cattle for the future, Cartwright (1970) believes that there must be specialized dam lines and/or breeds selected towards relatively small size, early maturing, milking qualities, freedom from calving difficulties, and twinning ability. These will be matched by the specialized sire lines and/or breeds which will be selected towards high rate of gain, efficient food conversion, high cut-out percentage, and tender, palatable beef. He is also convinced that there must be a shift towards special-purpose cattle not only in terms of breeds but by according recognition to the first generation of crosses so allowing them to be sold in a similar manner to registered pure-breds.

Dairy Cattle Breeding in the United Kingdom

The Milk Marketing Board is the most powerful body concerned with the testing and use of dairy bulls in the United Kingdom. The current testing and selection methods for A.I. bulls in Great Britain have been criticized by Hinks (1970a) as applying too weak a selection pressure for milk yields and by a low rate of tested bull utilization. This leads to the deliberate maintenance of a large proportion of the stud in an inactive and unproductive state. The Milk Marketing Board has in fact established many bull resting properties where young sires are kept pending the results of progeny tests. The British methods contrast forcibly with those favoured in Scandinavia where semen is collected from young bulls on test and then the bulls themselves slaughtered at an early age, leading to a bigger turnover of bulls. Hinks suggests that there should be a change of policy to make more use of bulls by increasing the semen collected and stored from 10,000 semen doses per annum as at present, to the New Zealand Dairy Board's figure of 15,000 doses per tested sire per annum. If this is done then we can increase our selection rate of up to 1 in 6 bulls for essentially the same cost.

He found that the cost of adopting the Scandinavian system would be high because of the massive costs involved in the collection, processing, and storage of large quantities of semen, much of which is obtained from bulls which subsequently prove to be of inferior breeding merit. The advantages to be gained from the adoption of a semen-storage programme appeared small in relation to the benefits to be obtained from improved bull utilization. It would mean that the cost of testing a bull, on the basis of one bull being selected in each 6 tested, would be increased by £142,000.

Since so much of our beef comes from the Friesian breed, now making up 76 per cent of the national dairy herd, there has been much discussion of combining performance testing for beef characters with the progeny tests for milk production in the testing programme of the A.I. Service. It is a fact, as has been shown in Norway (Soller, Bar-Anan, and Pasternak, 1966), that genetic advances can be made on both fronts simultaneously. The costs, however, are high, and Hinks (1970b) has shown that the capital investments in performance testing are likely to prove profitable, but less so than similar investments in the improvement of the dairy progeny test. Where performance testing is undertaken there appears to be little advantage to be gained from the application of selection rates in excess of 1 in 3, for the total cost involved is £35·5 thousand for each increase. On the basis of there being limited capital available, he says that the change in meat : milk price ratio necessary to justify the diversion of capital resources from the progeny test to the performance test is probably a change from the present 7 : 1 to approximately 12 : 1 to permit a performance test in which the best 50 per cent of bulls are selected for testing at A.I. centres.

NUTRITIONAL NOTES

Protein for Young Ruminants

The steady movement towards the greater use of intensive systems of raising calves and lambs has focused attention upon the best way to provide the right ratio of protein to energy. Apart from the suckler calf on the hill cow, the rearing of calves for beef, most of whom come from the dairy herd, necessitates making a decision about when to change from the relatively expensive milk-substitute diet to the cheaper cereal mixture and forage diet. Progress was made some years ago by the discovery that calves could be conveniently weaned from a liquid diet at about 5 weeks of age. In spite of a good deal of propaganda from the feedingstuffs industry, it would appear that large numbers of calves are given liquid diets beyond the age of 5 weeks (Roy, 1970). In this paper it is clearly shown that optimal weight-gains and the best food conversion will be obtained if calves are kept on liquid diets until they are approximately 100 kg. in weight. Nevertheless, this is much less profitable than the early weaning of calves.

Protein in Liquid Form.—Intensification of the sheep industry involves more lambs being born to each ewe, and thus the artificial rearing of lambs. Great progress has been made in the use of suitable milk substitutes but the optimum ratio of protein/energy has only recently been investigated. A series of studies undertaken by workers at the Rowett Rearch Institute has shed a lot of light upon this problem. In the lamb accustomed to suck from a teat it was found that the oesophageal groove reflex continues to operate. This allows suspensions of protein to pass directly into the abomasum, thus wholly avoiding degradation within the rumen (Ørskov and Benzie, 1969). When they gave a protein supplement in this manner to weaned lambs they found that there was increased nitrogen retention and decreased urinary nitrogen excretion when compared with lambs given the same protein in dry feed (Ørskov and Fraser, 1969).

In a more recent study from the same team (Ørskov, Fraser, and Corse, 1970), they used lambs 5–6 weeks of age that had been trained to drink milk from a bottle fitted with a teat but had also had free access to food consisting of dried grass and rolled barley. The protein supplements tested were casein, soya-bean meal, and white-fish meal. They were fed so as to achieve a final concentration of 16 per cent of crude protein in the dry matter of the diet. Each protein was given both dry as part of the concentrate mixture and as a liquid suspension. It was recognized that the level of 16 per cent was insufficient to allow maximal protein retention and below the requirements for growth of lambs of this weight. The results were striking in that there was a significantly greater nitrogen retention and lower urinary nitrogen excretion in the lambs that had the protein in liquid form. They also had a significantly higher weight-gain. In terms of the value of the different proteins given, the body-weight gain was greater with white-fish meal than with casein or soya-bean meal, whichever method of feeding was adopted. It was calculated that the improvement in retention of the protein supplement that occurred by giving it in liquid suspension was 31 per cent with casein, 27 per cent for fish meal, and 24 per cent for soya-bean meal.

Some more recent experiments (Ørskov, Fraser, and Corse, 1971) have added further to our understanding of this matter. It has been known for many years (Egan, 1965) that the voluntary intake of low nitrogen roughage is increased as a result of infusing casein into the duodenum of the mature sheep. This effect could not be explained as a result of greater quantity of endogenous nitrogen being recycled to the rumen since urea infusion had little or no effect. The Rowett workers had noted with concentrated diets an increase in voluntary intake by young lambs when the protein concentration of the diet was raised. The problem was to know whether this was due to an alteration in the rate of rumen digestion or to the effect of the protein *per se*. So they gave a rolled barley diet which included urea, vitamin, and mineral supplements and had a 13 per cent crude protein in the dry matter. It was given *ad libitum* to lambs which had been trained to receive milk from a bottle. Water was always available from a trough. They were given varying amounts from 0 to 51 g. of a fish-protein concentrate in 400 ml. of water which provided up to 6·9 g. of nitrogen per day. Another group of lambs received urea in the water to give 4·6 g. of nitrogen per day. They found that there was no difference between the lambs receiving only water and those receiving the urea in the water, but there was an increase in intake due to the protein supplementation amounting to about 15 per cent. There were no differences that were significant between the levels of fish supplementation. In other words, regardless of the rumen fermentation the protein intake of the young, fast-growing lamb has an effect on voluntary intake. As they say, in this respect the ruminant does not appear to behave differently to the non-ruminant animal. A most valuable summary of these interesting ideas about the part played by microbial nitrogen and dietary sources of nitrogen in the young ruminant is to be found in an article by Ørskov (1970) which was a contribution to the Fourth Nutrition Conference at Nottingham.

Formalin-treated Proteins.—Another carefully monitored and relatively large-scale experiment with varying protein levels fed to cross-bred lambs has just been published by Weston (1971). All the lambs were fed a basic pelleted diet composed of lucerne hay 40 parts, wheaten hay 10 parts, maize 30 parts, maize starch 20 parts, and minerals to give optimum input. Three diets of varying protein content were prepared by adding 0, 5, or 10 parts of formalin-treated casein to the basic ingredients. The diets contained on a dry-matter basis 11·7, 15·8, and 19·9 per cent crude protein respectively. The intake of the food was measured in all lambs and some 12 lambs of the 36 involved in the experiment were selected for digestion experiments and had fistulae inserted into their abomasa and into the intestines. By the use of suitable markers it was possible to monitor the flow of ingesta from the stomach and along the intestines and a large series of measurements was made.

The upshot of the work was that the lambs on the low-protein diet hardly increased their voluntary food intake at all during the experimental period, while the lambs getting the protein at the medium or high level both significantly increased their voluntary food intake, although there was no significant difference between the small increase attained by those on the highest level of protein. It was concluded that the optimum ratio between the digestible crude protein and the digestible organic matter of the diet for growing sheep of this age was approximately 18 g. of digestible crude protein per 100 g. of organic matter. This was another way of expressing the medium level of protein in the diet of 15·8 per cent. It proved adequate for the expression of maximum voluntary food intake. Any concentration of protein beyond this was unnecessary under *ad libitum* feeding and only increased urine excretion of nitrogen.

A useful summary of the present situation of feeding the very early weaned lamb by people at the Grassland Research Institute most closely associated with this method of intensifying fat lamb production has been published during the past year (Spedding, Treacher, and Penning, 1970). Under present conditions it has to be dampening in the final section where the economic viewpoint is confronted. Major costs and the value of the product are out of balance. At current values one has to minimize all costs, particularly those related to the high-price foods used in the early life of the lamb.

Pig Nutrition

The results of two co-ordinated trials have been published during the past year, the first being concerned with the way sows are fed during pregnancy and lactation. It involved seven research and teaching centres and involved 154 sows (Elsley and others, 1971). For a number of years there has been a difference of opinion upon whether it is better to feed pregnant sows at a higher level at the beginning of pregnancy than at the end, or to feed at a higher level just before farrowing. No general pattern has been agreed. This experiment compared the effect of feeding four different patterns of feed intake during pregnancy upon the reproductive performance of the sows. A balanced diet of 220 kg. was fed throughout the gestation to all sows. It was given either as a constant amount of 1·9 kg. per sow per day; a low/high system of 1·4 kg. for the first 3 weeks, gradually increasing throughout the pregnancy until at the 15th week it had reached 2·5 kg.; a high/low system which began by feeding at 2·5 kg., dropping during most of the pregnancy feeding to 1·8 kg. a day; and a final pattern of a high/low/high consisting of 2·5 kg. to begin with, dropping to 1·4 kg. during most of the pregnancy, and gradually increasing to 2·5 kg. again at the end.

During the lactation all the sows were given a daily ration of 3·7 kg. of feed for litters of 5 pigs or less and 0·4 kg. for each additional piglet. At most centres it was possible to have the sows given the same nutritional régime for three parities. The upshot was that although the pattern of feed intake slightly affected the live-weight changes of the sows during the course of pregnancy, the treatments had no significant affect on overall change in weight of the sows, either in pregnancy or lactation in any of the three parities. The live-weights of the sows at the end of the third parity were similar for all treatment groups. The feeding régimes had no appreciable or significant affect on the numbers of pigs born, their average weight at birth, or on the number of pigs that survived to weaning at 6 weeks, or their live-weight. The health and breeding regularity of the sows were also unaffected by the treatments. This is a very interesting vindication of the belief that it is not important how the sows are fed during their pregnancy. It is important to have a level which allows the sow slightly to increase its body-weight and, of course, to have the ration properly balanced.

The other co-ordinated trial was a very large-scale one organized by the A.R.C. in co-operation with many farms (Braude and Lerman, 1970). It involved twenty-one centres. Its purpose was to discover whether the addition of synthetic lysine to a 'standard' ration which is widely used in this country had any beneficial effect upon the performance of growing pigs. This standard ration contained less crude protein and total lysine than the levels recommended in the A.R.C. *Nutrient Requirement of Pigs*. The 'standard' ration consisted of 7 per cent fish meal, supplying 16·2 per cent crude protein, and 0·72 per cent total lysine, reducing to 14 per cent crude protein and 0·57 per cent total lysine in the second half of the growth period, compared with 17·6 per cent crude protein and 0·82 per cent total lysine of the A.R.C. recommended ration, reducing to 15 per cent crude protein and 0·64 per cent total lysine in the second half of the growth period. At each of the twenty-one centres, 9–11-week-old pigs were allocated to the four experimental treatments at random, except that initial weight, sex, and litter distribution were equalized as far as possible. The pigs were weighed once weekly and were fed wet, twice daily, according to live-weight and to scale. As soon as possible after a pig exceeded 89·5 kg. (197 lb.) live-weight at the weekly weighing it was dispatched for slaughter. On the day of dispatch the pig was weighed at a specified time and a similar slaughter régime was followed at each of the slaughterhouses. Carcass measurements were taken according to another prescribed routine.

The result of this elaborate trial was to establish that the standard ration produced slightly lower performance but about the same profit. The performance of the pigs on the standard ration could be improved by the addition of synthetic lysine, but such supplementation would not be profitable unless the cost of synthetic lysine was less than £1·05 per kg. The response to the added synthetic lysine was similar on rations in which the source of supplementary protein was either white-fish meal or soya-bean meal.

Growth Additives.—Braude, Mitchell, and Pittman (1970) examined the usefulness of Payzone (a guanidine derivative produced by Cyanamid of Great Britain Ltd.) as a supplement in relation to the known growth-promoting power of copper at 250 p.p.m. of the diet. They found that the daily live-weight gain and the feed per gain ratio were significantly and similarly improved by supplementation with either copper sulphate or Payzone. When both supplements were added to the diet the performance was further improved, and indeed was significantly better than that obtained with either supplement alone. This is of interest because when the synergistic effect of adding antibiotics and copper sulphate was tried some years ago there was no better growth response than with copper sulphate alone.

Zinc and Sex.—The fact that barrows, gilts, and, of course, boars grow at different rates and convert food with different efficiencies has been known for some time. A study has been made by a team at Michigan last year of sex influence upon the zinc requirement of growing pigs (Liptrap and others, 1970). They took 45 boars and the same number of barrows and gilts and randomly allotted them in two experiments where they received dietary zinc levels varying from 22 to 80 p.p.m. The dietary calcium intake was maintained at 0·7 per cent of the diet. All the pigs were fed and watered *ad libitum*. They found that the symptoms of zinc deficiency included reduced weight-gains, reduced feed consumption, as well as alterations in various blood constituents. Parakeratosis also appeared in a third of the boars and 27 per cent of the gilts when the level of zinc dropped to 30 p.p.m. There was no parakeratosis observed in the barrows at this level.

Oil-grown Yeast Supplementation.—There have been many newspaper reports of the growing of yeast upon crude-oil derivatives, with the hope expressed that the high-protein feed produced would offer an alternative to expensive fish meal or oil-seed meals in the feeding of livestock. The first account of the value of this hydrocarbon-grown yeast for growing pigs has just been published (Barber and others, 1971). The yeast, grown on normal paraffins (B.P. Proteins Ltd.), contained 62 per cent crude protein. Except for a lower content of methionine, its amino-acid content was similar to that of white-fish meal. They conducted two experiments: a feeding trial covering the live-weight range from 20 to 90 kg., and a metabolic trial in which the pigs were between 20 and 60 kg. live-weight, to study the extent of nitrogen retention and digestibility. They fed the two protein supplements of yeast plus methionine and white-fish meal at the standard level commonly used in practice, i.e., 7 per cent of white-fish meal for pigs up to 60 kg. live-weight, reducing to 3·5 per cent for pigs over 60 kg. to slaughter. The two protein supplements supplied the same amount of total nitrogen.

They found there was a small but significant difference in favour of the yeast treatment for growth-rate and feed-conversion ratio, but there was no consistent difference in the measurements of the carcasses due to the protein source. In the metabolic trial they found no significant difference in terms of performance, nitrogen retention, apparent nitrogen digestibility, or linear carcass measurements. It therefore appears that the new yeast protein with additional methionine is at least as good and possibly a better source of high-quality protein for growing and fattening pigs. The only point becomes that of cost.

REFERENCES

AGRICULTURAL RESEARCH COUNCIL (1967), *Nutrient Requirement of Farm Livestock, No. 3, Pigs*. London.
ANON. (1970), *N.A.A.S. Newsletter* 1970, No. 1, p. 4.
BADGER, G. D. (1970), *Experimental Husbandry, Farms and Experimental Horticultural Stations, 11th Progress Report*, p. 81. London: H.M.S.O.
BANNERMAN, M. M., and BLAXTER, K. L. (ed.) (1969) *The Husbanding of Red Deer*. Aberdeen University Press.
BARBER, R. S., BRAUDE, R., and MITCHELL, K. G. (1960), *Br. J. Nutr.*, **14**, 499.
— — — — — — and MYRES, A. W. (1971), *Ibid.*, **25**, 285.
BLAXTER, K. L. (1970), *Proc. Nutr. Soc.*, **29**, 244.
BOLTON, W. (1970), *Ibid.*, **29**, 253.
BORSTLAP, C. W. R. Z. (1968), Paper for *2nd Wld. Congr. Anim. Prod. Md.*
BRAUDE, R. (1970), *Proc. Nutr. Soc.*, **29**, 262.
— — and FOOT, A. S. (1942), *J. agric. Sci., Camb.*, **32**, 70.
— — and LERMAN, P. (1970), *Ibid.*, **74**, 575.
— — MITCHELL, K. G., NEWPORT, M. J., and PITTMAN, R. J. (1970), *Proc. Nutr. Soc.*, **29**, 10A.
— — — — and PITTMAN, R. J. (1970), *Ibid.*, **30**, 11A.
— — — — and ROBINSON, K. L. (1950), *J. agric. Sci., Camb.*, **40**, 84.
CARTWRIGHT, T. C. (1970), *J. Anim. Sci.*, **30**, 706.
CLARK, C. (1970), in *Change in Agriculture* (ed. BUNTING, A. H.), p. 11. London: Butterworth.
CLAUDIAN, J., and SERVILLE, Y. (1968), *Cah. Nutr. Diet.*, **3**, 29.
COPEMAN, G. (1971), *Grass To-day*, No. 10, p. 3.
CRABTREE, J. R. (1970), *J. Br. Grassld Soc.*, **26**, 63.
CUNDIFF, L. V. (1970), *J. Anim. Sci.*, **30**, 694.
DASMANN, R. F. (1963), *African Game Ranching*. Oxford: Pergamon.
DIRKS, (1926), *Conservation of Grasses and Forage Crops*, p. 288. Edinburgh: Oliver and Boyd.
EGAN, A. R. (1965), *Aust. J. agric. Res.*, **16**, 451.
ELSLEY, F. W. H., BATHURST, E. V. J., BRACEWELL, A. G., CUNNINGHAM, J. M. M., DENT, J. B., DODSWORTH, T. L., MACPHERSON, R. M., and WALKER, N. (1971), *Anim. Prod.*, **13**, 257.
FOOD AND AGRICULTURAL ORGANIZATION (1969), *St. Fd Agric.*
HENDERSON, A. R., and MACDONALD, P. (1971), *J. Sci. Fd Agric.*, **22**, 157.
HILL FARMING RESEARCH ORGANISATION (1969–70), *Fifth Report*. Edinburgh.
HINKS, C. J. M. (1970a), *Anim. Prod.*, **12**, 569.
— — (1970b), *Ibid.*, **12**, 577.
HOLMES, W. (1970), *Proc. Nutr. Soc.*, **29**, 237.
KAY, R. N. B. (1970), *Ibid.*, **29**, 271.
VON LA CHEVALLERIE, M. (1970), *Proc. S. Afr. Soc. Anim. Prod.*, in the press.
LIPTRAP, D. O., MILLER, E. R., ULLREY, D. E., WHITENAK, D. L., SCHOEPKE, B. L., and LUECKE, R. W. (1970), *J. Anim. Sci.*, **30**, 736.
MINISTRY OF AGRICULTURE, FISHERIES, AND FOOD: NATIONAL FOOD SURVEY COMMITTEE (1969), *Household Food Consumption and Expenditure*, 1967, with a supplement giving Preliminary Estimates for 1968. London: H.M.S.O.
MASON, I. L. (1971), *Anim. Breed. Abstr.*, **39**, 1.
MEAT AND LIVESTOCK COMMISSION (1971), *Beef Improvement*. Scientific Study Group Report.
MORAN, J. B. (1970a), *J. agric. Sci., Camb.*, **74**, 315.
— — (1970b), *Ibid.*, **74**, 323.
NATURE CONSERVANCY (1967), *Red Deer Research in Scotland: Progress Report* 1. Edinburgh.
ØRSKOV, E. R. (1970), *Proc. 4th Nutr. Conf. Fd Manrs* (ed. SWAN, H., and LEWIS, D.). London: Churchill.
— — and BENZIE, D. (1969), *Br. J. Nutr.*, **23**, 415.
— — and FRASER, C. (1969), *Proc. Nutr. Soc.*, **28**, 55A.

ØRSKOV, E. R., FRASER, C., and CORSE, ELIZABETH L. (1970), *Br. J. Nutr.*, **24**, 803.
— — — — — — (1971), *Proc. Nutr. Soc.*, **30**, 25A.
PIRIE, N. W. (1969), *Ibid.*, **28**, 85.
RAYMOND, W. F. (1971a), *Grass To-day*, No. 10, p. 20.
— — (1971b), *Ibid.*, No. 10, p. 55.
ROY, J. H. B. (1970), *Proc. 4th Nutr. Conf. Fd. Manrs* (ed. SWAN, H., and LEWIS, D.). London: Churchill.
SKINNER, J. D. (1970), *Trop. Anim. Hlth Prod.*, **2**, 151.
SOLLER, M., BAR-ANAN, R., and PASTERNAK, H. (1966), *Anim. Prod.*, **8**, 109.
SPEDDING, C. R. W., TREACHER, T. T., and PENNING, P. D. (1970), *Proc. 4th Nutr. Conf. Fd Manrs* (ed. SWAN, H., and LEWIS, D.). London: Churchill.
WATSON, J. N. (1971), *Grass To-day*, No. 10, p. 13.
WESTON, R. H. (1971), *Aust. J. agric. Res.*, **22**, 307.
WILLIAMS, D. O. (1971), *Experimental Husbandry Farms and Experimental Horticultural Stations, 11th Progress Report*, p. 73. London: H.M.S.O.
WOODFORD, E. K. (1971), *J. Br. Grassld Soc.*, **26**, 1.

THE HUSBANDRY OF LABORATORY ANIMALS

Roger Ewbank, B.V.Sc., M.R.C.V.S.

The veterinary surgeon with his training and experience in animal surgery, disease, husbandry, and anaesthesia would seem to be well equipped to provide a technical service not only to assist the scientific investigator at the experimental level but also to plan and maintain reliable laboratory animal production units. Until recently this service has been little asked for or offered. Nowadays, however, a growing number of veterinarians are beginning to take a full or part responsibility for the health, welfare, productivity, and use of laboratory animals.

It is difficult to get a reliable estimate of the present involvement of the profession with this type of work, but there are a few relevant facts which can be quoted. At the time (1963–5) of the inquiries made by the Departmental Committee on Experiments on Animals (Littlewood Committee), the results of a private survey indicated that more than 100 veterinary surgeons in private practice were being regularly consulted about the health, etc., of laboratory animals. In 1963 the British Laboratory Animal Veterinary Association, a professional group limited in membership to veterinarians, was started and soon attracted some 60 or so members, a number which has remained fairly constant over the years. The Laboratory Animal Science Association was founded in the U.K. in 1964 with 132 members (12 per cent of whom were veterinarians) and this has increased to 316 in 1970 (18 per cent of whom are veterinary surgeons).

A number of contributions to the veterinary journals support the case that the veterinary profession has become more involved with the care and management of laboratory animals. There is a paper by Stevenson (1963) on the role of the veterinarian in laboratory animal medicine and an editorial and a review (Anon., 1965a, b) covering the Report of the Littlewood Committee together with a resulting series of letters in the correspondence column of the *Veterinary Record* (**77**, 768, 825, 888, 911, 969, 970, and 1030). A symposium on the implications of the increasing importance of laboratory animals for the veterinary profession (Bleby, 1966; Paterson, 1966; Seamer,

1966) was held at the British Veterinary Association's 1966 Congress and was published together with the resulting discussion in the *Veterinary Record* for that year. A letter in the *Veterinary Record* (Ewbank, 1970) on laboratory animal husbandry in the undergraduate veterinary curriculum stimulated further correspondence (**87**, 670, 700, 764, 812, and **88**, 26) on professional education in laboratory animal science.

This increase in veterinary involvement with laboratory animal science will probably continue as a result of pressure from both outside the profession as the number of animal experiments per year increases, and it is realized that the veterinarian has much to contribute to the health, welfare, productivity, and efficient utilization of laboratory animals, and from inside the profession as it becomes recognized that laboratory animal production and care can be a rewarding use of professional knowledge and skill. A considerable boost to professional commitment to laboratory animal science would probably result if the recommendations of the Littlewood Committee (Report, 1965) are ever implemented. Whether this increase will match that which has occurred in the United States is, however, open to dispute. In that country it has been predicted that by 1975 there may be as many veterinarians engaged in laboratory animal medicine as are working in farm livestock practice (Pritchard, 1966).

'Quality' in Laboratory Animals

Nowadays it is being increasingly realized that precise experimental methods need animals which are defined just as much in their disease (or absence of disease) status as in their genetic form (Bleby, 1970). Schemes have been set up for the production and testing of animals of standard genetic make up and varying degrees of absence of intercurrent disease (Laboratory Animals Centre 1969; Townsend, 1969; Parrott and Festing, 1971). This approach to the production of relatively disease-free stock demands that the husbandry system should be designed from the start with disease control in mind (Jonas, 1965; Ruys, 1969). The veterinarian may, by training and outlook, be the person who can most readily design and supervise this kind of enterprise. In some ways laboratory animal production systems could be an ideal teaching model for veterinary preventive medicine.

Training in Laboratory Animal Husbandry

The main core of the veterinary syllabus, pathology (in its widest meaning), is probably a sufficient base upon which the average veterinarian can, if necessary, build for himself a knowledge of the pathological aspects, diagnosis, and control of laboratory animal disease. The chief limiting factor to his efficient utilization of this knowledge might be his limited acquaintance with the husbandry of the laboratory animals. Information on laboratory animal husbandry should, ideally, first be made available at the undergraduate level (Ewbank, 1970) in the form of a short course of lectures and practical classes on the husbandry of, say, mouse, rat, guinea-pig, hamster, rabbit, and quail. If given after the extensive nutrition, housing, genetics, and breeding sections of the main animal husbandry course it can act as an adequate introduction both to laboratory animal husbandry itself and to the veterinarians' career possibilities in laboratory animal science. A side benefit of a course of this nature is that future research workers become acquainted, at an early stage of their careers, with the care and management of the laboratory species. It can be argued that an accurate knowledge of the characteristics and welfare of the laboratory animal can be just as important to the success of a research project as an appreciation of the workings of bench apparatus.

A further advantage of instruction in laboratory animal care could be that the broadening of the veterinary undergraduate curriculum to cover species other than the traditional horse, ox, sheep, pig, dog, cat, and fowl could make the immediate postgraduate worker better able to cope with problems in general biological research and in the diseases of exotic pets, zoo, and wild animals.

This undergraduate introductory coverage must, of course, be supplemented by a self-imposed, 'in-job' training supported by studying the extensive literature available, and wherever possible by the taking of appropriate postgraduate degree or diploma courses.*

Literature on Laboratory Animal Husbandry, etc.

The published material is very extensive. Useful annoted bibliographies (with indexes) of the literature on the production, care, and use of laboratory animals up to 1962 have been prepared by Cass, Campbell, and Lange (1960, 1963). Lengthy lists of books, monographs, pamphlets, and collected papers on all aspects of laboratory animal production, health, and care are given in the U.S. Public Health Service Publication No. 1024 (1968) *Guide for Laboratory Animal Facilities and Care* and in the International Committee on Laboratory Animals Bulletin No. 20 (March, 1971). The four key texts in English, however, are probably *The U.F.A.W. Handbook on the Care and Management of Laboratory Animals* (U.F.A.W., 1967), *Animals for Research—Principles of Breeding and Management* (Lane-Petter, 1963), *The I.A.T. Manual of Laboratory Animal Practice and Techniques* (Short and Woodnott, 1969), and *The Principles of Humane Experimental Technique* (Russell and Burch, 1959). The best way to keep up with the scientific literature is probably to systematically look through current issues of the following English language journals: *Laboratory Animal Science* (formerly *Laboratory Animal Care*, published by the American Association for Laboratory Animal Science), *Journal of the Institute of Laboratory Animal Technicians* (published by the U.K. Institute of Laboratory Animal Technicians), and *Laboratory Animals* (published on behalf of the U.K. Laboratory Animal Association). This last publication conveniently lists the contents of other laboratory animal science journals—notably *Laboratory Animal Science*, *Expérimentation Animale* and *Zeitschrift für Versuchstierkunde*. *The Journal of Small Animal Practice* has started including, about every third month, a useful annotated list of laboratory animal literature compiled by a member of the Medical Research Council's Laboratory Animal Centre. The latest news and developments in the laboratory animal world are probably most easily followed in the twice-yearly *News Letter of the (U.K.) Laboratory Animal Centre*, in the twice-yearly *Bulletin of the International Committee on Laboratory Animals*, and in the (U.S.) Institute of Laboratory Animal Resource's *I.L.A.R. News*, which is published four times a year.

The veterinary surgeon has much to contribute to the welfare and productivity of laboratory animals. It would be a great pity if the profession failed to realize its potential in this increasingly important field. It is hoped

---

* The Royal Veterinary College (University of London) has an M.Sc. course in laboratory animal science in the advanced planning stage.

that this paper does, at least, indicate (1) the profession's increasing involvement with laboratory animal science, (2) its special contribution to the subject, (3) the importance of professional education in laboratory animal husbandry, and (4) routes of access to the extensive literature.

REFERENCES

ANON. (1965a), *Vet. Rec.*, **77**, 579.

— (1965b), *Ibid.*, **77**, 580.

BLEBY, J. (1966), *Ibid.*, **79**, 869.

— — (1970), *Veterinary Annual*, 11th Issue, p. 140. Bristol: Wright.

CASS, J. S., CAMPBELL, I. R., and LANGE, L. L. (1960), *Fed. Proc. Fedn Am. Socs exp. Biol.*, **19**, No. 4, Part 3. (Suppl. 6.)

— — — — — — (1963), *Ibid.*, **22**, No. 2, Part 3. (Suppl. No. 13.)

EWBANK, R. (1970), *Vet. Rec.*, **87**, 637.

JONAS, A. M. (1965), *J. Am. vet. med. Ass.*, **146**, 600.

LABORATORY ANIMALS CENTRE (1969), L.A.C. Manual Series, No. 1, London.

LANE-PETTER, W. (ed.) (1963), *Animals for Research—Principles of Breeding and Management*. New York: Academic.

PARROTT, R. F., and FESTING, M. F. W. (1971), L.A.C. Manual Series, No. 2, London.

PATERSON, J. S. (1966), *Vet. Rec.*, **79**, 864.

PRITCHARD, W. R. (1966), *Can. vet. J.*, **7**, 55.

REPORT (1965), *Report of the Departmental Committee on Experiments on Animals*, Cmnd. 2641. London: H.M.S.O.

RUSSELL, W. M. S., and BURCH, R. L. (1959), *The Principles of Humane Experimental Technique*. London: Methuen.

RUYS, T. (1969), *Lab. Anim. Care*, **19**, 489.

SEAMER, J. (1966), *Vet. Rec.*, **79**, 874.

SHORT, D. J., and WOODNOTT, D. P. (eds.) (1969), *The I.A.T. Manual of Laboratory Animal Practice and Techniques*, 2nd ed. London: Crosby Lockwood.

STEVENSON, D. E. (1963), *Vet. Rec.*, **75**, 1188.

TOWNSEND, G. H. (1969), *Ibid.*, **85**, 225.

UNIVERSITIES FEDERATION FOR ANIMAL WELFARE (1967), *The U.F.A.W. Handbook on the Care and Management of Laboratory Animals*, 3rd ed. Edinburgh: Livingstone.

NEW DRUGS AND APPLIANCES

RECENT PHARMACEUTICAL PREPARATIONS, APPLIANCES, ETC.

In this Section we give short descriptions of new Drugs and Appliances of the past year. It should be understood that the information is supplied by the Makers. We invite all those concerned with the Veterinary Manufacturing Industries to co-operate with us in making this Section valuable for present and permanent reference.

NEW DRUGS

Aureomycin 2000.—A highly soluble powder formulation of Aureomycin chlortetracycline hydrochloride specifically designed for administration to poultry at high concentration in the drinking water. Each 150 g. contain 30 g. (20 per cent) chlortetracycline hydrochloride in a stabilizing fungistatic base. Indicated as an aid in prevention and for the treatment of the following diseases: Respiratory, enteric, and systemic infections of monovalent or mixed aetiology caused by mycoplasmas, *E. coli*, and other sensitive bacteria. Dose: 1 jar (150 g.) per 15 gal. (68·19 litres) drinking water providing a stable concentrate of 2 g. chlortetracycline hydrochloride per gallon. Pack: 6 × 150 g. jars. (Agricultural Division, Cyanamid of Great Britain Ltd., Gosport, Hampshire.)

Aurex Liquid.—Contains: neomycin sulphate 0·5 per cent, sulphacetamide 9·0 per cent, sodium octoate 10·0 per cent, sevin 1·0 per cent, and tetracaine hydrochloride 0·5 per cent. For the treatment of otitis externa and otoacariasis. Pack: 12 ml. and 22 ml. (Smith Kline & French Laboratories Ltd., Welwyn Garden City, Hertfordshire.)

Aurofac MA.—A soluble formulation of Aureomycin chlortetracycline hydrochloride for addition directly to liquid milk or reconstituted milk-replacer on the farm, or for incorporation in dried milk or milk-replacer products either on the farm or at the time of manufacture. May also be given in a small volume of liquid as a drench. Each 0·5 kg. additive contains 100 g. chlortetracycline hydrochloride. Indicated for the treatment and prevention of bacterial enteritis and of primary or secondary bacterial pneumonia; for the control of bacterial infections during periods of stress. Dose: 3·0 g. (approx. 1 teaspoonful) per 100-lb. (45·5-kg.) calf daily or per 1 lb. dried milk or milk-replacer powder; 7·0 kg. (15·5 lb.) per 1 ton dried milk or milk-replacer powder. Dosage may be varied according to severity of the disease. Continue treatment for a period of 5–7 days or until signs of disease are no longer apparent in calves no longer at risk. Not recommended for adult ruminants. Pack: 500 g. and 10 kg. (Agricultural Division, Cyanamid of Great Britain Ltd., Gosport, Hampshire.)

Candizine Tablets.—Each tablet contains: piperazine phosphate 250 mg. For the treatment of roundworm infestations in small animals. Pack: 250 ml. (Smith Kline & French Laboratories Ltd., Welwyn Garden City, Hertfordshire.)

Dinol Injectable.—Each millilitre contains: dienoestrol 5 mg. For the treatment of functionable sterility in cows and mares caused by low oestrogen production. Pack: 10 ml. (Smith Kline & French Laboratories Ltd., Welwyn Garden City, Hertfordshire.)

Emtryl Premix and Emtryl Soluble.—Premix contains 22·5 per cent w/w dimetridazole; Soluble contains 40 per cent w/w dimetridazole. For the prevention and treatment of blackhead in turkeys and the control of swine dysentery. Premix should be used at rate of 2 lb. per ton of feed. Medicated feed should be given after weaning for 4 weeks. For control of swine dysentery medication of drinking water is recommended. Soluble is given at rate of 1 oz. per 10 gallons of drinking water for 3–7 days. Premix in containers of 2½ and 25 lb.; Soluble in containers of 1 oz., 4 oz., and 1 lb. (Pharmaceutical Specialities (May & Baker) Ltd., Dagenham, Essex.)

Enduracell d.—Live virus vaccine, canine-tissue culture origin. For immunization of healthy dogs against canine distemper. Pack: 10 individual doses. (Smith Kline & French Laboratories Ltd., Welwyn Garden City, Hertfordshire.)

Enduracell dh.—Live virus vaccine, canine-tissue culture origin. For immunization of healthy dogs against canine distemper and hepatitis. Pack: 10 individual doses. (Smith Kline & French Laboratories Ltd., Welwyn Garden City, Hertfordshire.)

Enduracell dhl.—Live virus vaccine, canine-tissue culture origin. Killed *Leptospira canicola* and *icterohaemorrhagiae* vaccine. For immunization of healthy dogs against canine distemper, hepatitis, and leptospirosis. Pack: 10 individual doses. (Smith Kline & French Laboratories Ltd., Welwyn Garden City, Hertfordshire.)

Felocine.—Killed virus vaccine, feline-tissue culture origin. For immunization of healthy cats against feline infectious enteritis (panleucopenia). Pack: 10 individual doses. (Smith Kline & French Laboratories Ltd., Welwyn Garden City, Hertfordshire.)

Fulcin Feed Additive.—A premix containing 10 per cent griseofulvin for the treatment of ringworm in cattle and horses. Available in 3·5-kg. and 1-kg. packs. One-kg. pack contains sufficient additive to treat 5×5-cwt. cattle. (I.C.I. Pharmaceutical Division, Alderley Park, Macclesfield, Cheshire.)

Fungidex Cream.—Contains: zinc undecylenate 12 per cent, undecylenic acid 5 per cent, copper undecylenate 3 per cent, and dichlorophen 2 per cent. A powerful antimycotic agent with anti-pruritic action. Pack: 49 g. (1¾ oz.). (Smith Kline & French Laboratories Ltd., Welwyn Garden City, Hertfordshire.)

Game Bird Wormer.—A formulation containing 10 per cent of tetramisole hydrochloride for treatment of gapesworm and other important roundworms. Administered in the drinking water. Available in packs of 10×34-g. containers. Each container will treat 300 birds of ½ lb. or 150 birds of 1 lb. live weight. (I.C.I. Pharmaceutical Division, Alderley Park, Macclesfield, Cheshire.)

Grofas.—A non-antibiotic growth promoter for pigs and non-laying poultry. Available as 4 per cent quindoxin premix in 5-kg. and 25-kg. sacks. Recommended rates of use are 50 g. of active compound per ton of feed for weaner and grower-pig rations and 20 g. of active compound per ton of feed for fattening pig, broiler, and turkey rations. (I.C.I. Pharmaceutical Division, Alderley Park, Macclesfield, Cheshire.)

Horseguard Antiseptic Healing Cream.—Contains cod liver oil B.P., selected vegetable oils, 0·5 per cent 4-chloro-3:5-xylenol (P.C.M.X.), 0·75 per cent 2:2′-dihydroxy-5:5′-dichlorodiphenyl monosulphide (fenticlor), and 5 per cent zinc oxide. For the treatment of wounds, scratches, scurf, saddle-sores, cracked heels, and all minor skin conditions. Pack: 200-g. containers. (British Cod Liver Oils (Hull and Grimsby) Ltd., Hedon Road, Hull, Yorkshire.)

Horseguard Antiseptic Hoof Oil.—Contains: neatsfoot oil, cod liver oil, castor oil, linseed oil, thin pine tar, 0·5 per cent 4-chloro-3:5-xylenol (P.C.M.X.), and 0·75 per cent 2:2′-dihydroxy-5:5′-dichlorodiphenyl monosulphide (fenticlor). For the treatment of brittle hooves, sand cracks, corns, seedy toe, thrush, canker, and all fungal and bactericidal infections of the hoof. Improvement of healthy growth of horn of the wall and frog. Pack: 1-pint tins, 1-gallon tins, and 5-gallon drums. (British Cod Liver Oils (Hull and Grimsby) Ltd., Hedon Road, Hull, Yorkshire.)

Horseguard Antiseptic Hoof Ointment.—Contains neatsfoot oil, cod liver oil, castor oil, linseed oil, thin pine tar, 0·5 per cent 4-chloro-3:5-xylenol (P.C.M.X.), and 0·75 per cent 2:2′-dihydroxy-5:5′-dichlorodiphenyl monosulphide (fenticlor). For the treatment of thrush, sand crack, and other minor conditions of the hoof and frog in horses and ponies, also hoof conditions involving fungal and bacterial attack. Pack: 200-g. containers. (British Cod Liver Oils (Hull and Grimsby) Ltd., Hedon Road, Hull, Yorkshire.)

Horseguard Nutritional Supplement and Health Conditioning Oil.—Supplies the important principles of selected vegetable oils, wheat-germ oil, and cod-liver oil and a balanced range of polyunsaturated glycerides. Contains: vitamin A 76,000 I.U. per 100 g., vitamin D 7600 I.U. per 100 g., vitamin E 100 I.U. per 100 g., linoleate 15 per cent, docosahexaenoate 7 per cent, and eicosapentaenoate 8 per cent. Total polyunsaturates 34 per cent. For the promotion of healthy skin and coat condition, healthy joints, strong teeth, and bones. Builds natural resistance to disease. Particularly effective in encouraging a healthy, natural, glossy, and protective coat on all horses and ponies. Pack: 1-pint tins, 1-gallon tins, and 5-gallon drums. (British Cod Liver Oils (Hull and Grimsby) Ltd., Hedon Road, Hull, Yorkshire.)

Kaogel.—For all scours, diarrhoeas, and enteritis. Contains 3 g. kaolin providing adsorption, protection for the intestinal mucosa, increases faecal bulk. Pectin 65 mg. per

15 ml. is supposed to render the colonic environment hostile to the growth of pathogens. Simple to use alone or in combination. Big 4-litre pack has ample space to allow addition of any water-soluble antibiotic. Available in plastic containers of 150 ml., 360 ml., and 4 litres. (Parke, Davis & Co., Pontypool, Monmouthshire.)

Lept ci.—Killed *Leptospira canicola* and *icterohaemorrhagiae* vaccine. For immunization of healthy dogs against canine leptospirosis. Pack: 10 individual doses. (Smith Kline & French Laboratories Ltd., Welwyn Garden City, Hertfordshire.)

Micralax Micro-enema.—Each dispenser contains: sodium citrate 450 mg., sodium alkyl sulphoacetate 45 mg., and sorbic acid 5 mg. For use where an enema is necessary. Pack: 12 dispensers. (Smith Kline & French Laboratories Ltd., Welwyn Garden City, Hertfordshire.)

Nemicide.—A 7·5 per cent injectable solution of levamisole hydrochloride for treatment and control of lungworm and stomach and bowel worms—including *Nematodirus*—in cattle and sheep. Available in 500-ml. bottles. One bottle contains sufficient doses for 25×4-cwt. cattle or 166×75-lb. sheep. (I.C.I. Pharmaceutical Division, Alderley Park, Macclesfield, Cheshire.)

Netrosylla.—Broad-spectrum antimycotic for the topical treatment of ringworm in horses, dogs, and cats. The active ingredient is 10 per cent Etisazole solution which is diluted with water in the ratio of 1 : 10 and then applied topically to the affected areas daily for 3–5 consecutive days. Healing of the lesions occurs from a few days to three weeks after the last application of the product. Has a fungicidal action against *Trichophyton, Microsporum, Aspergillus, Candida*, and *Torulopsis* species. It is also effective against *Penicillium commune, Mucor mucedo, Blakeslea trispora*, and *Saccharomyces cerevisiae*. In addition, it has antibacterial activity against Gram-positive and Gram-negative bacteria, except *Pseudomonas, Proteus, Klebsiella*, and *Mycobacterium* species. (Bayer Agrochem Ltd., Eastern Way, Bury St Edmunds, Suffolk.)

Nilverm in-feed Wormer.—A feed additive containing 2·5 per cent levamisole hydrochloride for routine control of roundworms in cattle and sheep. Available in 900-g. packs—one pack will dose 15×4-cwt. cattle or 120×60-lb. sheep. (I.C.I. Pharmaceutical Division, Alderley Park, Macclesfield, Cheshire.)

Nilverm Injection.—A 7·5 per cent solution of levamisole hydrochloride for treatment and control of lungworm and stomach and bowel worms—including *Nematodirus*—in cattle and sheep. Available in 500-ml. packs, designed for use with the I.C.I. Superjector. One pack contains sufficient doses for 25×4-cwt. cattle or 166×75-lb. sheep. (I.C.I. Pharmaceutical Division, Alderley Park, Macclesfield, Cheshire.)

Nilzan in-feed Wormer.—A feed additive containing 2·5 per cent levamisole hydrochloride and 5 per cent oxyclozanide for routine control of roundworms and fluke in cattle and sheep. Available in 900-g. packs—one pack will dose 15×4-cwt. cattle or 120×60-lb. sheep. (I.C.I. Pharmaceutical Division, Alderley Park, Macclesfield, Cheshire.)

Norderm.—Each millilitre contains: total unsaturated fatty acids 729 mg., lecithins (source of choline) 10·8 mg., vitamin A 230 I.U., vitamin D_2, 54 I.U., polyoxyethylene sorbitan mono-oleate 3·0 mg., and sorbitan mono-oleate 37·0 mg. For the prevention and treatment of skin and coat conditions in small animals caused by diets deficient in unsaturated fatty acids. Pack: 133 ml. and 3·8 litres. (Smith Kline & French Laboratories Ltd., Welwyn Garden City, Hertfordshire.)

'Nortran' Tablets.—Each tablet contains: trifluomeprazine (as the maleate) 10 mg. For stress conditions in small animals where a tranquillizer is indicated. Pack: 250. (Smith Kline & French Laboratories Ltd., Welwyn Garden City, Hertfordshire.)

Paracide Capsules.—Each capsule contains: dichlorophen 125 mg.–4·0 g. and toluene 150 mg.–4·8 g. For the removal of ascarids and hookworms and an aid to removal of tapeworms in dogs. Pack: 25, 50, and 100. (Smith Kline & French Laboratories Ltd., Welwyn Garden City, Hertfordshire.)

Parentrovite Multidose Injection.—A highly concentrated injectable preparation of the B-complex vitamins, together with vitamin C, in ready-to-use 50-ml. multidose vials, for intravenous or intramuscular administration. Action depends on a rapid increase of the intracellular concentrations of the B-complex, where stress, toxic, or deficiency conditions have interfered with normal cell metabolism, or in conditions of increased demand for detoxication. Ascorbic acid is concerned in all reactions associated with physiological stress. (Beecham Veterinary Products, Beecham House, Brentford, Middlesex.)

Penbritin Soluble Powder.—Specifically for use in poultry disease in a stabilized form to add to drinking water. Indicated for the treatment of bacterial infections due to susceptible Gram-positive and Gram-negative organisms. In bottles containing 5·5 g. of ampicillin. (Beecham Veterinary Products, Beecham House, Brentford, Middlesex.)

Pragmatar Shampoo.—Contains: cetyl alcohol–coal tar distillate 0·5 per cent, lauryl isoquinolinium bromide 0·2 per cent, and hexachlorophene 2·0 per cent. For the treatment of a wide range of skin disorders. Pack: 177 ml. and 3·8 litres. (Smith Kline & French Laboratories Ltd., Welwyn Garden City, Hertfordshire.)

Rabiffa Rabies Vaccine (Inactivated).—A novel type of inactivated vaccine produced by tissue-cell culture. It possesses high antigenicity and is free from anaphylactic and toxic side-effects. For use in all carnivores including domestic dogs and cats and wild Canidae and Felidae. (Pharmaceutical Specialities (May & Baker) Ltd., Dagenham, Essex.)

Ranizole.—A drench containing thiabendazole B. Vet. C. and rafoxanide, for the treatment and control of mixed infestations of gastro-intestinal nematodes and liver fluke in sheep and cattle. Supplied in 1050-ml. or 4·2-litre bottles. (Merck Sharp & Dohme Ltd., Hertford Road, Hoddesdon, Hertfordshire.)

Rompun Dry Substance.—A sedative and analgesic for horses and certain species of zoo animals. The active ingredient is Xylazine which is presented as a powder for dissolving in distilled water to make an injectable solution of either 5 or 10 per cent. Indicated in all cases where sedation is required including the handling of fractious animals, medical examinations, treatment, and for transporting animals. For major surgery additional anaesthesia should be used. Contra-indicated in the last month of pregnancy except at the time of parturition. The dose-rate in the horse is 2·0 mg. per kg. body-weight by intramuscular injection. The maximum effect is produced within 15 minutes of injection. In zoo animals the dose-rate varies according to species and the degree of wildness. The full effect is usually obtained within 20–30 minutes of injection. (Bayer Agrochem Ltd., Eastern Way, Bury St. Edmunds, Suffolk.)

Sulkamycin—S Bolettes.—Each bolette contains: sulphadimidine 2·0 g., phthalylsulphacetamide 1·0 g., neomycin sulphate 250 mg., and powdered ext. belladonna (equivalent to 0·2 mg. belladonna alkaloids) 16·0 mg. For the treatment of the bacterial pneumonia/enteritis complex in calves and other young animals. Pack: Strip pack 50, and bulk pack 50. (Smith Kline & French Laboratories Ltd., Welwyn Garden City, Hertfordshire.)

Sulkamycin—S Powder.—Each 28 g. contains: sulphadimidine 8·0 g., phthalylsulphacetamide 4·0 g., powdered ext. belladonna (equivalent to 0·7 mg. belladonna alkaloids) 64 mg., neomycin sulphate 1·0 g., and kaolin+base to 28 g. For the treatment of the bacterial pneumonia/enteritis complex in calves and other young animals. Pack: 2 oz. and 1 lb. (Smith Kline & French Laboratories Ltd., Welwyn Garden City, Hertfordshire.)

Sulkamycin Tablets.—Each tablet contains: phthalylsulphacetamide 325 mg., neomycin sulphate 50 mg., and powdered ext. belladonna (contains 0·0375 mg. belladonna alkaloids) 3·0 mg. For the treatment of enteric infections in small animals. Pack: 250. (Smith Kline & French Laboratories Ltd., Welwyn Garden City, Hertfordshire.)

Sulphadimidine Spanbolet.—Each sustained-release tablet contains: sulphadimidine 22·5 g. For sustained-release treatment for infectious diseases in non-lactating cattle, caused by sulphonamide-sensitive organisms. Pack: 5×10. (Smith Kline & French Laboratories Ltd., Welwyn Garden City, Hertfordshire.)

Sulphatose Parenteral.—Each ml. contains: sulphamerazine 65 mg. and sulphathiazole 65 mg. For the treatment of general infections and calf scours sensitive to combined sulphonamide therapy. Pack: 250 ml. (Smith Kline & French Laboratories Ltd., Welwyn Garden City, Hertfordshire.)

Telodron Spansule Capsules.—Each capsule contains: chlorpheniramine maleate 8·0 mg. in sustained release form. For the prompt and prolonged relief of allergic manifestations in small animals. Pack: 250. (Smith Kline & French Laboratories Ltd., Welwyn Garden City, Hertfordshire.)

Tiguvon—Warble-fly and louse dressing for cattle in a formulation that is ready for use. The active ingredient is 2 per cent fenthion. The product is poured along the backs of cattle in the autumn or spring. When applied in this fashion a proportion of active ingredient passes through the skin and is absorbed into the circulation so that all stages of warble-fly larvae present in the body are destroyed. Animals also usually remain free from lice infestation for several weeks. (Bayer Agrochem Ltd., Eastern Way, Bury St. Edmunds, Suffolk.)

Tri-Sulpha-G.—Each ml. contains: sulphadimidine 45 mg., sulphathiazole 45 mg., and sulphapyridine 20 mg. For the treatment of infections in large animals caused by sulphonamide-sensitive organisms. Pack: 3·8 litres. (Smith Kline & French Laboratories Ltd., Welwyn Garden City, Hertfordshire.)

Vi-Sorbin.—Each 5 ml. contains: cyanocobalamin 8·34 mcg., vitamin B_6 2·0 mg., ferric pyrophosphate 100·0 mg., folic acid 0·5 mg., and sorbitol solution 4·4 ml. For the prevention and treatment of vitamin and iron deficiencies in small animals. Pack: 133 ml. and 900 ml. (Smith Kline & French Laboratories Ltd., Welwyn Garden City, Hertfordshire.)

Vi-Sorbits Tablets.—Each chewable tablet contains: ferrous fumarate 50 mg., cyanocobalamin 8 mcg., vitamin B_6 10·2 mcg., folic acid 0·2 mg., vitamin B_1 1·0 mg., vitamin B_2 1·0 mg., nicotinamide 10·0 mg., calcium pantothenate 0·5 mg., vitamin A 125 I.U., vitamin C 12·5 mg., vitamin D_2 125 I.U., vitamin E 2 I.U., D-sorbitol 665 mg., calcium (as calcium phosphate) 41·5 mg., phosphorus (as calcium phosphate) 31·8 mg., and magnesium (as magnesium stearate) 1·0 mg. For the treatment of iron and vitamin deficiencies in small animals. Pack: 50. (Smith Kline & French Laboratories Ltd., Welwyn Garden City, Hertfordshire.)

Vitament, Multi-Vitamin Miscible Powder.—A water-miscible formulation of 13 ingredients for use with cattle, pigs, poultry, lambs, foals, etc., for increasing the supply of vitamins under many conditions with consequent improvement to health, disease resistance, or speed of recovery. A 500-g. tin will fortify 250 gallons of water, sufficient for 13,000 chicks, 7500 growers, 5000 layers or breeders, 500 lambs or growing pigs (50 lb. liveweight), 250 12-week calves or foals. Suitable for use in troughs or drinkers and automatic systems. In tins of 500 g. (Beecham Veterinary Products, Beecham House, Brentford, Middlesex.)

Vitapet.—Supplies the important principles of selected vegetable oils, wheat-germ oil, and cod-liver oil, and a balanced range of polyunsaturated glycerides. Contains: vitamin A 76,000 I.U. per 100 g., vitamin D 7600 I.U. per 100 g., vitamin E 100 I.U. per 100 g., linoleate 15 per cent, docosahexaenoates 7 per cent, and eicosapentaenoates 8 per cent. Total polyunsaturates 34 per cent. For the promotion of healthy skin and coat condition, healthy joints, strong teeth, and bones. Builds natural resistance to diseases. Particularly effective in encouraging a healthy, natural, glossy, and protective coat on all small animals and pets. Pack: 1-gallon cans and 5-gallon drums. (British Cod Liver Oils (Hull and Grimsby) Ltd., Hedon Road, Hull, Yorkshire.)

Zanil in-feed Granules.—A feed additive containing 5 per cent oxyclozanide for routine control of fluke in cattle and sheep. Available in 900-g. packs—one pack will dose 22 × 4-cwt. cattle or 120 × 60-lb. sheep. (I.C.I. Pharmaceutical Division, Alderley Park, Macclesfield, Cheshire.)

Zumax.—Nutritional supplement and health conditioning oil with added calcium and phosphorus. Supplies the important principles of selected vegetable oils, wheat-germ oil, and cod-liver oil, and a balanced range of polyunsaturated glycerides, together with the important minerals calcium and phosphorus. Contains: vitamin A 38,000 I.U. per 100 g., vitamin D 3800 I.U. per 100 g., vitamin E 50 I.U. per 100 g., linoleate 7·5 per cent, eicosapentaenoate 4 per cent, calcium 12 g. per 100 g., docosahexaenoate 3·5 per cent, phosphorus 9 g. per 100 g. Total polyunsaturates 17 per cent. For the general improvement of healthy condition and vitality of dogs, cats, and other pets, particularly older animals, and for vitamin-A and vitamin-D deficiency diseases. Promotes healthy skin and coat condition, firm bones, and strong teeth. Pack: 150-ml. bottles. (British Cod Liver Oils (Hull & Grimsby) Ltd., Hedon Road, Hull, Yorkshire.)

NEW PUBLICATIONS

A List of English Veterinary Works and New Editions published during the Preceding Twelve Months

For the convenience of our readers, works in this list can be ordered through the publishers' retail book selling department, 44 *Triangle West, Bristol BS*8 1*EX.*

The Afghan Hound. By Charles Harrisson. Pp. 239. 30 illus. *Popular Dogs* £2·00

The Alsatian. 6th ed. By Joseph Schwabacher and Thelma Gray. Pp. 242. 31 illus. *Popular Dogs* - - - - - - - - - - - £2·00

Anatomical Techniques. 2nd ed. By D. H. Tompsett. Pp. 304. 107 illus. *Churchill Livingstone* - - - - - - - - - - - £5·00

Animal Cell Culture Methods. By G. D. Wasley and J. W. May. Pp. 192. 60 illus. *Blackwell Scientific* - - - - - - - - - £2·50

Atlas of Topographic Anatomy of the Domestic Animal. By Peter Popesko. Pp. 622. 609 illus. *Saunders* - - - - - - - - - £21·05

The Beagle. 2nd ed. By Thelma Gray. Pp. 224. 20 illus. *Popular Dogs* - £1·75

The Beagle as an Experimental Dog. By A. C. Andersen. Pp. 616. 722 illus. *Baillière Tindall* - - - - - - - - - - - - £9·70

Biological Chemistry. 2nd ed. By Henry R. Mahler and Eugene H. Cordes. Pp. 1009. *Harper & Row* - - - - - - - - - - - £4·50

The Biology of Affluence. Ed. G. Smith and J. C. Smyth. Pp. 156. Illustrated. *Oliver & Boyd* - - - - - - - - - - - £2·00

Bovine Mastitis. By Schalm, Carroll and Jain. Pp. 360. 261 illus. *Baillière Tindall* £7·50

Canine Cardiology. By Stephen J. Ettinger. Pp. 616. 329 illus. *Saunders* - £13·85

Canine Neurology. 2nd ed. By B. F. Hoerlein. Pp. 593. 614 illus. *Saunders* £13·85

Cattle Fertility and Sterility. By S. A. Asdell. Pp. 288. 50 illus. *Churchill Livingstone* - - - - - - - - - - - - £4·50

Cell Biology. By J. D. Burke. Pp. 276. 102 illus. *Churchill Livingstone* - £4·50

Cell Biology. By Robert A. Dowben. Pp. 570. *Harper & Row* - - £6·05

Cell Respiration. By W. O. James. Pp. 144. Illustrated. *English Universities* £1·95

The Cocker Spaniel. 6th ed. By Veronica Lucas-Lucas. Pp. 160. 26 illus. *Popular Dogs* - - - - - - - - - - - - £2·00

Colourpoint Longhair and Himalayan Cats. By S. M. Manton. Pp. 142. 32 illus. *Allen & Unwin* - - - - - - - - - - - £3·00

The Complete Herbal Book for the Dog. By Juliette de Bairacli Levy. Pp. 207. 29 illus. *Faber & Faber* - - - - - - - - - - £2·50

The Control of Injurious Animals. By J. M. Chevrett, J. B. Ford, I. V. Herbert, and A. J. Probert. Pp. 200. Illustrated. *English Universities* - - - £1·75

Current Veterinary Therapy—4. By Robert W. Kirk. Pp. 830. Illustrated. *Saunders* £11·90

Dictionary of Comparative Pathology and Experimental Biology. By Robert W. Leader and Isabel Leader. Pp. 238. Illustrated. *Saunders* - - £5·95

A Dictionary of Immunology. Ed. W. J. Herbert and P. C. Wilkinson. Pp. 208. 12 illus. *Blackwell Scientific* - - - - - - - - £2·25

Dog Training My Way. By Barbara Woodhouse. Pp. 112. 16 illus. *Faber & Faber* £1·80

The Embryonic Pig: A Chronological Account. By A. W. Marrable. Pp. 144. *Pitman Medical* - - - - - - - - - - - £2·25

Energy Transformations in Mammals. By Frederic L. Hoch. Pp. 217. Illustrated. *Saunders* - - - - - - - - - - - - £4·25

The Farm Business. By L. Norman and R. B. Coote. Pp. 304. *Longman* - £3·75

The Farmer's Dog. 4th ed. By John Holmes. Pp. 160. 15 illus. *Popular Dogs* £1·75

Fish Culture. By C. F. Hickling. Pp. 317. 71 illus. *Faber & Faber* - £4·50

Goat Husbandry. By David Mackenzie. Pp. 368. 70 illus. *Faber & Faber* £3·75

The Great Dane. By Jean Lanning. Pp. 192. 30 illus. *Popular Dogs* - £2·00

A Guide to the Birds of South America. By R. M. de Schauensee. Pp. 484. Illustrated. *Oliver & Boyd* - - - - - - - - - - - - £7·00

Hammond's Farm Animals. 4th ed. By John Hammond, I. L. Mason, and T. F. Robinson. Pp. 320. *Arnold* - - - - - - - - - - - £6·00

Handbook of the Birds of Cyprus and Migrants of the Middle East. By David A. Bannerman and W. Mary Bannerman. Pp. 248. Illustrated. *Oliver & Boyd* £3·00

Immunology for Students of Medicine. 3rd ed. By J. H. Humphrey and R. G. White. Pp. 768. 119 illus. *Blackwell Scientific* - - - - - - £3·00

INFECTIOUS DISEASES OF WILD MAMMALS. By Davis, Karstad, and Trainer. Pp. 419. Illustrated. *Baillière Tindall* - £10·50

INFECTIOUS AND PARASITIC DISEASES OF WILD BIRDS. By Davis, Karstad, Trainer, and Anderson. Pp. 344. Illustrated. *Baillière Tindall* - £7·50

INTERNATIONAL TRADE IN TEMPERATE ZONE PRODUCTS. Ed. F. O. Grogan. Pp. 288. Illustrated. *Oliver & Boyd* - £2·50

INTRODUCTION TO EVOLUTION. 3rd ed. By Paul Moody. Pp. 527. Illustrated. *Harper & Row* - £5·60

IRISH AGRICULTURE IN A CHANGING WORLD. Ed. I. F. Baillie and S. J. Sheehy. Pp. 272. Illustrated. *Oliver & Boyd* - £2·50

THE LIFE PUZZLE. By A. G. Cairns-Smith. Pp. 192. Illustrated. *Oliver & Boyd* £1·95

LIVING SYSTEMS. By James M. Ford and James E. Monroe. Pp. 444. Illustrated. *Canfield Press* (*Harper & Row*) - £4·30

MAMMALIAN BIOCHEMISTRY. By I. R. Falconer. Pp. 368. 80 illus. *Churchill Livingstone* £3·75

MEAT PRODUCTION FROM ENTIRE MALE ANIMALS. By D. N. Rhodes. Pp. 352. 32 illus. *Churchill Livingstone* - £3·00

MEDICAL AND VETERINARY PROTOZOOLOGY. By K. M. G. Adam, J. Paul, and V. Zaman. Pp. 208. 186 illus. *Churchill Livingstone* - £6·00

METHODS OF TERATOLOGICAL STUDIES IN EXPERIMENTAL ANIMALS AND MAN. Ed. H. Nishimura and R. J. Miller. Pp. 250. *Pitman Medical* - £12·00

MICROBIOLOGY. By B. D. P. Davis and R. Dulbecco. Pp. 1476. Illustrated. *Harper & Row* £4·90

MILLER'S GUIDE TO THE DISSECTION OF THE DOG. By Howard E. Evans and Alexander de Lahunta. Pp. 291. 199 illus. *Saunders* - £5·10

ORTHOPEDIC SURGERY OF THE DOG AND CAT. 2nd ed. By Ellis P. Leonard. Pp. 351. 286 illus. *Saunders* - £6·60

THE OVARIAN CYCLE OF MAMMALS. By J. S. Perry. Pp. 232. *Oliver & Boyd* - £3·00

PAPERS ON THE REGULATION OF GENE ACTIVITY. By William Loomis. Pp. 420. Illustrated. *Harper & Row* - £3·15

PARASITIC DISEASES OF WILD MAMMALS. By Davis and Anderson. Pp. 364. Illustrated. *Baillière Tindall* - £10·50

PATHOLOGY OF PROTOZOAL AND HELMINTHIC DISEASES. By R. A. Marcial-Rojas. Pp. 1028. 984 illus. *Churchill Livingstone* - £30·00

PHARMACOLOGICAL EXPERIMENTS ON INTACT PREPARATIONS. By the staff of the Pharmacology Department, University of Edinburgh. Pp. 128. 67 illus. *Churchill Livingstone* £1·50

PHARMACOLOGICAL EXPERIMENTS ON ISOLATED PREPARATIONS. 2nd ed. By the staff of the Pharmacology Department, University of Edinburgh. Pp. 150. 80 illus. *Churchill Livingstone* - £1·50

RADIOIMMUNOASSAY METHODS. Ed. K. E. Kirkham and W. M. Hunter. Pp. 704. 350 illus. *Churchill Livingstone* - £6·00

THE REMOTER RURAL AREAS OF BRITAIN. Ed. J. Ashton and W. H. Long. Pp. 288. Illustrated. *Oliver & Boyd* - £2·50

THE SHETLAND SHEEPDOG. 4th ed. By Margaret Osborne. Pp. 245. 46 illus. *Popular Dogs* £1·75

THE SPRINGER SPANIEL. 2nd ed. By Dorothy Morland-Hooper and Ian B. Hampton. Pp. 229. 30 illus. *Popular Dogs* - £2·00

THE STAFFORDSHIRE BULL TERRIER. By John F. Gordon. Pp. 192. 29 illus. *Popular Dogs* £1·75

TERMITES, THEIR RECOGNITION AND CONTROL. 2nd ed. By W. V. Harris. Pp. 240. Illustrated. *Longman* - £4·50

UFAW HANDBOOK ON THE CARE OF FARM ANIMALS. Pp. 344. 139 illus. *Churchill Livingstone* - £5·00

FOURTH UNIVERSITY OF NOTTINGHAM NUTRITION CONFERENCE FOR FEED MANUFACTURERS. Ed. H. Swan and D. Lewis. Pp. 176. *Churchill Livingstone* - £1·25

VETERINARY CLINICAL PARASITOLOGY. By Sloss. Pp. 250. 298 illus. *Baillière Tindall* £4·75

VETERINARY CLINICAL PATHOLOGY. By Doxey. Pp. 356. 115 illus. *Baillière Tindall* £3·75

VETERINARY MICROBIOLOGY. By A. Buxton and G. Fraser. Pp. 450. 250 illus. *Blackwell Scientific* - About £7·50

THE VETERINARY PHYSICIANS INDEX. 5th ed. By T. G. Hungerford. Pp. 600. *Angus & Robertson* - £14·00

INDEX

The more important articles are in heavy type

PRELIMINARY LIST

Veterinary Physiology

Edited by **Professor John Phillis,** *Department of Physiology, University of Manitoba.*

About 500 *pages* (*illustrated*). *Price about* **£7·50.**

Professor Phillis is editing the first comprehensive textbook of veterinary physiology. Each section covering a particular aspect of the subject is contributed by a specialist in that field and this multi-author approach overcomes the difficulties arising from the complexity of the subject.

The Electrogenic Sodium Pump

Professor G. A. Kerkut and Dr. Barbara York, *Department of Physiology and Biochemistry, University of Southampton.*

192 *pages.* 105 *illustrations. Price* **£4·50.**

This monograph reviews our current knowledge on this increasingly fascinating cellular mechanism. As well as presenting biochemists, physiologists, and biologists with an account of the electrogenic sodium pump in nerve-axons, motoneurons, and muscle-fibres, the authors discuss the significance of this mechanism, which links neurochemistry and electrophysiology and will eventually contribute to our complete understanding of the central nervous system.

Tremors and Tremorogenic Agents

Dr. R. W. Brimblecombe, *Medical Division,* **and Dr. R. M. Pinder,** *Chemical Division, Chemical Defence Establishment, Porton Down.*

206 *pages,* 12 *illustrations.* **£5·00.**

Anyone involved in the study of tremor, whether neurochemists, biochemists, pharmacologists, or clinicians, will be interested in this discussion of our present knowledge of the phenomenon and its chemical induction. It is a book to stimulate argument and promote research.

Fish Genetics

Dr. C. E. Purdom, *Ministry of Agriculture, Fisheries and Food Fisheries Laboratory, Lowestoft.*

About 200 *pages* (*illustrated*). *Price about* **£5·00.**

The subject of fish genetics is discussed at a level which will interest not only those actively involved in research but also anyone interested with the breeding of tropical fish.

Predictive Toxicometrics

Professor E. M. Boyd, *Department of Pharmacology, Queen's University, Ontario.*

About 380 *pages,* 116 *illustrations.* **£9·00.**

The prediction of toxic reactions and the safety of chemical agents are discussed, together with the question of what is the minimal amount of laboratory information which must be obtained before a new drug may safely be tested in man. Any doctor or scientist involved with the effects of drugs, pesticides, and herbicides on man and his environment will be interested in this book.

Diseases of Poultry 2nd Edition

ISBN 0 7236 0223 9

P. SENEVIRATNA, *B.V.Sc. (Madras), Ph.D. (Lond.), F.R.C.V.S.*
Dean of the Faculty of Agriculture and Veterinary Science and Head of the Department of Veterinary Science, University of Ceylon

CONTENTS OF THE BOOK

Section A.—DISEASES OF THE DOMESTIC FOWL. I, General. II, Diseases caused by Viruses and Related Organisms. III, Bacterial Diseases. IV, Fungal Diseases. V, Parasitic Diseases. VI, Deficiency Diseases. VII, Miscellaneous Diseases. VIII, Non-specific Diseases. IX, Tumours and Neoplastic Diseases. X, Lethal Factors and Influence of Heredity on Disease and Production. XI, Diagnosis of Poultry Disease.

Section B.—COMMON DISEASES OF TURKEYS. XII, Viral Diseases. XIII, Bacterial Diseases. XIV, Fungal Diseases. XV, Parasitic Diseases. XVI, Miscellaneous Diseases.

Section C.—DISEASES OF DUCKS, GEESE, AND MISCELLANEOUS BIRDS. XVII, Diseases of Ducks. XVIII, Diseases of Geese and Miscellaneous Birds.

Section D.—DISEASES OF CAGE BIRDS. XIX, Diseases of Cage Birds.

Section E.—MISCELLANEOUS. XX, Common Drugs used in Avian Medication. XXI, Defects of Incubation. XXII, Poisons and Toxins. XXIII, Elementary Poultry Surgery.

References. Index.

Price **£2·60,** post **15p.** $9\frac{1}{4} \times 6\frac{1}{8}$ in. (23·5×15·6 cm.) 240 Pages 20 Illustrations

WRIGHTS BRISTOL